Radiology of the Postoperative GI Tract

Springer
New York
Berlin
Heidelberg
Hong Kong
London
Milan
Paris
Tokyo

Bruce R. Javors, MD

Department of Radiology, Saint Vincent's Hospital,
New York, New York, USA

Ellen L. Wolf, MD

Department of Radiology, Montefiore Medical Center,
Bronx, New York, USA

Radiology of the Postoperative GI Tract

With 320 Illustrations

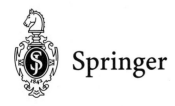

Springer

Bruce R. Javors, MD
Department of Radiology
Saint Vincent's Hospital
New York, NY 10003
USA
bjxraydoc@aol.com

Ellen L. Wolf, MD
Department of Radiology
Montefiore Medical Center
Bronx, NY 10467
USA
ewolf@montefiore.org

Cover illustrations: *Top*: Intraoperative film from a cystic duct cholangiogram performed during a laparascopic cholecystectomy. *Middle*: Transverse sonogram demonstrates the encrusted tip of a ventriculoperitoneal shunt catheter surrounded by a sonolucent area with a hyperechoic rim. This represents a CSF pseudotumor or so-called "CSF'oma." *Bottom*: CT section through the mid-abdomen reveals a markedly dilated transverse duodenum in a patient who has undergone a Billroth II procedure (not shown). This is part of the spectrum of findings in afferent loop syndrome. *Back cover*: Frontal film from a double contrast upper GI series shows a marginal ulcer in a patient who has undergone a partial gastrectomy and gastrojejunostomy (Billroth II procedure).

Library of Congress Cataloging-in-Publication Data
Javors, Bruce R.
　　Radiology of the postoperative GI tract / Bruce R. Javors, Ellen L. Wolf.
　　　p. ; cm.
　　Includes bibliographical references and index.
　　ISBN 0-387-95200-4 (h/c : alk.paper)
　　1. Gastrointestinal system—Radiography. 2. Gastrointestinal
system—Surgery—Complications—Diagnosis. I. Wolf, Ellen L. II. Title.
　　[DNLM: 1. Digestive System—radiography. 2. Digestive System
Diseases—radiography. 3. Digestive System Surgical Procedures—adverse effects.
4. Postoperative Complications—radiography. WI 141 J4lr 2002]
　　RC804.R6 J38 2002
　　617.4'301—dc21

2002019467

ISBN 0-387-95200-4　　　　　　　Printed on acid-free paper.

Printed in the United States of America.

9 8 7 6 5 4 3 2 1　　　　　　SPIN 10790657

www.springer-ny.com

Springer-Verlag　New York Berlin Heidelberg
A member of BertelsmannSpringer Science+Business Media GmbH

Preface

The focus of this book is on the normal postoperative appearance of the gastrointestinal tract and the abnormalities specific to various surgical techniques. The authors have generally avoided the topics of abscesses, leaks, and other fluid collections unless specific attention was warranted. The imaging of recurrent neoplasm was also not included unless rather unique imaging characteristics were involved. The problem of recurrent Crohn's disease was, however, included because of the controversies regarding its clinical and radiographic features. Organ transplantation was not addressed because such procedures are performed and followed at only a few centers.

Over the last two decades the number of routine upper and lower gastrointestinal examinations has markedly decreased. More and more, the focus of conventional barium studies has shifted to the examination of the postoperative patient. The last text dedicated to the postoperative appearance of the gastrointestinal tract was published more than 30 years ago, prior to the advent of computerized tomographic and magnetic resonance imaging. Although a few review articles and several chapters in major radiology textbooks have dealt with this subject, we felt there was a need for a more comprehensive approach.

Our experience in teaching many residents has led us to realize that a knowledge of the surgical procedures themselves was at the heart of radiological comprehension, hence the emphasis on the basic principles of surgical technique in the chapters that follow. The line drawings that accompany the text were simplified to emphasize the anatomy and are not meant to be precise renditions of the actual surgical technique.

Bruce R. Javors, MD
Ellen L. Wolf, MD

Acknowledgments

The authors gratefully acknowledge the financial support of the E-Z-Em Corporation. Morton Meyers, MD, was instrumental in the birth of this book. Most of all we would like to thank our residents, who have over the years performed and monitored so many of the studies that follow. They have also asked the questions that pushed us to seek answers that at times were not readily available. From those basic questions, the need for this book arose. We hope that what follows does justice to their quest for knowledge.

We would like to thank Rob Albano at Springer-Verlag, for his patience. The authors would also like to thank Lourdes Guzman, Eleanor Murphy, and Seymour Sprayregen, MD, for their assistance.

Bruce R. Javors, MD
Ellen L. Wolf, MD

Contents

1

The General Abdomen

Free Intraperitoneal Air

Free intraperitoneal air is expected in the immediate postoperative period. The frequency and duration of its detection may vary with the diagnostic modality utilized. The clinical importance of its detection may depend on whether the patient is receiving mechanical ventilation. Free intraperitoneal air may result from the dissection of air from a ruptured alveolus, back along the tracheobronchial tree, through the mediastinum, and either transdiaphragmaticly or via the retro- and subperitoneum into the abdominal spaces [1]. This can lead to a false positive diagnosis with resultant unnecessary exploration of the patient [1].

Free air may also result from peritoneal dialysis. Faulty bag exchange or exterior line exchange may allow air entry into the abdomen. Chest x-rays may show free air in 4% of patients [2]. However, up to 11% of cases of free air in patients undergoing peritoneal dialysis may be secondary to gastrointestinal (GI) tract perforation. The amount of the air cannot be used to differentiate mechanical causes from pathological ones [2].

Conventional (plain film) radiographs of the abdomen may reveal free air in 30 to 77% of patients immediately after surgery [3–7]. This decreases to 38% on day 3 and 17% on day 17 [8]. The left lateral decubitus film, which allows air to rise and be highlighted between the liver and the parietal peritoneum, is positive in 53% of patients on postoperative day 3 and in 8% on day 6. As would be expected, these results compare unfavorably with the use of computerized tomography (CT) to detect free air. On postoperative day 3, 87% of CT images are positive for free air, and fully half are positive on day 6 [8]. Serial examinations in 10 patients showed a decrease in the amount of free air in six patients during the same examination period, and a complete disappearance in the other four [8].

An area of some controversy is whether body habitus affects the rate at which free air is absorbed. Two older studies, based on plain films, detected a higher rate of free air in asthenic individuals [3,5]. A more

recent study utilizing both CT and plain films led to markedly different findings [8]. The plain film showed that obese individuals had a
significantly lower rate of free air than others. Surprisingly, CT examinations showed no difference between asthenic and obese individuals
in the detection of free air. The differences between these two techniques may be explained by the susceptibility of the plain film to degradation by increased scattered radiation and decreased penetration and
density secondary to obesity.

The plain film findings of free air are numerous and are enumerated
in Table 1.1 [9] (Fig. 1.1). The optimal film and phase of respiration for
the detection of free air are the end inspiratory chest x-ray, and the end
expiratory left lateral decubitus films of the abdomen [10]. Besides the
usual findings on plain films, computed tomography has shown two
new areas, both along the undersurface of the anterior abdominal wall,
in which free air may be detected. Above the level of the umbilicus, air
may collect in the recess between the two rectus abdominal muscles
(along the linea alba). Similarly, below the umbilicus, air may collect
along the lateral margins of the rectus sheath [8].

Barium or Water-Soluble Contrast Media

The question of which contrast medium to use in cases of suspected or
known perforation is a difficult one to answer. The response depends
on what level of the GI tract is involved, whether the patient is at risk
of aspirating the contrast medium, and whether there is a risk of fecal
contamination. Each of these possible scenarios is further complicated
by personal preferences, demands of the referring physician, local prac-
tice, dogma, and somewhat contradictory and often outdated experimental evidence.

Based on experimental work done on cats, James and his colleagues
published two often cited works on the effects of water-soluble contrast medium, barium sulfate, oral pharyngeal flora, and mixtures of
flora and contrast media on the feline mediastinum [11,12]. Post-
mortem examinations were done over time intervals reaching 90 days.

Barium was initially evenly distributed in the mediastinum, but
clumps were noted by 3 to 5 days postinstallation. Even after 90 days
an estimated 50% of the barium remained but was not detected in the
draining lymph nodes of the mediastinum. Histological sections
revealed that the barium was incorporated into reactive surface
mesothelial cells and large macrophages after 2 to 5 days. By one
month, fibrous connective tissue surrounded nodules of barium-filled
macrophages. Some inflammatory cells were present along with
foreign body giant cells. The addition of esophageal flora comprising
coliform, *Proteus*, Gram-positive aerobic spore-forming bacilli, micro-
aerophilic and anaerobic streptococci, and lactobacilli did not significantly change these findings [11,12].

Pure Gastrografin injected into the cat mediastinum led to no gross
pathologic changes. A few inflammatory cells were noted 7 days later.
The addition of oral pharyngeal flora led to no significant change in

TABLE 1.1. **Signs of pneumoperitoneum on a supine radiograph.**

I. Upper abdomen
    A. Right upper quadrant
        1. Anterior to liver (subtle)
            a. Anterior–superior bubble
            b. Ill-defined periduodenal lucency
            c. Right upper quadrant slit
            d. Lucent liver
        2. Anterior to liver (gross)
            a. Falciform ligament sign
            b. Ligamentum teres sign
            c. Diaphragm muscle slip sign
        3. Within liver
            a. Ligamentum teres sign
        4. Posterior to liver
            a. Morrison's pouch—doge's cap sign
        5. Inferior to liver
            a. Hepatic edge sign
            b. Ligamentum teres notch sign
            c. Visible gallbladder
    B. Paramedian
        1. Lesser sac gas
        2. Cupola sign
        3. Visible lower cardiac border
    C. Left upper quadrant—left-sided pneumoperitoneum

II. Midabdomen
    A. Free gas
        1. Rigler's sign
        2. Triangle sign
        3. Football sign
        4. Visible transverse mesocolon
        5. Visible small bowel mesentery
    B. Air confined in intraperitoneal ligaments
        1. Pneumo-omentum
        2. Pneumomesocolon

III. Lower abdomen
    A. Urachus
    B. Medial umbilical folds
    C. Later umbilical folds
    D. Visible bladder roof
    E. Pneumoscrotum
    F. Isolated lower abdominal free air

IV. Extra-abdominal intraperitoneal free air
    A. Free air in hiatal hernia sac
    B. Free air in ventral hernia sac

V. Unrecognized plain film signs
    A. Midrectus sign
    B. Pararectus sign

Source: Ref. 9.

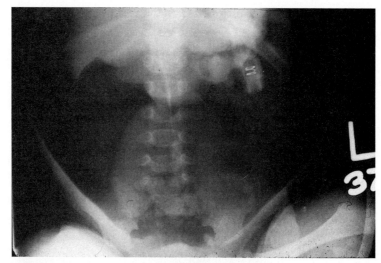

A

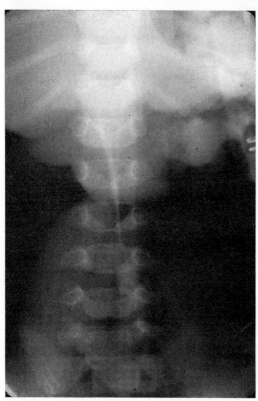

B

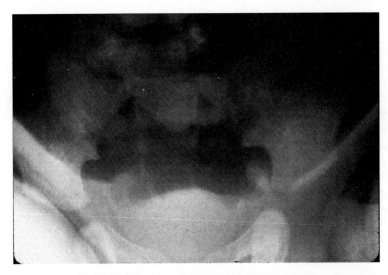

C

FIGURE 1.1. Plain film findings of free air. (A) Massive free air. Supine film of the abdomen reveals a massive pneumoperitoneum following misplaced gastrostomy tube. (B) Falciform ligament sign. Coned-down view of the same patient shows the falciform ligament as a linear density obliquely oriented in the midabdomen. (C) Incomplete inverted V sign. Coned-down view of the pelvis in the same patient reveals the soft tissue densities of the medial collateral ligaments, as well as remnants of the umbilical arteries. When these converge upon the umbilicus they form the inverted V sign of pneumoperitoneum.

histological appearance. Surprisingly, the injection of pharyngeal flora alone did not lead to significant mediastinitis. This may have been secondary to the use in the experiment of too dilute a concentration. Severe mediastinitis could be produced by using a more concentrated mixture, but this led to so many experimental deaths that the results were meaningless. Experience in humans with esophageal perforation leads us to conclude that oral pharyngeal flora leads to severe and potentially fatal mediastinal infections.

When contrast medium is aspirated into the tracheobronchial tree, or enters via an esophageal airway fistula, the lungs' reaction is very different from that seen in the mediastinum. Huston et al. instilled a commercial preparation into rat airways and defined four major patterns of histologic response [13].

The first was that of the initial inflammatory response. In this stage, the alveoli and smaller bronchioles are filled with the barium suspension and large numbers of polymorphonuclear leukocytes. Little fluid (exudate) was seen in the alveolus. These changes developed within 12 hours but by 24 hours the white blood cells had started to degenerate.

The next phase, mononuclear infiltration, developed within 48 hours and lasted up to 15 days. This stage was characterized by mononuclear cells containing phagocytosed barium suspension. Other mononuclear cells had replaced the lining epithelium of the smaller airways. Two weeks later, many of these mononuclear cells had fused together. Retractile masses filled with barium were noted, secondary to rupture of some of these mononuclear cells. This stage was entitled mononuclear disintegration.

The last phase was that of tissue reaction. At 90 to 120 days after the administration of barium, installation the lung tissue looked grossly normal. A few small areas, related to the retractile masses noted earlier, showed early giant cell formation. No fibrosis was yet noted.

At no stage was barium noted in either draining lymph nodes or the liver or spleen. Most aspirated barium is cleared either by coughing or by mucociliary action [13].

In a more recent study, published in 1984, Ginai et al. [14] compared pure barium sulfate with Gastrografin, a commercial preparation of barium sulfate, and two nonionic water-soluble contrast agents. Both pure barium sulfate and the commercial preparation led to patchy bronchopneumonia by the eighth day, accompanied by epithelioid cell granulomas in the lung. By 6 weeks intramural granulomas were noted within the bronchial walls as well. Many of these changes seen by both Huston and Ginai may be secondary to mechanical plugging of the smaller airways by the ingested barium with subsequent atelectasis and inflammatory reaction [13,14].

In contrast to the barium preparations, and their long-lasting and long-standing mechanical effect, water-soluble contrast media are rapidly absorbed from the lungs as evidenced by their faint visualization just minutes after instillation and total disappearance by 24 hours. The severely hypertonic Gastrografin (its osmolality of 1900 is approximately six times that of plasma) causes a shift of fluid from the intravascular compartment to perivascular spaces and the lung parenchyma that may result in pulmonary edema or death [15,16]. Gastrografin also leads to the early development of perivascular infiltrates with mononuclear cells. Collapse and minimal alveolar infiltrates were also noted. By the fourth day, swelling and desquamation involving the alveolar lining was noted. The low osmolar contrast invoked very minimal changes in the perivascular spaces as well as within the alveolus.

Experimental evidence of the effects of barium sulfate or water-soluble contrast agents on the pleural surface is not available to the best of our knowledge. Given the similarity of the mesothelial lining of the chest and abdomen, it is reasonable to assume that these effects would mimic those discussed shortly [17].

Below the diaphragm, consideration of which contrast to use is complicated by the interaction of the contrast agent and enteric flora, especially fecal material. Cochran and colleagues examined the effects in dogs of pure barium sulfate [U.S. Pharmacopeia (USP) grade] and commercial barium preparations with and without the addition of fecal material [18]. When commercial barium sulfate was injected into the peritoneal cavity it almost immediately disbursed widely throughout over the next 2 to 5 days; clumping, most likely secondary to water resorption and the effect of fibrinous exudates, was noted. Extensive adhesions with severe hemorrhagic or purulent peritonitis developed, resulting in the death of most of the experimental animals. Sterilizing the barium did not significantly change these results.

When feces alone were injected into the peritoneal cavity, diffuse peritonitis ensued with multiple adhesions. When the fecal material was sterilized, no deleterious effects were noted. When barium and unsterile feces were mixed, a rapidly fatal hemorrhagic peritonitis resulted. Retroperitoneal infusion of barium led to granuloma formation [19]. However, in the absence of infection, extravasated barium led to no significant complications.

The conclusion the authors reached, which seems justifiable to this day, is that barium and feces are synergistic in their effects [18]. In addition, the additives to pure barium sulfate, used to stabilize the suspension and add to its properties (mucosal coating ability, palatability), adversely affect the peritoneal membranes. The negative effects of the fecal material are due to the accompanying infection, rather than the physical nature of the bacteria.

Ferrante and colleagues injected water-soluble contrast into rat abdomens [20]. They found no significant difference in the various ionic and nonionic contrast agents used. This was in marked distinction to barium injections, which resulted in adhesions and ascites.

Tubes and Lines

Nasogastric and nasoenteric tubes may be placed for a variety of diagnostic and therapeutic reasons. A whole host of mishaps and complications may be associated with their use, however, despite the usually benign nature of their insertion and usage.

Complications associated with insertion include perforation and malpositioning within the tracheobronchial tree. Complications arising from positioning in the GI tract include those related to obstruction, rupture of the mercury bag, perforation, and local irritating effects [21].

Perforation by a nasogastric or nasoenteric tube often occurs at the level of the pharynx, where the tip of the tube is often directed laterally into the piriform sinus. Exiting the piriform sinus, the tube may tract inferiorly, alongside the esophagus for a variable distance. Resistance may be encountered at multiple levels as it passes various mediastinal components (Fig. 1.2). When contrast is injected, it outlines a

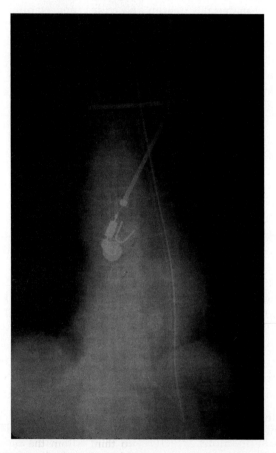

FIGURE 1.2. **Misplaced NG tube.** Chest film shows nasogastric tube misplaced in the mediastinum secondary to a perforation in the neck. No return was obtained from this tube. A CT image of the neck, not shown, demonstrated its path in the neck, lateral to the esophagus and trachea.

nonmotile tract that is slightly irregular and does not usually communicate with the GI tract. Multiple tracts may be seen in association with multiple attempts at tube placement (Fig. 1.3). The esophagus itself may be perforated with a greater potential for mediastinitis secondary to reflux and entrance of gastric secretions and flora into the mediastinum [22–24].

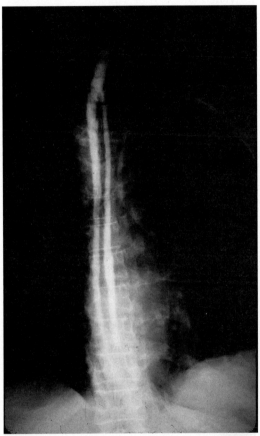

A

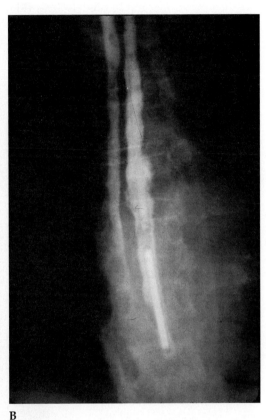

B

FIGURE 1.3. Unsuccessful attempts at feeding tube insertion. (A) False tracks of a feeding tube. Single-contrast esophagogram shows two thin, parallel tracks of barium in the chest, neither of which represents the esophagus. Both are false lumens secondary to unsuccessful attempts at passing a metallic-tipped feeding tube. (B) Feeding tube within a false track. Another film from the subsequent study shows the feeding tube in one of the false lumens. (Courtesy of K. Cho, MD, Newark, NJ)

Patients with impaired neurological status are most at risk for inadvertent tube placement in the tracheobronchial tree. Depending on how
far the tube is inserted, it may lie within a major bronchus (Figs. 1.4–1.6)
or even be pushed through smaller and smaller airways, eventually
perforating the visceral pleura to lie within the pleural space itself (Fig.
1.7A). Obviously, initiating feeding through such a malpositioned tube
would have dire consequences. A pneumothorax may also be the
sequela of such a malpositioned tube [25,26] (Fig. 1.7B). Some authors
have advocated the use of a routine chest x-ray before any nasogastric
(NG) tube is utilized [24]. They believe that clinical tests of tube
placement are inadequate. The American College of Radiology, in its
Appropriateness Criteria, also cites the value of obtaining a routine
postprocedure film [27].

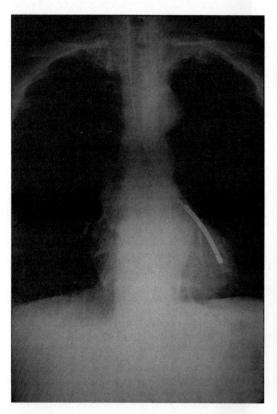

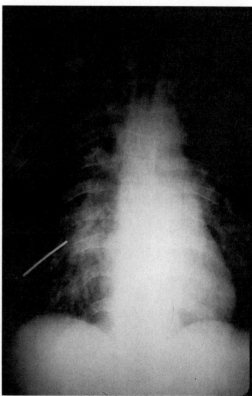

FIGURE 1.4. Feeding tube in a left-sided bronchus. Chest film demonstrates a metallic-tipped
feeding tube in the left lower lobe bronchus. Since
the right main stem bronchus has a more oblique
takeoff at the carina, most tubes go there.

FIGURE 1.5. Feeding tube in a right-sided
bronchus. Chest film with a feeding tube in a
right lower lobe bronchus.

FIGURE 1.6. Unusual NG tube placement. Chest film reveals a circuitous path taken by a feeding tube. It traverses the esophagus, reaches the stomach, doubles back to the pharynx, enters the trachea, and ends in the bronchus intermedius. (Courtesy of R. Lautin, MD, New York, NY)

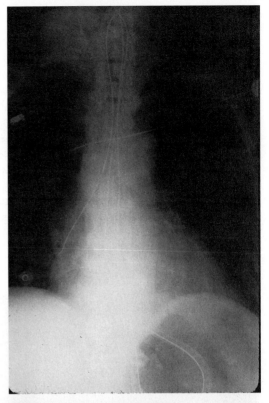

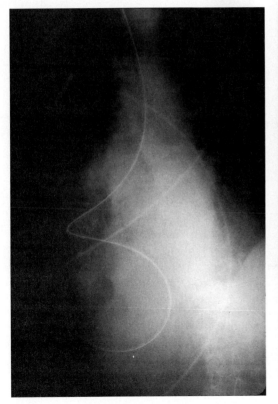

A

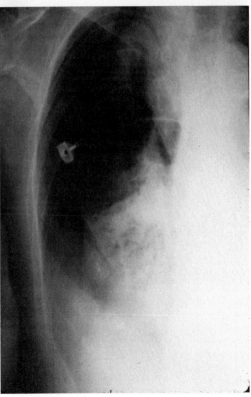

B

FIGURE 1.7. Malpositioned feeding tube and sequela. (A) Feeding tube within the right pleural cavity. Chest film demonstrates a feeding tube that has been advanced through the tracheobronchial tree and lies coiled in the pleural space. (B) Pneumothorax following chest tube removal. Another chest film taken of the same patient after removal of the feeding tube shows a pneumothorax.

Poly(vinyl chloride) tubes that are exposed to gastric acidity harden over time. This may lead to either perforation or difficulty in removal [21,28,29]. Thus long-term usage should be avoided. Other local complications of short- and long-term NG tube intubation include nasopharyngeal irritation and ulceration, sinusitis, serous otitis, and pharyngitis [21]. The polyvinyl NG tube may also predispose a patient to gastroesophageal reflux and ulceration (Fig. 1.8). Rapid onset of a stricture may ensue (Fig. 1.9), although it is not clear whether this effect is due to reflux, the presence of the tube, or both [30].

Two of the more commonly used long intestinal decompression tubes are the Cantor and Miller–Abbott. Both utilize a mercury-filled bag at the proximal end to facilitate passage distally through the GI tract. A Miller–Abbott tube has a venting channel alongside the decompression lumen.

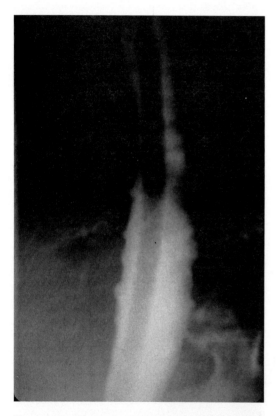

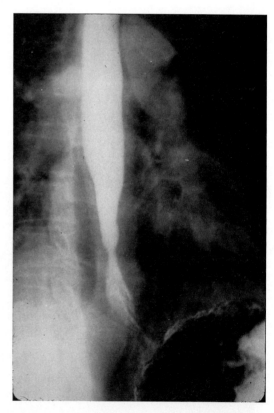

FIGURE 1.8. **Ulcerations induced by an NG tube.** Single-contrast esophagogram shows multiple ulcerations secondary to the placement of an NG tube.

FIGURE 1.9. **Stricture induced by an NG tube.** Esophagogram demonstrates a distal esophageal stricture, caused by previous NG tube placement.

The latex balloon may act as a semipermeable membrane, allowing intestinal gaseous contents (predominantly carbon dioxide and hydrogen sulfide) [31] to enter the bag [32] (Fig. 1.10). This may occur in 0.3% of patients according to Cantor, as cited by others [32]. This gaseous accumulation may lead to increasing distention of the balloon until the partial pressures within it and the intestinal lumen equilibrate. At that point the balloon no longer distends [33]. Other factors affecting the gaseous distention include the surface area and thickness of the balloon wall and the length of time it is exposed to intestinal gases [34]. Ten days is often cited as the point in the time at which the distention reaches a critical diameter [34]. The dilated air- and mercury-filled balloon may cause considerable clinical problems.

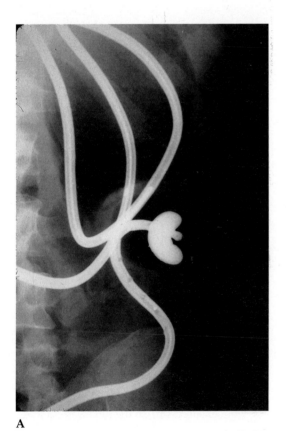
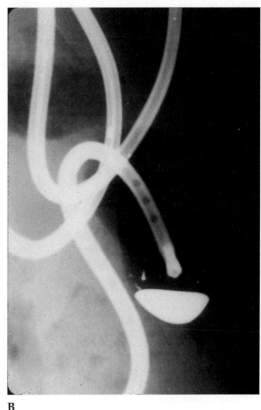

A   B

FIGURE 1.10. **Air-distended mercury bag of a Cantor tube.** Supine (A) and upright (B) films of the abdomen with a Cantor tube in place. Note the large amount of air in the mercury-filled bag.

First, it may cause obstruction of the lumen of the small bowel, thus creating or exacerbating the very condition it is intended to treat [21,33–35]. When this occurs, gentle retraction is usually tried. If this is not successful, decompression of the balloon may be attempted before laparotomy is necessitated [34]. Cutting of the tube hoping for its eventual expulsion is another but often unsuccessful therapeutic maneuver [32] (Fig. 1.11). Yet another possibility is placing another long intestinal tube, proximal to the offending tube, attempting to decompress the small-bowel lumen as an aid in the reverse flow of gas across the latex membrane [32].

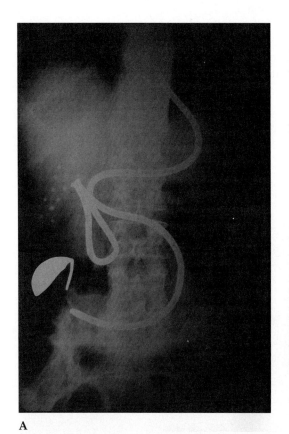
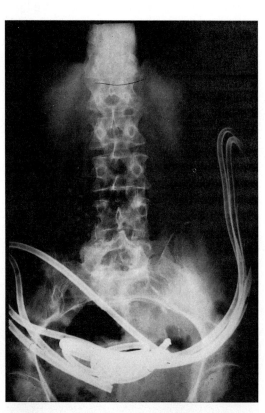

A   B

FIGURE 1.11. **Incarcerated Cantor tube.** (A) Supine film of the abdomen (A) showing a Cantor tube in the distal small bowel. Attempts at withdrawing the tube were unsuccessful, so the tube was cut loose and allowed to pass distally (B).

Percutaneous puncture of the balloon is a relatively safe and well-tolerated option. Use of a small-gauge needle allows safe passage through the small-bowel wall without undue risk of injury and leakage of intestinal contents even in the face of obstruction [34]. CT guidance helps to avoid the transgression of the colon or other organs, but some authors found fluoroscopy a better alternative [33] (Fig. 1.12). A more esoteric, but not readily available method of decompressing the balloon is that of placing the patient in a hyperbaric chamber [36]. This allows successful reduction in the size of the balloon and subsequent removal.

Even nonballoon catheters may be prone to similar problems. One case report involves a single-lumen mushroom catheter that had its nipple balloon to an obstructive degree [33]. In the manufacture of this device, a small amount of gauzelike material is introduced into the nipple to occupy the potential space between the leaves of latex. This potential space eventually acted like the latex balloons just discussed and becomes filled with intestinal gas. Percutaneous puncture successfully decompressed this catheter as well.

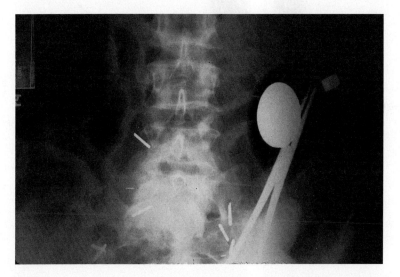

FIGURE 1.12. **Decompression of air-filled mercury bag of a Cantor tube.** Spot film of the lower abdomen during a fluoroscopic attempt at decompressing the air-filled mercury bag of a Cantor tube. This was necessitated by a small-bowel obstruction caused by the dilated mercury bag.

Other complications secondary to the presence of long intestinal tubes have also been reported. Some of these are well known to clinicians and radiologists, while others are unusual (Fig. 1.13) and may warrant inclusion in the medical literature.

Overly vigorous attempts at advancing a soft nasoenteric tube may also cause buckling and loop formation of the tube. Eventually a knot may form. This presents a major problem when the tube has to be removed. Gentle retraction may allow uneventful removal [37], or an endoscopist may have to assist [38]. Another possible remedy is to insert another tube, perhaps a stiffer one, through the loop of the knot. This is similar to the angiographic approach to knotted catheters. Retracting over the stiffer tube may allow unknotting of the problematic tube.

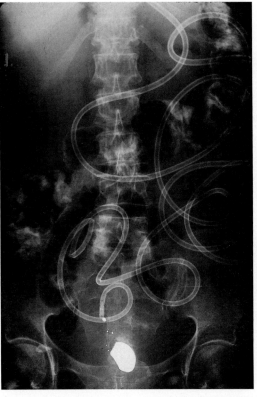

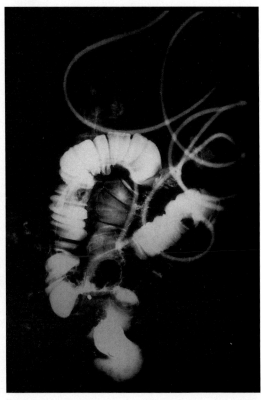

A   B

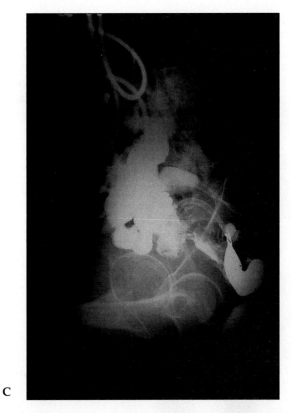

C

FIGURE 1.13. **Unusual course of Cantor tube through ileocolic fistula.** Abnormal course of a Cantor tube is demonstrated on this supine abdominal radiograph (A). It apparently reaches the rectum, but does not enter the proximal colon. Anteroposterior (B) and lateral (C) films from a contrast exam reveal that the tube has transited an ileocolic fistula to reach the rectum.

Foreshortening of the small bowel over a nasoenteric tube is frequently demonstrated at contrast studies. This may progress to frank intussusception (Fig. 1.14). One article has suggested that when this foreshortening and pleating effect becomes fixed by adhesions, it may predispose the patient to the development of intussusception, even after the tube has been removed [39]. Even retrograde intussusceptions have been described [40].

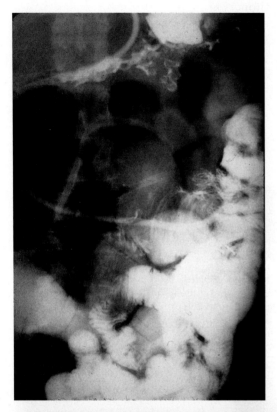

A

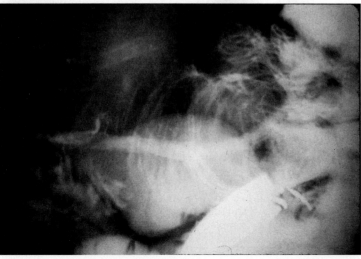

B

FIGURE 1.14.
Intussusception about a Cantor tube. Overhead film from a small-bowel series (A) shows a filling defect in the jejunum. A spot film from the same exam (B) reveals the coiled-spring appearance of an intussusception about the Cantor tube.

When multichannel long intestinal tubes are used for decompression, care must be taken that medications and contrast media are placed in the proper lumen. If not, inadvertent overdistention of the balloon can occur.

Not without their own set of problems are tubes placed directly into the jejunum for feeding purposes. These may be inserted incidentally during more extensive intra-abdominal procedures or as a separate procedure. The overall complication rate is approximately 10% [41]. These problems may include infarction, intraperitoneal leaks and perforation, and even volvulus [41,42]. Tube jejunostomies were found to have more frequent complications than needle catheter jejunostomies [41]. These may include kinking or adhesions at the insertion site, leading to bowel obstruction (Fig. 1.15), pleating and foreshortening of the bowel over the tube (Fig. 1.6A,B), frank intussusception, or obstruction from the balloon tip of a tube (Fig. 1.16C).

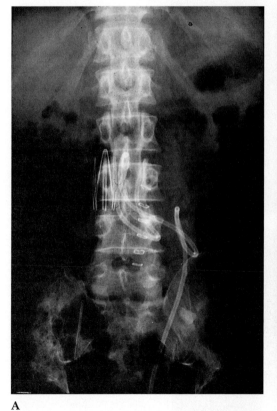

A

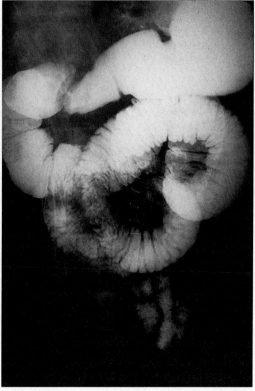

B

FIGURE 1.15. Small-bowel obstruction secondary to a jejunostomy tube. Supine radiograph of the abdomen (A) reveals dilated loops of small bowel in the left upper quadrant. A jejunostomy catheter is present. A small-bowel series on the same patient (B) demonstrates an abrupt transition in the caliber of the small bowel (incomplete small-bowel obstruction) at the insertion site of the jejunostomy tube.

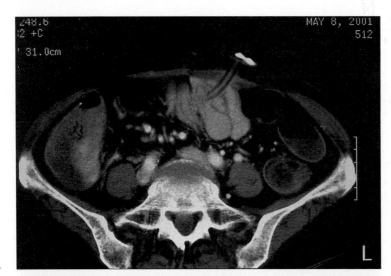

FIGURE 1.16. Small-bowel pleating and obstruction due to jejunostomy tube. Three sections from a CT series of the abdomen and pelvis demonstrate a jejunostomy tube as it enters the abdomen (A), causes pleating of the small bowel over the tube (B), and shows an abrupt transition from dilated to normal bowel at the balloon tip of the catheter (C). The patient was clinically obstructed and improved after the tube had been removed.

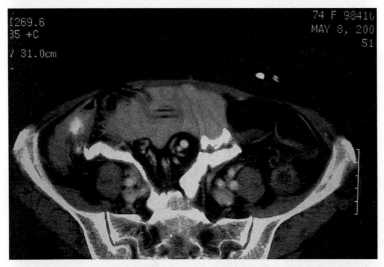

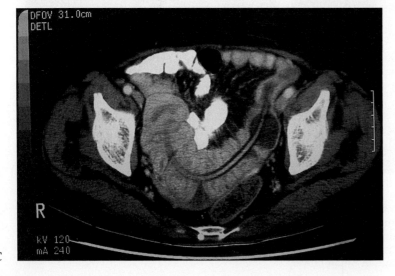

Although not strictly a procedure that involves the gastrointestinal tract, placement of ventriculoperitoneal (VP) shunts may cause problems that manifest themselves in the abdomen. VP shunts are usually placed to decompress hydrocephalus due to both benign and malignant conditions. Complications may be related to migration of the shunt catheter with or without subsequent infection, abnormal fluid collections, spread of neoplasm, and other miscellaneous mechanical problems.

When a VP shunt is placed in the abdomen, it is not sutured in place. Therefore it can migrate. Since the catheter is nonreactive, fibrous tissue does not form about its tip, leading to some complications discussed later. When the catheter does shift in position, it may migrate through various intra-abdominal passageways, perforate hollow viscera, or penetrate solid ones. An example of the first type is passage via a patent processus vaginalis resulting in a scrotal hydrocele [43]. Another congenital anomaly associated with tube migration was a patent foramen of Bochdalek [44]. In this instance, a patient developed a hydrothorax filled with cerebrospinal fluid (CSF) as the catheter transitted from the abdomen to the chest across the abnormal pleuroperitoneal communication. In another instance, the tip of the shunt catheter migrated through the foramen of Winslow, resulting in a CSF collection within the lesser sac [45]. The latter was detected on a scintigraphic examination.

Perforation, even through the thick wall of the stomach, may occur during placement of the shunt catheter [46] or many months later [47]. Perforation through the colonic wall has resulted in a VP shunt presenting per rectum during defecation [48]. The shunt was subsequently removed via a sigmoidoscope.

Multiple cases of liver [49–52] or even splenic [53] abscesses have been reported. These have an appearance similar to other pyogenic abscesses except for the presence of a VP shunt in the abdomen or liver proper. Liver lesions were described at CT imaging as a hypodense cyst with multiple septations. On sonography the lesion was cystic with internal echoes and septations, and the shunt tip was seen within the pseudocyst [50]. In all cases the shunt catheter had to be externalized, the abscess drained, and systemic antibiotics used to treat the infection. In at least one case a perforation of the colonic wall by the VP shunt catheter led not to an abdominal infection but retrograde spread to the head [54]. This resulted in an *E. coli* meningitis.

In rare instances, fibrous tissue may form around the abdominal portion of the ventriculoperitoneal shunt. As CSF continues to drain into the abdomen, it may be encapsulated by the fibrous tissue without an epithelial lining [55]. This gives rise to a peritoneal pseudocyst or CSF pseudocyst, also anecdotally called a CSF'oma (Fig. 1.17). These occur in slightly less than 2% [56] or as many as 4.5% of all shunts [55], developing as soon as 3 weeks postoperatively [57]. Predisposing factors for their development include previous shunt placement [55,57] and infection [57]. Following VP shunt placement, intraperitoneal surgery, either open [58] or laparoscopic [59], may lead to an increased incidence of pseudocyst formation.

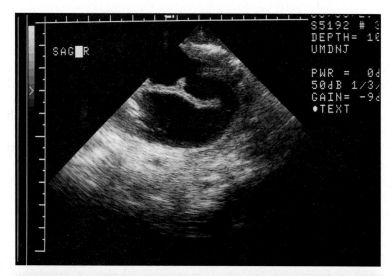

A

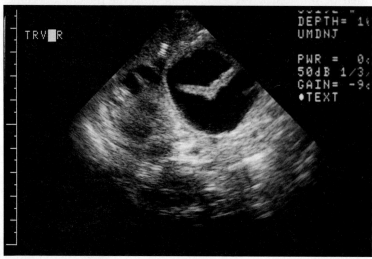

B

FIGURE 1.17. **CSF'oma.** Sagittal (A) and transverse (B) scans of the midabdomen show a sonolucent structure with a slightly echogenic wall, consistent with a CSF'oma. The debris-coated VP shunt is well seen inside this pseudocyst. (Courtesy of R. Wachsberg, MD, Newark, NJ)

The presence of a pseudocyst may be associated with either local abdominal signs or symptoms or related to increased intracranial pressure [55]. According to most authors, abdominal signs and symptoms predominate in children [56–58], although one study also included increased intracranial pressure among the clinical presentations [55]. The same authors also stated that abdominal signs and symptoms predominate in adults.

The diagnosis of a CSF pseudocyst is made most often on ultrasound [55–57]. A sonolucent mass may be identified in the area of a palpated abnormality. Sizes of up to 2 L have been reported [59]. Treatments include shunt revision and repositioning [55–58,60]. Aspiration of the pseudocyst contents can be performed under CT [58] or ultrasound guidance [56,60] or intraoperatively (with or without cyst wall resection) [55,56,58–61]. In one series of 27 patients, 15 of the abdominal CSF pseudocyst resolved spontaneously [60].

Infection rates of the pseudocyst may range as high as 77% in children under the age of 4 years [60]. Overall, the infection rate is approximately 30% [55,60]. No difference in the imaging characteristics between infected and sterile pseudocysts has been described.

Just as the shunt catheter can act as a conduit for abdominal flora to reach the central nervous system, so can central nervous system neoplasms seed down the shunt catheter to enter the peritoneal cavity. This complication arises on average approximately 17 months after shunt surgery, and the patients often die (73%) [62,63]. The time from the diagnosis of the abdominal symptoms to the patient's demise was only 2 months [62]. Germinomas were the most common lesion in pediatric patients over the age of 10 years, while in the under-10-year-old group medulloblastomas were the most common primary lesion [62].

Unusual mechanical problems related to the presence of the catheter itself have also been reported. The VP shunt in the abdomen may accidentally be detached from the intracranial portion and retract into the abdomen (Fig. 1.18). In another case, a VP shunt catheter formed a knot

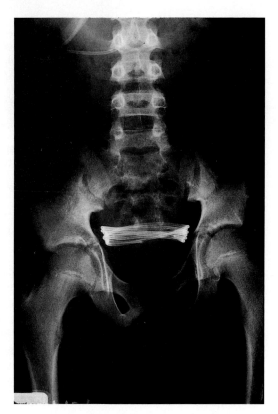

FIGURE 1.18. **Broken VP shunt.** Supine film of the abdomen shows a long fragment of a VP shunt catheter that had become detached from the more proximal portion. It lies folded back upon itself in the supravesical region.

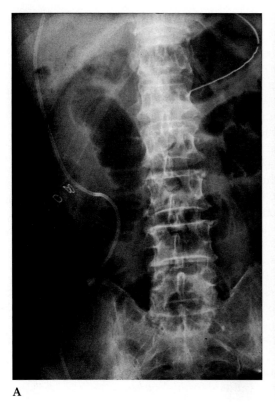

A

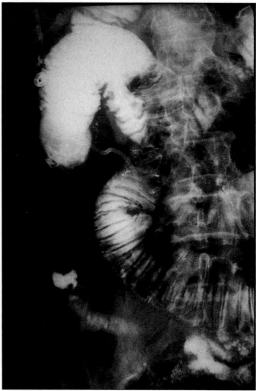

B

FIGURE 1.19. Small-bowel obstruction secondary to VP shunt. Supine film of the abdomen (A) reveals the presence of a VP shunt on the left. Dilated loops of small bowel indicate a small-bowel obstruction. Small-bowel series on the same patient (B) shows an abrupt change in small-bowel caliber, with the VP shunt wrapped around the transition point.

around a loop of small bowel, resulting in a strangulated obstruction [64]. The authors recommended attempting to remove the knot by straightening the shunt catheter over a guide wire. In another patient, the catheter provided the axis about which a small-bowel volvulus occurred [65]. In a similar fashion, the small bowel may be acutely wrapped about a VP shunt with resultant obstruction (Fig. 1.19).

Ingested Mercury

Metallic mercury may enter the GI tract secondary to accidental or purposeful ingestion or rupture of a mercury-filled balloon of a small intestinal tube (Miller–Abbott or Cantor) (Fig. 1.20). Accidental ingestion is usually secondary to breakage of a thermometer in the mouth. Encountered much less often is swallowing of an oral thermometer (Fig. 1.21) with subsequent breakage and mercury spillage. Obviously in medical facilities the use of electronic instruments has greatly

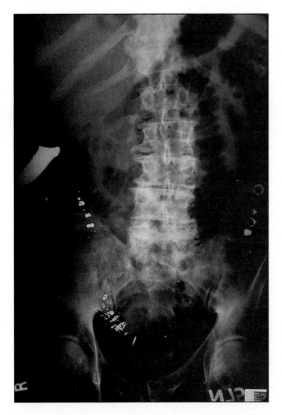

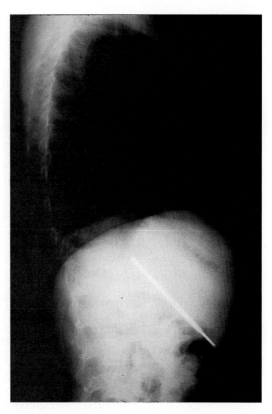

FIGURE **1.20. Mercury spill from a Cantor tube.**
Supine film of the abdomen reveals a Cantor tube
in the small bowel. Although most of the mercury
is still in the bag, multiple small globules have
escaped and lie within the intestines.

FIGURE **1.21. Swallowed thermometer.** Lateral
film of the chest shows an accidentally ingested
oral thermometer inside the stomach.

decreased the risk of such accidents, but they may still occur in the
home setting.

Elemental mercury (valence = 0) is poorly absorbed from the gastrointestinal tract [66]. Therefore, large doses are necessary to cause
toxicity. When inorganic mercury (valence = +1, +2) is placed in the GI
tract, 7 to 15% of the dose is absorbed. This is the principal danger
following the swallowing of a mercury "button" or disc battery by children. Organic mercury poisoning is usually associated with fungicides
or other industrial contamination.

The risk to patients who have elemental mercury in the GI tract is
related to its oxidation to inorganic mercury. This does not usually
occur within the GI tract, partially because the mercury is fairly rapidly
eliminated in the stool. However, if and when mercury extravasates,
especially into the retroperitoneum, conditions are favorable for its
oxidation. Retention within a diverticulum or the appendix may lead
to local inflammation and systemic effects [67].

Another, and much more rare complication of mercury-filled balloons of Miller–Abbott tubes is that of aspiration. In one case, the balloon ruptured during removal and the patient aspirated approximately 5 mL of mercury [68]. Acute mercurialism resulted in the patient's death 5 days later.

Retained Surgical Implements

The problem of the retained surgical implement is an old one that is not infrequently encountered. Estimates range from 1 in 1000 to 1 in 1500 laparotomies [69–72]. The true incidence of the problem may be more difficult to ascertain because "a foreign body problem is rarely discussed as there is an understandable tendency not to advertise one's errors" [73].

Surgeons have been using, and losing, sponges, and presumably other implements as well, since 1884 [74] (Figs. 1.22 and 1.23). By 1929, abdominal roentgenograms were recommended and used to detect inadvertently retained sponges [75] (Fig. 1.24). Markers of barium-impregnated threads were introduced after 1933 [76] (Fig. 1.25). Yet the problem continues to this day.

There are many interconnected factors leading to the ongoing problem. During laparotomy, changes in the operative field and in the positions of intestines that are displaced and packs (laparotomy or lap pads) that are moved for better visualization can lead to the obscuring of the sponge or "lap" pad. The pelvis, because of its many recesses, is the area most frequently involved in cases of "lost" sponges [70]. However, in our personal experience, widespread oncological resection is by far the most common procedure in which this happens. Long and difficult procedures in which it is easy to lose count of placed sponges and pads may also contribute to losing track of implantables, as does the patient's overall condition [77]. Changeovers in nursing and other ancillary personnel may also contribute to miscounts of the sponges and pads. Lastly, lack of familiarity with the x-ray, CT, and ultrasound appearance of retained sponges may lead to a failure to recognize their presence promptly on postoperative examinations [70,78].

The natural history the retained surgical sponge ranges from simple extrusion along surgical planes to erosion into an adjacent hollow viscus. Superimposed infection may lead to abscess formation and the need for drainage and/or reexploration. Four stages of the body's reaction to a retained surgical spine, namely, foreign body reaction, secondary infection, mass formation, and remodeling, were documented in an experimental study [79].

Detection during the first postoperative month is usually related to inflammation [70]. Aseptic reaction is usually without any significant symptoms. An exudative reaction leads to early but nonspecific symptoms [80]. Afterward, discovery is related to mass effect, bowel obstruction, erosion, and/or fistula formation [69,70,78,81]. Symptoms may include abdominal pain, postoperative ileus, bladder disturbances, or rectal tenesmus [78].

FIGURE 1.22. **Retained surgical clamp.** Antero-posterior (A) and lateral (B) films from an upper GI series show a large metallic clamp, retained in the abdomen. The patient was asymptomatic and had not had surgery in at least 20 years; this was an incidental finding.

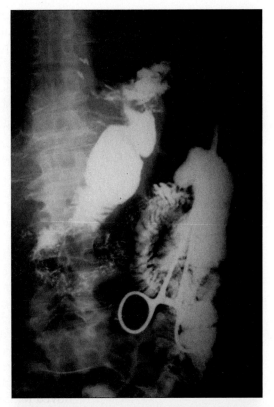

A

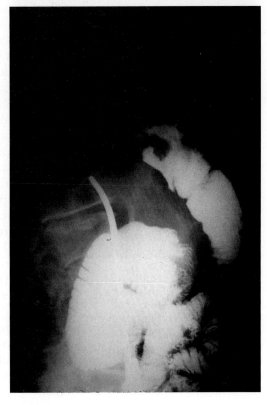

B

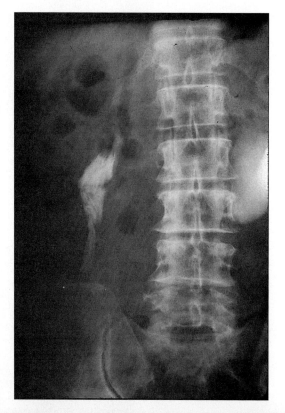

A

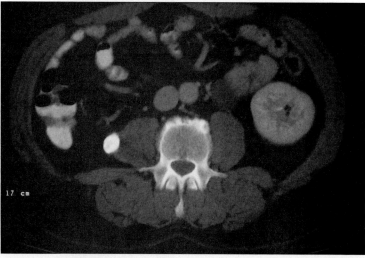

B

FIGURE 1.23. Retained Penrose drain. Supine film of the abdomen (A), CT image of the abdomen at "soft tissue" window settings (B), and the same section at " bone" window settings (C) show a calcified Penrose drain folded back upon itself alongside the psoas muscle. The folded nature is best appreciated on the extrawide window width afforded by the "bone" settings.

FIGURE 1.23. (*Continued*)

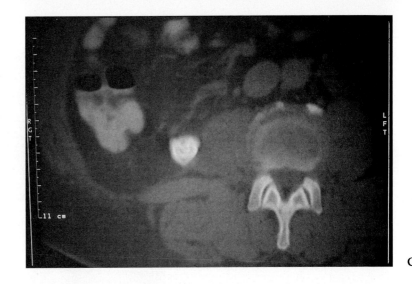

C

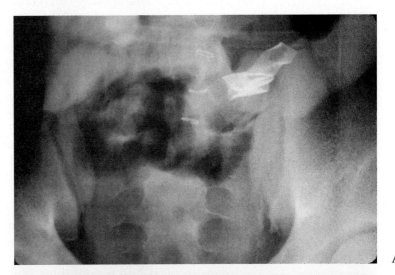

A

FIGURE 1.24. **Retained laparotomy pad.** Supine film of the pelvis (A) and CT scan through the same region (B) reveal a radiopaque marker of a lap pad surrounded by a sterile fluid collection (seroma).

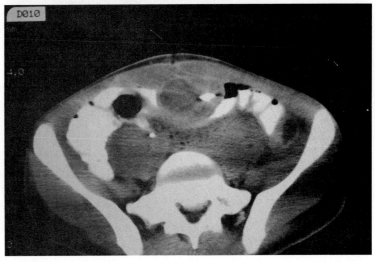

B

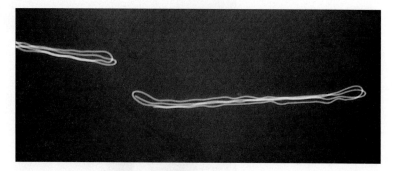

FIGURE 1.25. **Sponge marker.** X-ray image of the barium-impregnated thread used as a marker for a surgical sponge.

Chorvat et al. reported that more than 50% of sponges were discovered more than 5 years postoperatively [82]. At least one third of these patients were asymptomatic, and the sponges were found and removed incidental to other reasons for reexploration. These findings must be tempered by the observation that Chorvat's work predates the use of abdominal CT, modern ultrasound techniques, or MR imaging.

As already noted, sponges used in the operating room contain a barium-impregnated thread that makes them readily identifiable on postoperative plain films [83]. Lap pads have a wide radiopaque tape and often a large metallic ring attached (Fig. 1.26). With a rare exception of thoracotomy dressings and those used in vaginal packing [personal experience of one of the authors (BJ)], the detection of a marker should be presumed to represent a retained sponge [83]. Unfortunately, if the marker has been distorted, it may not appear as a curvilinear density in sponges that have been folded or otherwise compressed. A marker that has deteriorated over time may not be readily detectable [84]. A cadaver study revealed a 25% false negative rate of detecting the markers on plain films [85].

Liessi described the following three different presentations of retained sponges on plain films [86]: the detection of the marker, a calcified mass, and a "whirl-like" pattern due to the sponge itself (Figs. 1.27–1.32).

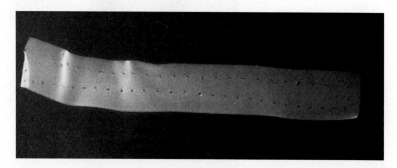

FIGURE 1.26. **Lap pad marker.** X-ray image of the radiopaque lap pad marker.

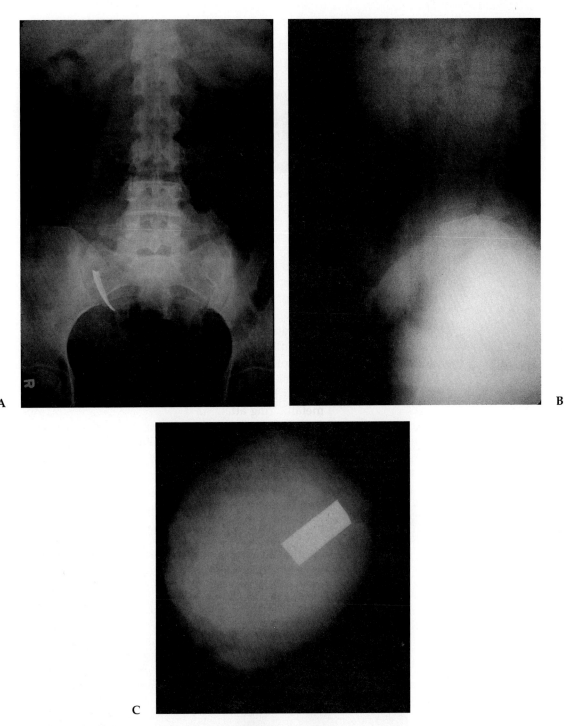

FIGURE 1.27. **Gossypiboma.** Supine (A) and lateral (B) plain films of the abdomen demonstrate the marker for a lap pad surrounded by a soft tissue mass (best seen on the lateral film). A specimen radiograph (C) demonstrates the retained lap pad encompassed by a large fibrous mass.

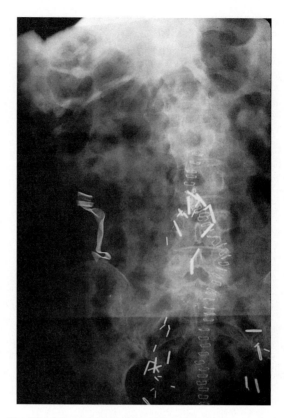

FIGURE 1.28. **Retained lap pad.** Supine film of the abdomen demonstrates a retained lap pad in the right midabdomen. The multiplicity of surgical clips serves as a visual distractor, making the diagnosis more difficult.

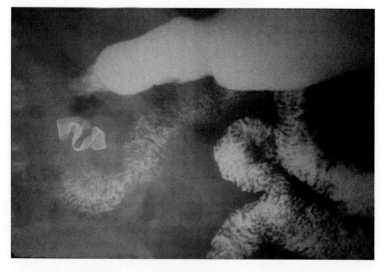

FIGURE 1.29. **Retained lap pad.** Frontal film from an upper GI series shows a retained lap pad projecting into the duodenal "C" loop.

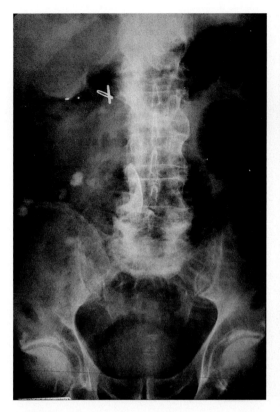 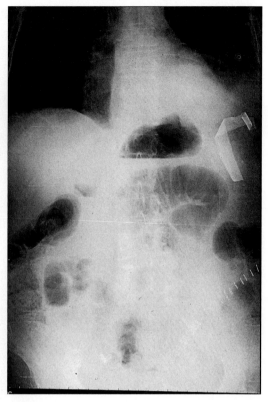

FIGURE 1.30. **Retained lap pad that is difficult to see.** Supine film of the abdomen reveals a hard-to-find lap pad marker superimposed over the lumbar spine.

FIGURE 1.31. **Remote retained lap pad.** Upright film of the abdomen reveals a lap pad marker in the left upper quadrant. Lap pads may often be found far from the actual site of the surgical procedure. When used to pack the bowel out of the surgeon's way, they may be forgotten and overlooked when the abdomen is being closed.

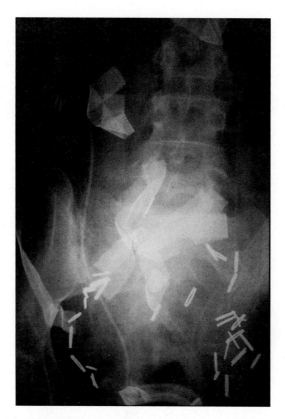

FIGURE 1.32. **Multiple retained lap pads.** Supine film of the abdomen showing multiple lap pads. The sheer number of markers should not dissuade one from reporting the possibility of retained implements.

On CT examination, many different patterns have also been described [80,81,84,86]. One sign is that of a cystic mass with high density contents representing a hematoma containing a retained sponge [81]. A second pattern is that of a well-defined mass containing multiple gas bubbles [80,81]. Another possible appearance is that of a cystic mass (with or without a calcified rim) that contains multiple thin linear densities in an folded or zigzag configuration [81]. This represents the folded nature of a "lap" pad or towel. A variant on this appearance is a whorled or spokelike configuration of the cyst contents [69,80,84,86]. When these appearances are noted, it can be very difficult to differentiate a gossypiboma from an abscess [80,87] (Fig. 1.33). At times, differentiation from other intra-abdominal masses, including recurrent or even primary neoplasms, may also be difficult [69,71,77,86,88].

Although this effect is rarely encountered, the inflammatory response to a retained surgical sponge may cause erosion into adjacent bowel. When a barium enema is performed in that instance, the irreg-

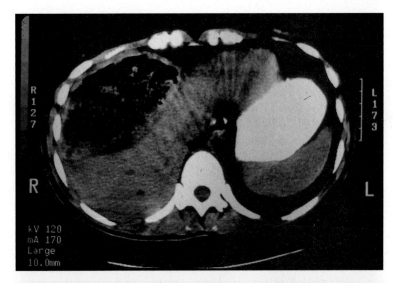

A

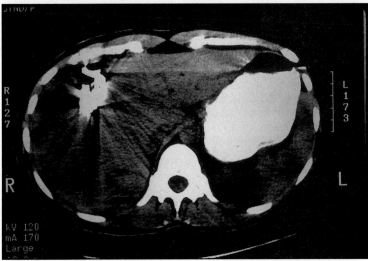

B

FIGURE 1.33. **Abscess secondary to retained lap pad.** Two CT sections reveal a large perihepatic abscess (A) secondary to a retained lap pad (B).

ular retained mass presents as multiple polypoidal defects in the bowel lumen as barium insinuates itself into the sponge matrix [78].

Sonography may also detect gossypibomas, either as an incidental finding or as the focus of the examination. When encountered, they present as an echogenic mass with acoustic shadowing [86,89]. The echogenicity is secondary to the numerous interfaces within the sponge [89]. When the acoustic shadowing is related to a palpable mass, the finding is considered diagnostic and appropriate therapy should be instituted [90].

The features of the gossypiboma that become visible on magnetic resonance imaging (MRI) depend on the protein content and nature of the fluid trapped within the sponge matrix [77]. Usually T1- and T2-weighted images will have low signal intensity representing a fibrous rim [77].

Oxidized Cellulose (Surgicel)

Another foreign body that can cause an imaging dilemma, but one that is deliberately left in the abdomen, is Surgicel (Johnson & Johnson Medical, Arlington, TX). This oxidized regenerated cellulose is a topical hemostatic agent that is bioabsorbable. The fiber is knitted into a gauze-like material. It is readily absorbed, chemically inert, and does not incite a foreign body reaction [91,92]. Thrombus forms when blood and the oxidized cellulose come into contact. It then may swell and increase in size. It is used to control capillary or venous bleeding [93]. Surgicel has a bactericidal effect on both aerobic and anaerobic bacteria. Although designed to be removed during surgery, it often is left in the surgical bed [93], especially during laparoscopic procedures [94].

On plain films the oxidized cellulose may be visualized as a linear band of increased density or as a mottled lucency secondary to air being trapped within its gauzelike structure [95] (Fig. 1.34). The latter configuration allows it to mimic an abscess in the surgical bed. A similar feature with a mixed attenuation mass containing a central air collection may be seen in a CT image [94].

Sonography reveals findings similar to those with a retained surgical spine with a highly echogenic mass with posterior reverberation artifact [96]. Some surrounding fluid may also be seen. The mass may mimic a recurrent ovarian malignancy [93] or other neoplasms [97,98].

The MR appearance is variable, depending on the stage of resorption during which the oxidized cellulose is imaged. In the early postoperative period, air trapped between the gauze fibers may result in signal void on both T1- and T2-weighted images [94]. In addition, T1-weighted images reveal a slightly increased signal intensity, while the signal on T2-weighted images is hypointense [94]. This latter finding is important in differentiating Surgicel from an abscess. The latter is markedly intense on T2-weighted images, whereas a Surgicel mass is not enhanced after gadolinium administration [93,94]. One-month follow-up studies revealed a marked decrease in size in half of patients, and complete resolution in a third. In patients in whom the mass decreased in size, the T2-weighted images showed markedly increased signal intensity, while masses were isointense on T1-weighted images [94].

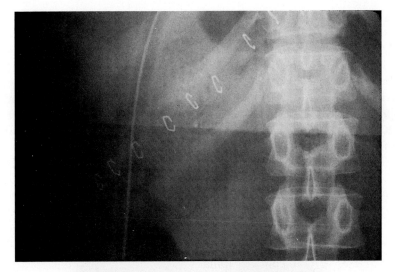

A

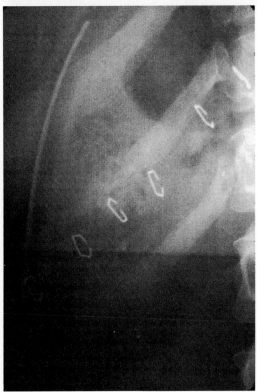

B

FIGURE 1.34. **Surgicel mimicking an abscess.** Supine film of the right upper quadrant (A) and a close-up of the same region (B) reveal multiple small air bubbles in a mottled pattern in this immediately postoperative patient. Although the anomaly could be mistaken for an abscess, the timing suggests a more benign etiology. In this case, the surgeon had implanted Surgicel to aid in hemostasis.

Meshes

Hernia repairs, especially for large recurrent hernias, aim at reestablishing abdominal wall substance and restoring the interaction of the abdominal wall musculature [99]. Various substances have been used to reinforce or reestablish the abdominal wall. These include fascia lata, stainless steel and tantalum metal meshes (Figs. 1.35–1.37), knitted monofilament polypropylene (Marlex) mesh, and an expanded polytetrafluoroethylene (Gore-Tex) patch [99–101].

The constant flexing of the anterior abdominal wall may lead to weakening and fracturing of the wire mesh. Subsequent fragmentation may lead to migration. The mesh may be extruded externally or even erode into the intestines, causing chronic blood loss and anemia [101]. With newer synthetic meshes, the postoperative problems are more often related to detachment [102], seromas and hematomas [102], and infection [99,102].

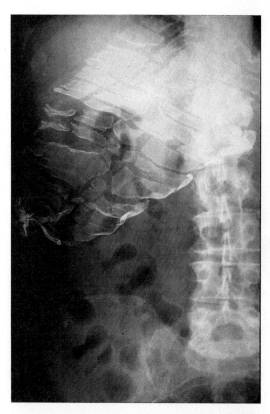

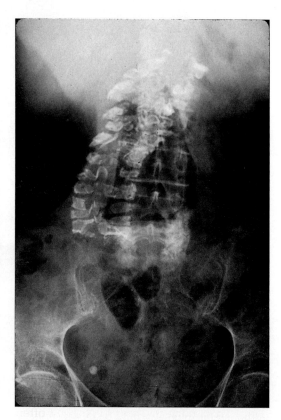

FIGURE 1.35. Metallic mesh for hernia repair. Supine film of the abdomen reveals a large metallic mesh in the right upper quadrant, stabilizing the anterior abdominal wall following a subcostal incision. This is an unusual location for an incisional hernia.

FIGURE 1.36. Metallic mesh. Supine film of the abdomen shows a metallic mesh used for the repair of a large ventral incisional hernia.

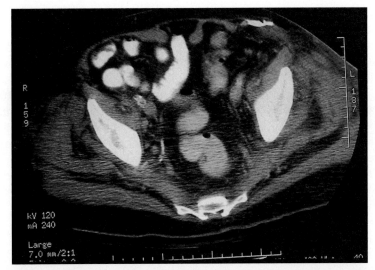

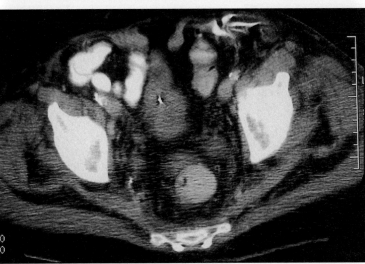

FIGURE 1.37. **Mesh for hernia repair.** Two adjacent CT sections (A, B) demonstrate a small metallic mesh used to reinforce an inguinal herniorrhaphy.

Scar Ossification

A very unusual complication of abdominal surgery is heterotopic ossification of midline abdominal scars. This variant of myositis ossificans may actually contain both bony and cartilaginous elements and, much more rarely, bone marrow [103]. Most often supraumbilical longitudinal incisions are involved, with a strong male preponderance (10:1) [104]. The scar lies between the two rectus muscles, bordered anteriorly by the abdominal wall fascia and posteriorly by the anterior parietal peritoneum [104]. No distinct linkage with the type of surgical procedure or the suture material used has been established.

Plain films reveal a calcific or bone density linear structure within the anterior abdominal wall, usually in a subxyphoid location (Figs. 1.38–1.40). Radionuclide studies show uptake of ^{99m}T-labeled pyrophosphate within the incision, even before the calcification or ossification is radiographically evident [105].

CT examination revealed rounded or flat linear ossification, or a combination of the two. When encountered, the rounded form is seen more proximally [103]. Central fat density was occasionally seen, consistent with the presence of bone marrow. Ossification can be noted as early as less than 3 weeks postoperatively and can be progressive.

The MR imaging characteristics were consistent with the underlying pathology [103]. A low intensity rim corresponded with fibrous tissue and/or calcium at the scar periphery. The central signal varies with the fat from marrow elements.

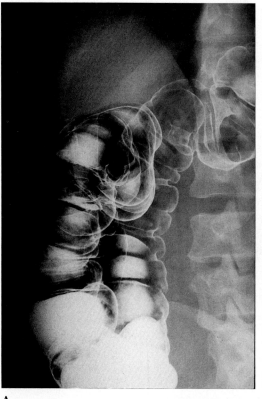

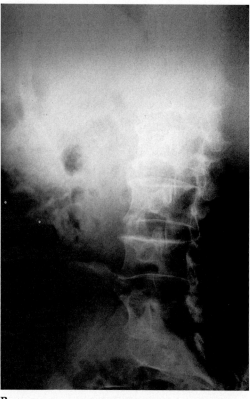

A   B

FIGURE 1.38. **Ossified scar.** Right posterior oblique abdominal film (A) and left anterior oblique film from a double-contrast enema (B) on the same patient show a linear calcific density in the upper abdomen. This represents an ossified scar.

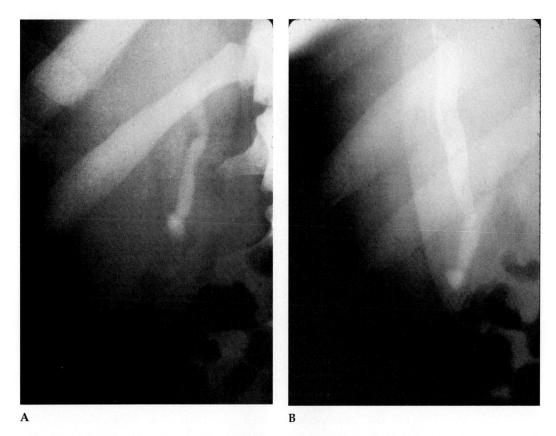

A   B

FIGURE 1.39. **Ossified scar.** Supine (A) and right posterior oblique (B) films of the right upper quadrant demonstrate an ossified scar in the upper abdomen. The oblique film (B) demonstrates the rather superficial location of the ossification.

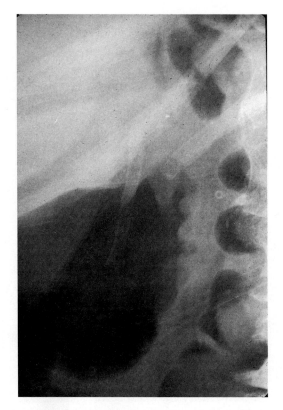

FIGURE 1.40. Ossified scar. Coned-down film of the right upper quadrant shows a linear density with a lucent center. The lucency may represent bone marrow elements within this ossified scar.

Intussusception

Intussusception may occur during the immediate postoperative period without a lead point; Agha reported abnormal bowel motility, electrolyte imbalances, and chronic dilatation of the bowel among these causes [106]. The coiled-spring appearance may be seen with either air [107] or barium [108] (Fig. 1.41) in the intussuscipiens outlining the intussusceptum. On CT examination, a target sign consists of contrast within the lumen of the intussusceptum surrounded by its mucosa. This is enveloped by the fat of the serosa or mesentery, which is further surrounded by contrast and the intestinal wall of the intussuscipiens [109–111]. When visualized longitudinally, the telescoping of the intussusceptum into the intussuscipiens is readily apparent. Much less frequently encountered is the unusual retrograde intussusception, where the intussusceptum is the distal small-bowel segment, and the intussuscipiens the more proximal part (Fig. 1.42).

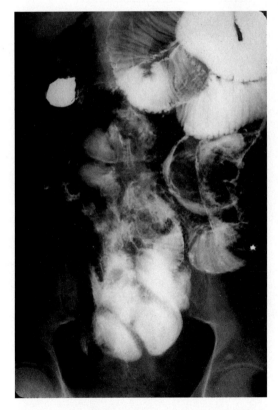

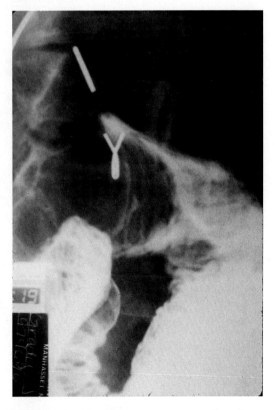

FIGURE 1.41. Postoperative intussusception. Small-bowel follow-through shows the coiled-spring appearance of an intussusception in the jejunum in the left midabdomen. No leading edge was evident in this recently postoperative patient.

FIGURE 1.42. Retrograde intussusception. Spot film from a small-bowel series shows a filling defect with a coiled-spring appearance in the proximal ileum. Fluoroscopic evaluation showed this to be changeable and functional in origin.

Herniation

Incisional hernias, also known as iatrogenic, postoperative, or cicatricial hernias, occur in a variety of clinical settings (Table 1.2) [112]. Like most hernias, incisional ones may incarcerate, with all the morbidity and mortality that accompanies that complication (Figs. 1.43 and 1.44).

TABLE 1.2. Etiology of incisional hernias.

Wound infection
Wound dehiscence
Increased intra-abdominal pressure in the early postoperative phase (e.g., coughing)
Atypical incision
Advanced age
Preexisting conditions
Collagen vascular diseases
Uremia
Obesity
Diabetes
Ascites

Source: Ref. 112.

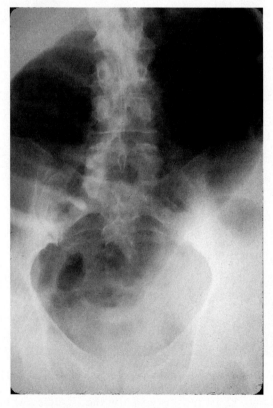

FIGURE 1.43. Small-bowel obstruction secondary to an incisional hernia. Supine film of the abdomen reveals markedly dilated loops of small bowel secondary to an incisional hernia.

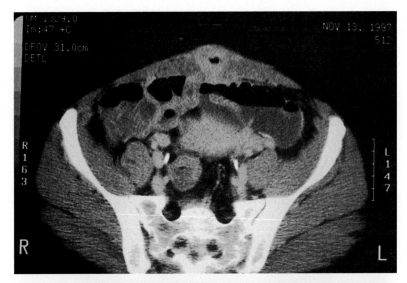

A

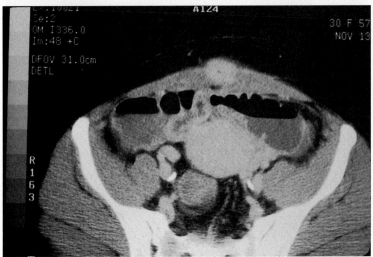

B

FIGURE 1.44. **Incarcerated incisional hernia.** Two adjacent CT sections (A, B) through the upper pelvis reveal a loop of small bowel incarcerated within a midline anterior abdominal wall incision. Note the thickened wall of the involved small bowel indicating vascular compromise. A small-bowel obstruction is also evident.

Although with the advent of laparoscopic surgery the size of the defects in the anterior abdominal wall (Fig. 1.45) has diminished greatly in comparison to those from conventional laparoscopy, incisional hernias may occur through the trochar sites (Fig. 1.46).

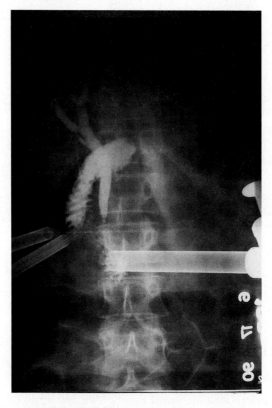

FIGURE 1.45. **Laparoscopic cholecystectomy instruments and insertion sites.** Single intraoperative film from a cystic duct cholangiogram performed during a laparascopic cholecystectomy demonstrates the various trochar insertion sites utilized in this technique.

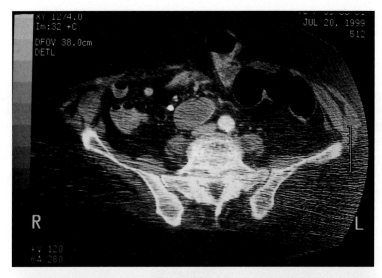

A

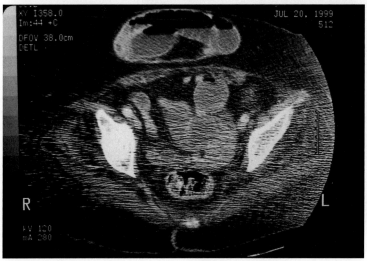

B

FIGURE 1.46. **Trochar hernia.** Two CT sections through the pelvis show a defect in the anterior abdominal wall adjacent to the umbilicus (A) through which the small bowel is herniating. This is due to prior puncture by a trochar for a laparoscopic cholecystectomy. The large extent of the hernia is evident on the more caudal section (B).

Internal postoperative hernias are not true hernias. Instead they represent a disordered clustering of bowel in an abnormally created peritoneal recess [112]. No hernia sac is present. These abnormalities may be seen on 0.2 to 2.9% of autopsies of patients who had undergone surgery [112,113]. They represent approximately half of all internal hernias. They may be seen going through the transverse mesocolon following Billroth II surgery, or other gastroenterostomy (Figs. 1.47 and 1.48). Other sites include the iliac bone through a bone graft donor site (Fig. 1.49), as well as other osseous defects. Following a nephrectomy, bowel may enter the now-empty renal fossa. Postoperative hernias are often asymptomatic [112]. When the herniation is intermittent, nonspecific abdominal complaints may be intermittent as well.

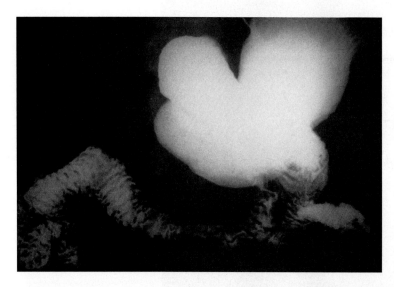

FIGURE 1.47. Internal postoperative hernia. Film from an upper GI series shows a dilated stomach superiorly, and dilated loops of small bowel adjacent to the greater curvature. The latter represent herniated small bowel through a postoperative defect in the transverse mesocolon.

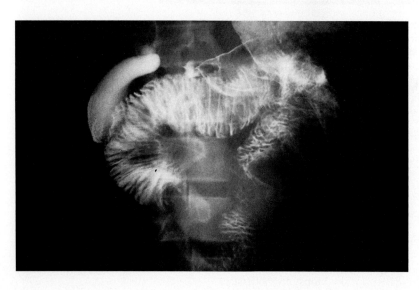

FIGURE 1.48. Postoperative transmesocolic hernia. Dilated small bowel is demonstrated in the upper abdomen as it is incarcerated within a transverse mesocolic defect. The defect, the result of a stab wound to the abdomen, was used to bring up a loop of small bowel for a complex diversion procedure.

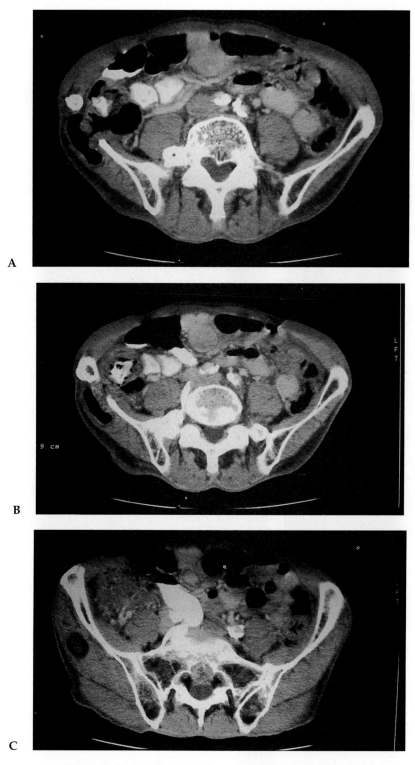

FIGURE 1.49. **Buttocks hernia through bony defect.** Three sections from a CT examination of the pelvis (A–C) reveal a bony defect in the right iliac wing through which loops of small bowel herniated into the buttocks. This was the result of an overly vigorous bone marrow biopsy in the past.

Postoperative hernias can easily be missed in the absence of provocative maneuvers and/or proper positioning of the patient [114]. Steep oblique and lateral films (Fig. 1.50) as well as a Valsalva maneuver may increase the diagnostic accuracy on routine contrast studies [115]. On conventional small-bowel studies as well as on enteroclysis, multiple small-bowel loops are encapsulated, crowded together, and fixed in

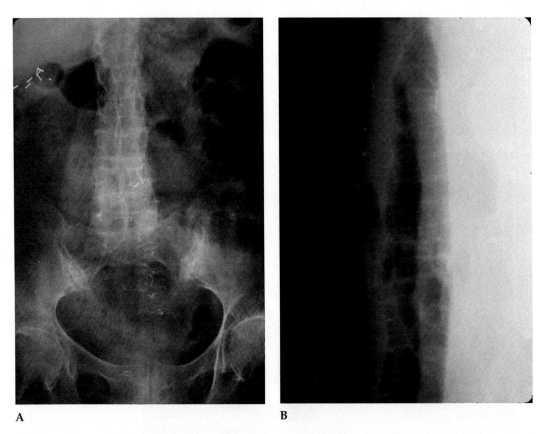

A   B

FIGURE 1.50. Incisional hernia. Supine (A) and cross-table lateral films (B) of the abdomen reveal dilated loops of small bowel consistent with a small-bowel obstruction. The lateral film (B) shows a herniated loop of small bowel entering an incisional defect in the anterior abdominal wall.

location [116] (Figs. 1.51 and 1.52). In addition, the proximal small bowel dilated while loops distally are collapsed (Fig. 1.53). Smooth symmetric tapering of the barium column may be noted at the neck of the internal hernia [117] (Fig. 1.54). CT and MR imaging have certainly improved our ability to diagnose both incisional and internal postoperative hernias [112,116].

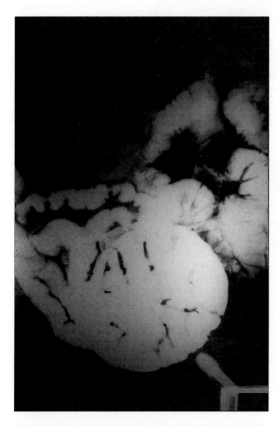

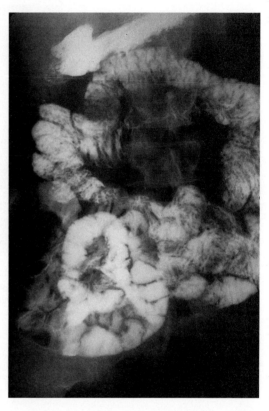

FIGURE 1.51. **Incisional hernia.** Film from a small-bowel series shows a large encapsulated group of small-bowel loops in the pelvis, an incisional hernia.

FIGURE **1.52. Incisional hernia.** Another small-bowel series, similar in appearance to that seen in Figure 1.47, this time in a right lower quadrant incisional hernia.

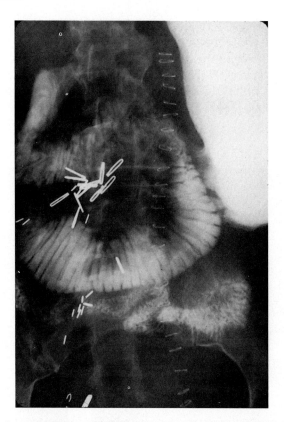

FIGURE 1.53. **Internal postoperative hernia.** Small-bowel series demonstrates a single dilated loop of proximal jejunum in the mid- and upper abdomen. Its fixed appearance on multiple films suggested that this was an internal hernia, not a simple adhesive small-bowel obstruction. This diagnosis was confirmed at surgery.

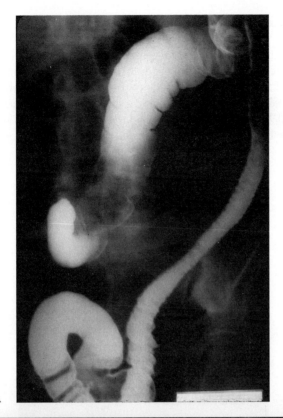

A

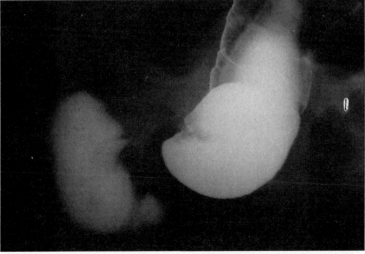

B

FIGURE 1.54. **Colon in incisional hernia.** Overhead film from a single-contrast barium enema (A) reveals obstruction to the retrograde flow in the proximal transverse colon. A spot film (B) of this area shows smooth concentric narrowing as the colon enters the incisional hernia.

Puckered Panniculus

It can be difficult to ascertain the postoperative status of some patients in the absence of surgical clips, staples, or suture material. One possible clue to a prior surgical history is the "puckered panniculus" sign. Baker and Cho described this sign as the retraction of the abdominal wall caused by a longitudinal incision [118]. This results in a bilobed appearance to the anterior abdominal wall as it overlies the pelvis (Fig. 1.55).

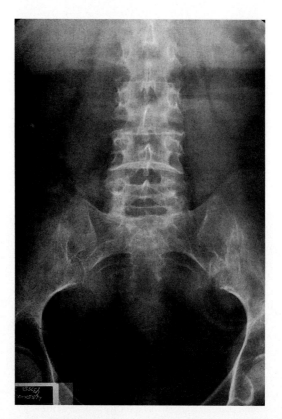

Figure 1.55. "Puckered panniculus." Supine film of the abdomen reveals the soft tissues of the anterior abdominal wall having a bilobate appearance, with retraction in the midline. This so-called puckered panniculus sign is an excellent indicator of prior surgery.

References

1. Summers B. Pneumoperitoneum associated with artificial ventilation. BMJ 1979;1(6177):1528–1530.
2. Cancarini GC, Carli O, Cristinelli MR, Manili L, Maiorca R. Pneumoperitoneum in peritoneal dialysis patients. J Nephrol 1999;12:95–99.
3. Bryant L, Wiot J, Kloecker R. A study of the factors affecting the incidence and duration of postoperative pneumoperitoneum. Surg Gynecol Obstet 1963;117:145–150.
4. Bevan PG. Incidence of postoperative pneumoperitoneum and its significance. BMJ 1961;2:605–609.
5. Harrison I, Litwer H, Gerwig W. Studies on the incidence of postoperative pneumoperitoneum. Ann Surg 1957;145:591–594.
6. Wiot JF, Benton C, McAlister WH. Postoperative pneumoperitoneum in children. Radiology 1967;89:285–288.
7. Felson B, Wiot JF. Another look at pneumoperitoneum. Semin Roentgenol 1973;8:437–443.
8. Earls JP, Dachman AH, Colon E, Garrett MG, Molloy M. Prevalence and duration of postoperative pneumoperitoneum: Sensitivity of CT vs left lateral decubitus radiography. AJR Am J Roentgenol 1993;161:781–785.
9. Baker SR, Cho SR. The Abdominal Plain Film with Correlative Imaging, 2nd ed. Stamford, CT: Appleton & Lange; 1999:87–175.
10. Miller RE, Becker GJ, Slabaugh RD. Detection of pneumoperitoneum: Optimum body position and respiratory phase. AJR Am J Roentgenol 1980;135:487–490.
11. James Jr AE, Montali RJ, Chaffee V, Strecker E-P, Vessal K. Barium or Gastrografin: Which contrast media for diagnosis of esophageal tears? Am J Gastroenterol 1975;68:1103–1113.
12. Vessal K, Montali RJ, Larson SM, Chaggee V, James Jr AE. Evaluation of barium and Gastrografin as contrast media for the diagnosis of esophageal ruptures or perforations. Am Roentgenol Radium Ther Nucl Med 1975;123:307–319.
13. Huston J, Wallack DP, Cunningham GJ. Pulmonary reaction to barium sulfate in rats. Arch Pathol 1952;54:430–438.
14. Ginai AZ, ten Kate FJW, ten Berg RGM, Hoornstra K. Experimental evaluation of various available contrast agents for use in the upper gastrointestinal tract in case of suspected leakage. Effects on lungs. Br J Radiol 1984;57:895–901.
15. Reich SB. Production of pulmonary edema by aspiration of water-soluble nonabsorbable contrast media. Radiology 1969;92:367–370.
16. Chiu CL, Gambach RR. Hypaque pulmonary edema. A case report. Radiology 1974;111:91–92.
17. Dodds WJ, Stewart ET, Vlymen WJ. Appropriate contrast media for evaluation of esophageal disruption. Radiology 1982;144:439–441. AJR Am J Roentgenol 1975;123:307–3319.
18. Cochran DQ, Almond CH, Shucart WA. An experimental study of the effects of barium and intestinal contents on the peritoneal cavity. AJR Am J Roentgenol 1963;89:883–887.
19. Sanders AW, Kobernick SD. Fate of barium sulfate in retroperitoneum. Am J Surg 1957;93:907–910.
20. Ferrante SL, Schreiman JS, Rouse JW, et al. Iopamidol as a gastrointestinal contrast agent. Lack of peritoneal reactivity. Invest Radiol 1990;25:141–145.

21. Hunter TB, Fon GT, Silverstein ME. Complications of intestinal tubes. Am J Gastroenterol 1981;76:256–261.
22. Tiller HJ, Rhea Jr WG. Iatrogenic perforation of the esophagus by a nasogastric tube. Am J Surg 1984;147:423–425.
23. Robinson P, Thomas NB. Intra-abdominal oesophageal perforation following nasogastric tube insertion. Eur Radiol 1999;9:1697–1698.
24. Jackson RH, Payne DK, Bacon BR. Esophageal perforation due to nasogastric intubation. Am J Gastroenterol 1990;85:439–442.
25. Hollimon PW, McFee AS. Pneumothorax attributable to nasogastric tube. Arch Surg 1981;116:970.
26. Fisman DN, Ward ME. Intrapleural placement of a nasogastric tube: An unusual complication of nasotracheal intubation. Can J Anaesth 1996; 43:1252–1256.
27. Tocino I, Westcott J, Davis S. Routine daily portable x-ray. In: The American College of Radiology Appropriateness Criteria. Reston, VA: The American College of Radiology; 1995:621–626.
28. Hayhurst EG, Wyman M. Morbidity associated with prolonged use of polyvinyl feeding tubes. Am J Dis Child 1975;129:72–74.
29. Drenick EJ, Lipset M. Difficulty with removal of plastic nasogastric tubes. JAMA 1971;218:1573.
30. Javors BR, Seeff J. The disrupted esophagus: Ulcers, holes and tears. J Postgrad Radiol 1993;13:1–27.
31. Cantor MO. Distension of the gastrointestinal tract. In: Cantor MO, Reynolds RP, eds. Gastrointestinal Obstruction. Baltimore: Williams & Wilkins; 1957:306–313.
32. Rozanski J, Kleinfeld M. A complication of prolonged intestinal intubation: Gaseous distention of the terminal balloon. Dig Dis 1975;20:1067–1070.
33. Paulson EK, Grant JP, Rice RP. Gaseous distension of a single-lumen mushroom-tip intestinal tube: An unusual cause of bowel obstruction. AJR Am J Roentgenol 1993;161:797–798.
34. Coleman SL, Miller E, Stroehlein JR, Hoffman HN. Nonoperative retrieval of an impacted long intestinal tube. Dig Dis 1977;22:462–464.
35. Yoshino MT, Boyle Jr RR. Strangulation of the colon caused by an intestinal decompression tube: Radiographic findings. AJR Am J Roentgenol 1987;149:735–736.
36. Lautin EM, Scheinbaum KR. Hyperbaric therapy for the removal of an obstructing intestinal tube balloon. Gastrointest Radiol 1987;12:243–244.
37. Otsuji E, Yamaguchi T, Sawai K, et al. Hepatogastroenterology 1999; 46:3172–3174.
38. Dinsmore RC, Benson JR. Endoscopic removal of a knotted nasogastric tube lodged in the posterior nasopharynx. South Med J 1999;92:1005–1007.
39. Redmond P, Ambos M, Berliner L, Pachter HL, Megibow A. Iatrogenic intussusception: A complication of long intestinal tubes. Am J Gastroenterol 1982;77:39–42.
40. Brown EO, Miller JM. Retrograde jejunal intussusception following the use of a Cantor intestinal tube. Am J Proctol Gastroenterol Colon Rectal Surg 1981;32:28–33.
41. Holmes 4th JH, Brundage SI, Yuen P, Hall RA, Maier RV, Jurkovich GJ. Complications of surgical feeding jejunostomy in trauma patients. J Trauma 1999;47:1009–1012.
42. Rai J, Flint LM, Ferrara JJ. Small bowel necrosis in association with jejunostomy tube feedings. Am Surg 1996;62:1050–1054.

43. Oktem IS, Akdemir H, Koc K, et al. Migration of abdominal catheter of ventriculoperitoneal shunt into the scrotum. Acta Neurochir (Wien) 1998;140:167–170.

44. Martin LM, Donaldson-Hugh ME, Cameron MM. Cerebrospinal fluid hydrothorax caused by transdiaphragmatic migration of a ventriculoperitoneal catheter through the foramen of Bochdalek. Child Nerv Syst 1997;13:282–284.

45. Eschelman DJ, Lee VW. Lesser sac cerebrospinal fluid collection. An unusual complication of a ventriculoperitoneal shunt. Clin Nucl Med 1990;15:415–417.

46. Christoph CL, Poole CA, Kochan PS. Operative gastric perforation: A rare complication of ventriculoperitoneal shunt. Pediatr Radiol 1995;25(suppl 1):S173–S174.

47. Alonso-Vanegas M, Alvarez JL, Delgado L, et al. Gastric perforation due to ventriculo-peritoneal shunt. Pediatr Neurosurg 1994;21:192–194.

48. Brown SR, Gourlay R, Battersby RD. Sigmoidoscopic neurosurgery? Treatment of an unusual complication of ventriculoperitoneal shunting. Br J Neurosurg 1996;10:419–420.

49. Huang LT, Chen CC, Shih TT, Ko SF, Lui CC. Pyogenic liver abscess complicating a ventriculoperitoneal shunt. Pediatr Surg Int 1998;13:6–7.

50. Peterfy CG, Atri M. Intrahepatic abscess: A rare complication of ventriculoperitoneal shunt. AJR Am J Roentgenol 1990;155:894–895.

51. Fisher RA, Rodziewicz G, Selman WR, White RJ, Vibhakar SD. Liver abscess: Complication of a ventriculoperitoneal shunt. Neurosurgery 1984;14:480–482.

52. Wang F, Miller JH. Cerebrospinal fluid pseudocyst presenting as a hepatic mass: A complication of ventriculoperitoneal shunt. Pediatr Radiol 1989; 19:326–327.

53. Mata J, Alegret X, Llauger J. Splenic pseudocyst as a complication of ventriculoperitoneal shunt: CT features. J Comput Assist Tomogr 1986; 10:341–342.

54. Ibrahim AW. E. coli meningitis as an indicator of intestinal perforation by V-P shunt tube. Neurosurg Rev 1998;21:194–197.

55. Rainov N, Schobess A, Heidecke V, Burkert W. Abdominal CSF pseudocysts in patients with ventriculoperitoneal shunts. Report of fourteen cases and review of the literature. Acta Neurochir (Wien) 1994;127:73–78.

56. Besson R, Hladky JP, Dhellemmes P, Debeugny P. Peritoneal pseudocyst—Ventriculo-peritoneal shunt complications. Eur J Pediatr Surg 1995;5:195–197.

57. Ersahin Y, Mutluer S, Tekeli G. Abdominal cerebrospinal fluid pseudocysts. Child Nerv Syst 1996;12:755–758.

58. White B, Kroop K, Rayport M. Abdominal cerebrospinal fluid pseudocyst: Occurrence after intraperitoneal urological surgery in children with ventriculoperitoneal shunts. J Urol 1991;146:583–587.

59. Brunori A, Massari A, Macarone-Palmieri R, Benini B, Chiappetta F. Minimally invasive treatment of giant CSF pseudocyst complicating ventriculoperitoneal shunt. Minim Invasive Neurosurg 1998;41:38–39.

60. Baskin JJ, Vishteh AG, Wesche DE, Rekate HL, Carrion CA. Ventriculoperitoneal shunt failure as a complication of laparoscopic surgery. J Soc Laparoendosc Surg 1998;2:177–180.

61. Roitberg BZ, Tomita T, McLone DG. Abdominal cerebrospinal fluid pseudocyst: A complication of ventriculoperitoneal shunt in children. Pediatr Neurosurg 1998;29:267–273.

62. Rickert CH. Abdominal metastases of pediatric brain tumors via ventriculoperitoneal shunts. Child Nerv Syst 1998;14:10–14.

63. Rickert CH, Reznik M, Lenelle J, Rinaldi P. Shunt-related abdominal metastasis of cerebral teratocarcinoma: Report of an unusual case and review of the literature. Neurosurgery 1998;42:1378–1382.

64. Starreveld Y, Poenaru D, Ellis P. Ventriculoperitoneal shunt knot: A rare cause of bowel obstruction and ischemia. Can J Surg 1998;41:239–240.

65. Bal RK, Singh P, Harjai MM. Intestinal volvulus—A rare complication of ventriculoperitoneal shunt. Pediatr Surg Int 1999;15:577–578.

66. Ellenhorn MJ, Barceloux DG. Medical toxicology. Diagnosis and treatment of human poisoning. New York: Elsevier; 1988:1007–1065.

67. Ernst E. Metallic mercury in the gastrointestinal tract. A case of ingested thermometer mercury. Acta Chir Scand 1985;151:651–652.

68. Zimmerman JE. Fatality following metallic mercury aspiration during removal of a long intestinal tube. JAMA 1969;208:2158–2160.

69. Rappaport W, Haynes K. The retained surgical sponge following intra-abdominal surgery. A continuing problem. Arch Surg 1990;125:405–407.

70. Hyslop JW, Maull KI. Natural history of the retained surgical sponge. South Med J 1982;75:657–660.

71. Jason R, Chisolm A, Lubetsky H. Retained surgical sponge simulating a pancreatic mass. J Natl Med Assoc 1979;71:501–503.

72. Parienty RA, Pradel J, Lepreux JF, Nicodeme CH, Dologa M. Computed tomography of sponges retained after laparotomy. J Comput Assist Tomogr 1981;5:187–189.

73. Jones A. The foreign body problem after laparotomy. Am J Surg 1971;122:785–786.

74. Wilson CP. Foreign bodies left in the abdomen after laparotomy. Gynecol Trans 1884;9:109–112.

75. Cahn N. Nachweis in der Bauchhohle verbleibener Stopftucher und Taupter. Zentralorgan Gesamt Chir 1929;45:759.

76. Greenhill JP. Foreign bodies left in the abdomen after operation. Am J Obstet Gynecol 1933;25:213–233.

77. Moyle H, Hines OJ, McFadden DW. Gossypiboma of the abdomen. Arch Surg 1996;131:566–568.

78. Gupta NM, Chaudhary A, Nanda V, Malik AK, Wig JD. Retained surgical sponge after laparotomy. Unusual presentation. Dis Colon Rectum 1985;28:451–453.

79. Wattanasirichaigoon S. Transmural migration of a retained surgical sponge into the intestinal lumen: An experimental study. J Med Assoc Thailand 1996;79:415–422.

80. Kalovidouris A, Kehagias D, Moulopoulos L, Gouliamos A, Pentea S, Vlahos L. Abdominal retained surgical sponges: CT appearance. Eur Radiol 1999;9:1407–1410.

81. Buy J-N, Hubert C, Ghossain MA, Malbec L, Bethoux J-P, Ecoiffier J. Computed tomography of retained abdominal sponges and towels. Gastrointest Radiol 1989;14:41–45.

82. Chorvat G, Kahn J, Camelot G, et al. Clinical course following retention of sponges left in the abdomen. Ann Chir 1976;30:643–646.

83. Williams RG, Bragg DG, Nelson JA. Gossypiboma—The problem of the retained surgical sponge. Radiology 1978;129:323–326.

84. Sheward SE, Williams Jr AG, Mettler Jr FA, Lacey SR. CT appearance of a surgically retained towel (gossypiboma). J Comput Assist Tomogr 1986;10:343–345.

85. Revesz G, Siddiqi TS, Buchheit WA, Bonitatibus M. Detection of retained surgical sponges. Radiology 1983;149:411–413.
86. Liessi G, Semisa M, Sandini F, Roma R, Spaliviero B, Marin G. Retained surgical gauzes: Acute and chronic CT and US findings. Eur J Radiol 1989;9:182–186.
87. Apter S, Hertz M, Rubinstein ZJ, Zissin R. Gossypiboma in the early postoperative period: A diagnostic problem. Clin Radiol 1990;42:128–129.
88. Zbar AP, Agrawal A, Saeed IT, Utidjian MR. Gossypiboma revisited: A case report and review of the literature. J R Coll Surg Edinb 1998;43:417–418.
89. Wan YL, Huang TJ, Huang DL, Lee TY, Tsai CC. Sonography and computed tomography of a gossypiboma and in vitro studies of sponges by ultrasound. Case report. Clin Imaging 1992;16:256–258.
90. Barriga P, Garcia C. Ultrasonography in the detection of intra-abdominal retained surgical sponges. J Ultrasound Med 1984;3:173–176.
91. Thaller SR, Kim S, Tesluk H, Kawamato H. The split calvarial bone graft donor site: The effects of Surgicel and hydroxyapatite impregnated with collagen. Ann Plast Surg 1990;25:435–439.
92. Pierce A, Wilson D, Wiebkin O. Surgicel: Macrophage processing of the fibrous component. Int J Oral Maxillofac Surg 1987;16:338–345.
93. Deger RB, LiVolsi VA, Noumoff JS. Foreign body reaction (gossypiboma) masking as recurrent ovarian cancer. Gynecol Oncol 1995;56:94–96.
94. Oto A, Remer EM, O'Malley CM, Tkach JA, Gill IS. MR characteristics of oxidized cellulose (Surgicel). AJR Am J Roentgenol 1999;172:1481–1484.
95. van Gelderen F. Appearance of oxidized cellulose (Surgicel) on abdominal radiographs. AJR Am J Roentgenol 1996;167:1593.
96. Melamed JW, Paulson EK, Kliewer MA. Sonographic appearance of oxidized cellulose (Surgicel): Pitfall in the diagnosis of postoperative abscess. J Ultrasound Med 1995;14:27–30.
97. Sandhu GS, Elexpuru-Camiruaga JA, Buckley S. Oxidized cellulose (Surgicel) granulomata mimicking tumor recurrence. Br J Neurosurg 1996;10:617–619.
98. Lang IM, Connolly B, Filler RM. Surgicel mimics possible recurrence of hepatoblastoma. Pediatr Radiol 1997;27:288.
99. Arnaud JP, Tuech JJ, Pessaux P, Hadchity Y. Surgical treatment of postoperative incisional hernias by intraperitoneal insertion of Dacron mesh and an aponeurotic graft: A report on 250 cases. Arch Surg 1999;134:1260–1262.
100. Keighley MR, Fielding JW, Alexander-Williams J. Results of Marlex mesh abdominal rectopexy for rectal prolapse in 100 consecutive patients. Br J Surg 1983;70:229–232.
101. Majeski J. Migration of wire mesh into the intestinal lumen causing an intestinal obstruction 30 years after repair of a ventral hernia. South Med J 1998;91:496–498.
102. Molloy RG, Moran KT, Waldron RP, Brady MP, Kirwan WO. Massive incisional hernia: Abdominal wall replacement with Marlex mesh. Br J Surg 1991;78:242–244.
103. Jacobs JE, Birnbaum BA, Siegelman ES. Heterotopic ossification of midline abdominal incisions: CT and MR imaging findings. AJR Am J Roentgenol 1996;166:579–584.
104. Lohela P, Orava S, Leionen A. Heteroptopic bone formation in abdominal midline scars. RORO Fortschr Roentgenstr 1983;139:412–415.
105. Pearson J, Clark OH. Heterotopic calcification in abdominal wounds. Surg Gynecol Obstet 1978;146:371–374.

106. Agha FP. Intussusception in adults. AJR Am J Roentgenol 1986;146:527–531.
107. Baker SR, Cho KC. The Abdominal Plain Film with Correlative Imaging, 2nd ed. Stamford, CT: Appleton & Lange; 1999:217–359.
108. Wiot JF, Spitz HB. Small bowel intussusception demonstrated by oral barium. Radiology 1970;97:361–366.
109. Curcio CM, Feinstein RS, Humphrey RL, et al. Computed tomography of entero-enteric intussusception. J Comput Assist Tomogr 1982;6:969–974.
110. Merine D, Fishma EK, Jones F, et al. Enteroenteric intussusception: CT findings in nine patients. AJR Am J Roentgenol 1987;148:1129–1132.
111. Balthazar EJ. CT of the gastrointestinal tract: Principles and interpretation. AJR Am J Roentgenol 1991;156:23–32.
112. Reeders JWAJ, Rosenbusch G. Clinical radiology and endoscopy of the colon. Stuttgart: Thieme; 1994:85–111.
113. Ghahremani GG. Internal abdominal hernias. Surg Clin North Am 1984;64:393–406.
114. Maglinte DDT, Miller RE, Lappas JC. Radiologic diagnosis of occult incisional hernias of the small intestine. AJR Am J Roentgenol 1984;142:931–932.
115. Javors BR. Manual of GI fluoroscopy. New York: Thieme; 1996:135–136.
116. Birnbaum BA, Maglinte DDT. Small bowel obstruction. In: Maglinte DDT, Herlinger H, Birnbaum BA, eds. Clinical Imaging of the Small Intestine, 2nd ed. New York: Springer-Verlag; 1998:467–506.
117. Herlinger H, Rubesin SE. Obstruction. In: Gore RM, Levine MS, Laufer I, eds. Textbook of Gastrointestinal Radiology. Philadelphia: WB Saunders; 1993:931–966.
118. Baker SR, Cho SR. The Abdominal Plain Film with Correlative Imaging, 2nd ed. Stamford, CT: Appleton & Lange; 1999:15–86.

2

The Esophagus

The development of the foregut and the resultant esophagus is rather straightforward in comparison to that of the mid- and hindgut. During the fourth week of development a median laryngotracheal groove forms at the caudal end of the primitive pharynx along its ventral surface [1]. Paired laryngotracheal folds bound this groove laterally [1]. This groove deepens and evaginates to eventually form the laryngotracheal diverticulum [1]. Growth between this zone and the developing stomach gives rise to the esophagus [2].

Longitudinal folds develop and form the tracheoesophageal septum, which divides the primitive foregut into a ventral, primitive respiratory apparatus and a dorsal definitive gastrointestinal tract [1]. The cranial part of the groove persists as the laryngeal additus, the opening into the larynx and trachea [2]. One unique feature of the developing esophagus is the failure of the surrounding mesenchyme to envelop the esophagus with a serosa. This has significant implications in the spread of disease from the esophagus into the surrounding tissue.

Anatomy

The esophagus extends from the region of the C6 to T11 vertebral bodies, traversing the neck and thorax on its way to the abdomen. In the neck, the esophagus lies just to the left of midline, posterior to the larynx and trachea, and anterior to the prevertebral fascia [1]. As it enters the chest, it curves slightly to the right, passing behind the carina or the left main stem bronchus to run posterior to the heart, where it maintains a close proximity to the left atrium. It bends to the left as it passes through the esophageal hiatus in the diaphragm. The intra-abdominal portion passes through the lesser sac for a distance of 2 to 4 cm before entering the stomach.

Similar to the rest of the gastrointestinal tract, the mucosa of the esophagus (squamous epithelium) overlies the lamina propria and muscularis mucosa. The inner circular and outer longitudinal muscular layers are not as strong as the intervening submucosa [3]. A serosal lining is also absent in the pharyngoesophageal segment, making suture retention more tenuous [4]. The submucosa comprises both elastic and fibrous tissue. The proximal esophagus is marked by the cricopharyngeus muscle, which functions as the upper esophageal sphincter, along with the inferior pharyngeal constrictors. The existence of a definable lower esophageal sphincter is more controversial.

The blood supply to the esophagus varies as one proceeds distally from the neck to the abdomen. Branches of the inferior thyroid arteries supply the esophagus in the neck. Bronchial arteries supply the upper thoracic esophagus, while direct branches from the thoracic aorta supply the lower thoracic region. Branches of the left gastric and inferior phrenic arteries supply the intra-abdominal esophagus as well as the most distal portion of the thoracic esophagus [3].

Venous drainage is via a submucosal plexus that pierces the muscular layer to connect with periesophageal veins that run parallel to the esophagus. The ultimate drainage in the neck is to the inferior thyroid veins and, in the chest, to the azygos and hemiazygos veins. More distally, the drainage is via the left gastric, caval, and portal veins and their tributaries [3].

Unlike the arterial supply and venous drainage, lymphatic drainage is not segmental [3]. This can lead to the longitudinal spread of disease a considerable distance from its site of origin, a phenomenon that helps account for the proximal spread of distal lesions as well as the distal spread of very proximal lesions.

The thoracic duct lies close to the esophagus as it traverses the posterior mediastinum from the diaphragm to the level of T5. There it crosses to the left, behind the esophagus, and eventually reaches the left subclavian artery at the level of the thoracic inlet before draining into the internal jugular vein [3].

The paired vagus nerves parallel the esophagus in the neck. In the thoracic region, they divide to form a racemose plexus. They return to a paired configuration as they approach the diaphragm. There the left vagus assumes a more anterior position and the right, a more posterior one, reflecting the rotation of the more distal, developing stomach. The left recurrent laryngeal nerve passes underneath the aortic arch to lie between the esophagus and the trachea. The right one lies in a similar groove in the neck [5].

Laryngectomy

Laryngeal carcinoma is often treated with surgical resection rather than radiotherapy. During laryngectomies, both partial and complete, the airway is completely separated from the pharyngeal–esophageal conduit. A tracheostomy assures proper respiratory function. The anterior wall of the pharyngoesophagus continuum (neopharynx) is closed, and drains are placed in the soft tissues of the neck [6].

In the immediate postoperative period, leaks (from the pharyngeal closure) and/or pharyngocutaneous fistulas are frequently encountered. Two predisposing factors for the development of fistulas are vomiting during the postoperative period [7] and gastroesophageal reflux [8]. The performance of a laryngectomy itself might actually cause to an increased incidence of gastroesophageal reflux [9]. Many of these fistulas can be observed, the patient's nutrition supported by enteral tube feedings, and surgery avoided [10].

In the late postoperative period, changes can be seen in both the form and function of the pharyngoesophageal region. Narrowing of the superior end of the surgical closure of this region can be seen in half of all patients and pseudodiverticula in almost half [11,12]. The latter represents an outpouching of the neopharyngeal lumen (Fig. 2.1). This outpouching is separated from the rest of the neopharynx by an oblique lucency that has been described as a pseudoepiglottis (Figs. 2.2 and

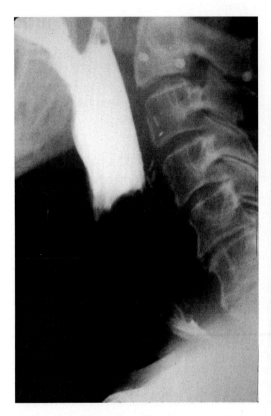

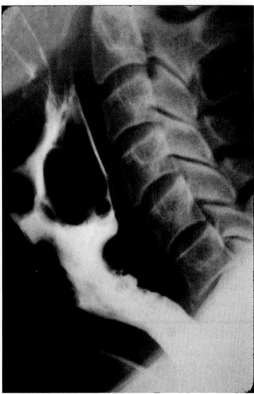

FIGURE 2.1. **Dilated neopharynx.** Lateral film from a cervical esophagram demonstrating a markedly dilated hypo- and neopharynx in a patient following total laryngectomy.

FIGURE 2.2. **Small pseudoepiglottis.** Lateral film from a cervical esophagogram demonstrating a small filling defect in the anterior neopharynx, the so-called pseudoepiglottis.

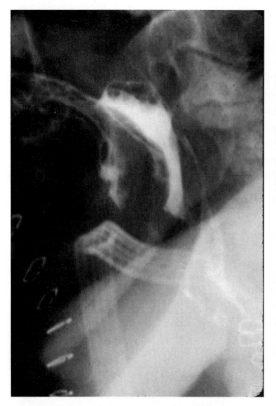

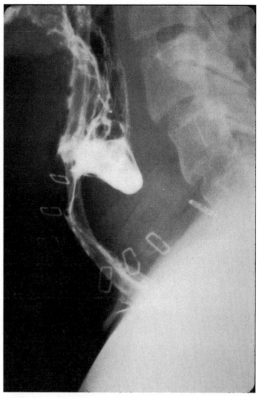

FIGURE 2.3. Larger pseudoepiglottis. Another, larger example of a pseudoepiglottis in the neopharynx of a postlaryngectomy patient.

FIGURE 2.4. Pseudodiverticulum of neopharynx. Lateral film from a cervical esophagogram demonstrating a large posterior bulge at the inferior end of the neopharynx.

2.3). The pseudodiverticulum is actually produced by the surgery itself and does not develop over time. However, it may enlarge secondary to increased intrapharyngeal pressure noted postoperatively, or because of food that becomes trapped in its lumen [12] (Fig. 2.4).

The retropharyngeal (prevertebral) soft tissues increase in thickness, but this does not necessarily indicate tumor recurrence [11] (Fig. 2.5). This finding may be secondary to detachment of the constrictor muscles from the prevertebral tissues. A prominent cricopharyngeus

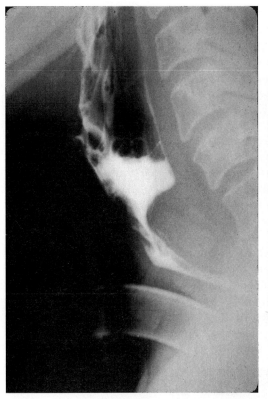 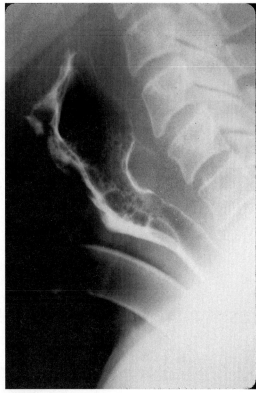

A   B

FIGURE 2.5. Typical prevertebral soft tissue
bulge following laryngectomy. (A) Lateral film
from cervical esophagogram demonstrating a
large posterior soft tissue bulge at the pharyngoesophageal junction. (B) Another lateral film,
taken a few seconds later, showing marked
changeability of the posterior soft tissue bulge,
which indicates its benign nature.

may be seen in approximately 15% of all patients. When recurrence
does occur, the neopharynx becomes narrowed and does not change
during swallowing, an important differential feature with respect to
the structural changes normally seen postoperatively [11]. Tumor
recurrence in regional lymph nodes may also be seen.

Various functional changes have also been described. When groups
with and without sectioning of the recurrent laryngeal nerve were compared, favorable swallowing results were, respectively, 70 and 88% [13].
Extension of the surgery to include resection of the base of the tongue
led to a significantly increased number of swallowing problems,
including decreased laryngeal elevation, loss of tongue propulsion of
the bolus, and increased oropharyngeal transit time [13]. Damage to or
sectioning of the pharyngeal branches of the vagus nerve may result in
cricopharyngeal muscle dysfunction. This problem is secondary to the
role these branches play in upper esophageal sphincter resting tone,
relaxation, and contraction [11]. More distally, esophageal motility is
usually unremarkable. However, when dysphagia is present postoper-

atively, it is critical to examine the entire esophagus to exclude distal strictures or even other foci of squamous cell carcinoma [11,12,14].

When a pharyngolaryngectomy has to be extended and the cervical esophagus is partially or completely resected, reestablishment of the continuity of the gastrointestinal tract is often attempted. One method is that of forming a tube from the pectoralis major muscle and its surrounding tissue (Fig. 2.6). This procedure may also be performed following serious complications and/or failure of a jejunal interposition [15], as discussed later. The major advantage of this type of reconstruction is that no laparotomy is needed [16]. Moreover, the anastomoses can be performed without using microvascular techniques. In one series of five cases, one patient had no complications, two had small anastomotic or suture line leaks, and one had a large breakdown of the flap requiring reoperation [16].

Much more commonly performed is interposition of a short segment of jejunum. In this procedure, a segment of jejunum is removed from the abdomen with a single supplying artery and draining vein. This segment is interposed (autotransplanted), with the blood vessels anastomosed to an external carotid artery branch and the internal jugular vein, respectively [17]. This surgery has the advantage over pectoralis

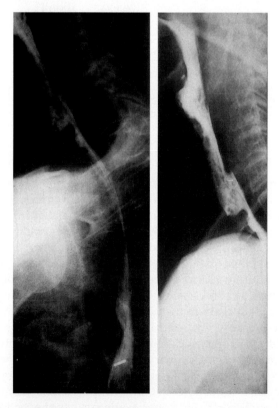

FIGURE 2.6. **Pectoralis muscle flap.** Two lateral films showing a long tubular conduit in the cervical region representing a pectoralis major muscle flap used to replace a portion of a resected esophagus.

major flaps and colonic interpositions of providing a propulsive conduit for food and saliva. When the blood supply is transplanted, there are fewer technical problems than are encountered when the stomach and/or colon is mobilized to reach the neck. The small bowel also more closely approximates the diameter of the esophagus and is more easily connected than those other wider conduits [17].

The radiographic appearance is just what would be expected from the description of the operative procedure. A short segment of jejunum is interposed between the hypopharynx and the distal cervical esophagus. End-to-end distal anastomoses are performed with either an end-to-side or end-to-end proximal one. The mucosal folds may be normal in appearance or thickened. Thickening may occur secondary to lymphedema and is seen in the first three postoperative months [15].

Complications include fistula formation and strictures. The former could be at either the proximal or distal anastomoses, affecting both sites equally [15]. Leaks may develop in 25% of patients. In almost half of these patients, the leak corresponded with clinically evident pharyngocutaneous fistulas [18]. In the remainder, no fistulas developed. However, there was the delayed appearance of fistulas (at 2 weeks) in slightly more than 10% of patients with no evidence of leak on their barium studies. Therefore, barium swallows offered only fair correlation with the immediate postoperative clinical course and should be considered an adjunct, not a definitive examination [18].

Strictures, when they develop, involve the proximal and distal anastomotic sites in equal numbers. Strictures, due either to benign causes or to recurrent disease, occurred much later in the postoperative course than fistulas (mean of 7 months vs 1–2 weeks, respectively [15]). Benign strictures could not be differentiated from malignant ones when they occurred late in the postoperative period [15].

Although some propulsive function is preserved when the jejunum is engrafted, it does not completely replace the resected esophagus in that regard. Instead, many patients need to "flush" solids down by swallowing liquids at the same time [19]. As opposed to normal esophageal function, the act of swallowing does not induce peristaltic contractions in the engrafted small bowel. However, distal to the graft, normal stripping action is observed, confirming that the latter is a local reflex action [19]. However, the graft does show evidence of regular contractile activity (phase III) of the migratory motor complex of the small intestine. This was observed in slightly less than half of all patients in one study [20] and in almost all patients in another [19].

A large retrospective review revealed that almost half of all patients were able to swallow a soft diet without difficulty postoperatively [15]. Dysphagia, when present (slightly more than half of all patients) was related to a myriad of causes, including recurrent disease, stricture, brainstem metastases, or the extent of the original surgical resection. Lymphedema and a redundant jejunal segment were additional causes noted by others [21,22].

Following laryngectomy some patients opt for the placement of a special prosthesis that allows them to regain speech without having to use an external device or to learn esophageal speech. This tracheo-

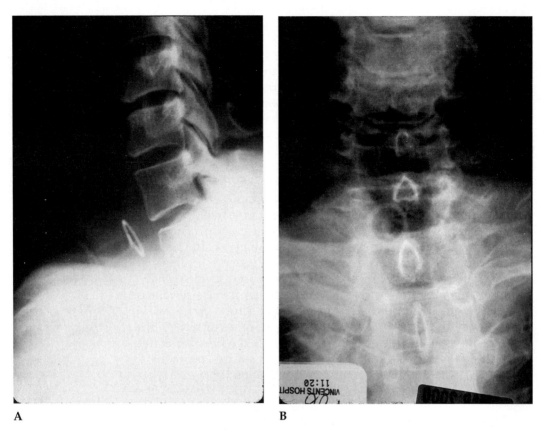

A   B

FIGURE 2.7. **Tracheoesophageal prosthesis.** Lateral (A) and frontal (B) views of the cervical esophagus showing the radiopaque marker for a tracheoesophageal prosthesis. Note on the lateral film that the air channel between the trachea and esophagus is readily identifiable.

esophageal prosthesis is implanted by creating a small fistula between the two lumina with a trochar. An introducer sheath is then placed to deliver the device itself. It can be recognized by a radiopaque ring at its base (Fig. 2.7). Occasionally the actual lumen within the device connecting the trachea and esophagus is visible (Fig. 2.7A).

Zenker's Diverticulum

A Zenker's diverticulum is an acquired outpouching of the pharyngoesophageal junction. It arises because of an inherent weakness in the posterior wall of the upper esophageal sphincter, the cricopharyngeus muscle. This area, called Killian's dehiscence, marks the junction of the oblique and transverse muscle fibers of that muscle. Zenker's diverticula may present with dysphagia, regurgitation of undigested ingested food, or aspiration pneumonia. Therapy is aimed at reducing or eliminating contents retained in the diverticulum and relieving the dysphagia.

Various surgical procedures have been proposed for the treatment of Zenker's diverticulum. The abalation of the diverticulum and/or its lumen is the aim of each. In very small diverticula, the performance of a cricopharyngeal myotomy may reduce the diverticulum to a small bulge in the mucosa, of no clinical significance [23]. When somewhat larger, the diverticulum may be suspended from the prevertebral fascia by a diverticulopexy. This procedure does not remove the diverticulum but, with the patient in the upright position, prevents the retention in its lumen of foodstuff and saliva. Therefore, there is little or no risk of overflow aspiration. A diverticulectomy actually removes the out-pouching. The base of a hand-sewn diverticular site is flat, while the use of a mechanical stapler often leaves a small mucosal outpouching (Fig. 2.8). The diverticulectomy is usually accompanied by a cricopharyngeal myotomy. In patients with contraindications for open surgery, there is an endoscopic alternative [24]. In this procedure an endoscopic stapler is placed with one limb in the diverticulum and the other in the esophageal lumen. When fired, the posterior wall between the diverticulum and esophageal lumen is stapled and divided, creating a wide open mucosal bulge that theoretically empties better and does not trap

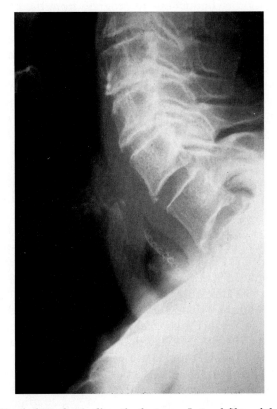

FIGURE 2.8. **Stapled Zenker's diverticulectomy.** Lateral film of the soft tissues of the neck following a stapled Zenker's diverticulectomy. Note the thin linear collection of air posterior to the staple line, a normal feature following a stapled procedure.

as much food as the original diverticulum. Some authors believe that this is actually the procedure of choice for most patients [25].

In the immediate postoperative period, small pharyngocutaneous fistulas from the cricopharyngeal myotomy site to the skin may be observed. Additional small areas of extravasation related to the myotomy may be seen without communication to the skin [4]. The pharyngoesophageal segment may be deviated anteriorly secondary to prevertebral soft tissue edema.

Follow-up exams many months to years later show no significant pharyngoesophageal deviation or residual fistulae [4]. A deformity along the left posterolateral aspect of the pharyngoesophageal segment may persist at the site of the cricopharyngeal myotomy [4]. A persistent posterior bulge, representing the cricopharyngeal muscle, may be seen protruding into the pharyngoesophageal segment despite the performance of an adequate myotomy. This was not evident in the immediate postoperative period and most likely is secondary to cricopharyngeal muscle regeneration.

Videofluoroscopic evaluation of patients after Zenker's diverticulectomy is not usually performed. However, one study of 15 patients revealed a marked array of swallowing abnormalities [26]. The most commonly identified problems included subepiglottic aspiration, failure of peristaltic contractions to progress from the pharynx to the esophagus, and dilatation or stenosis at the pharyngoesophageal junction, each in more than 90% of patients studied. Even in patients whose symptoms improved postoperatively, a large number of the same swallowing abnormalities were identified. Therefore, Zenker's diverticulectomy with cricopharyngeal myotomy is effective in improving or alleviating symptoms without correcting the underlying abnormal physiology of swallowing. This dichotomy of symptoms and objective findings hinders the evaluation and comparison of the techniques just described.

Esophageal Atresia/Tracheo Esophageal Fistula (EATEF)

A complex of disorders that range from variable degrees of narrowing to complete obliteration of the esophageal lumen with an associated airway fistula, EATEF is often seen in the setting of prematurity and low birth weight [27]. Surgery has two main aims, to close the fistula and to reestablish continuity of the gastrointestinal tract with a relatively normal luminal diameter. Various options include a primary repair with an esophagoesophageal anastomosis, a free jejunal graft to bridge the gap between esophageal segments, and colonic interposition. These would all be coupled with fistula closure.

Although jejunal grafts and colonic interposition are discussed in more detail in the section of esophageal surgery, they are briefly discussed here because the patients involved are very young, present some different postoperative complications, and often have other associated congenital anomalies; perhaps most importantly, the corrective surgery for these patients must last a lifetime.

There is a fivefold increase in complications encountered in patients in whom the original airway fistula and esophageal narrowing are at the level of the carina [28]. The gap between the esophageal pouches is usually greatest at this level, and either jejunal grafts or colonic interposition may be necessary to bridge this separation. Gastroesophageal reflux is also 10 times more commonly encountered in patients with a wide gap than in those without [28]. These patients may need an associated Nissen fundoplication to prevent reflux and its associated risk of aspiration. Severe reflux has been associated with a higher risk of recurrent anastomotic strictures. However, antireflux surgery is not as successful in patients with EATEF as it is in those patients with otherwise uncomplicated gastroesophageal reflux disease GERD [29].

Strictures are encountered in 18 to 40% of patients and are at the level of the anastomosis [27,28,30] (Fig. 2.9). They are often the sequelae of anastomotic leaks or reflux, as noted earlier. Although esophago-esophageal and esophagocolonic strictures were encountered with equal frequency, the latter led to surgical revision in most cases, while the former could be handled conservatively with dilatation(s) [27]. Leaks may be found in 17 to 21% of patients [27,28,30,31]. Recurrence of the fistula may occur in 5 to 12% of all patients [27,28,30].

Tension on the anastomosis was considered to be the primary cause and predictor of complications in patients undergoing EATEF repairs

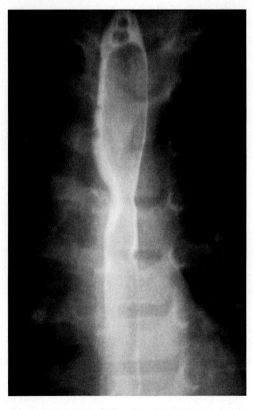

FIGURE 2.9. **Esophageal stricture following EATEF repair.** Single frontal film of the thoracic esophagus in a child following previous primary repair of an esophageal atresia–tracheoesophageal fistula. A mild degree of stricture is noted at the site of the repair. Peristaltic contractions were interrupted at this level during fluoroscopic evaluation.

[28]. However, the use of braided silk sutures was also noted to be a significant risk factor, especially for anastomotic leaks [30,31]. In critically ill children with pulmonary complications, emergency ligation of the fistula, without correction of the accompanying esophageal disorder, was considered to be preferable to gastrostomy alone [30].

Intramural Lesions

Although rare, leiomyomas are the most common benign esophageal neoplasm. When they must be removed, they are usually enucleated. For lesions of the upper and middle thirds of the esophagus, a right thoracotomy is most often used to avoid the aortic arch [32,33]. Videothorascopic enucleation is a new alternative to open thoracotomy [34]. When the distal esophagus is involved, a left thoracotomy is preferred [35]. Usually, when the esophageal muscle fibers are exposed, they are thinned and splayed out over the tumor [35]. An extramucosal defect may be left behind. This resultant weakness in the wall can result in a mucosal bulge, an acquired pseudodiverticulum (Fig. 2.10).

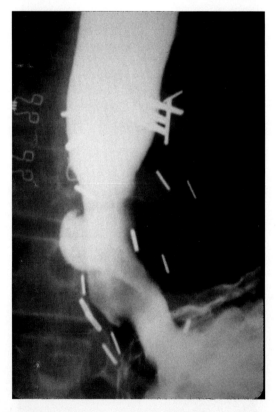

FIGURE 2.10. **Pseudodiverticulum following extramucosal lesion resection.** Oblique film from an esophagogram showing a bulge from the distal esophagus in a patient with previous resection of a leiomyoma. This collection is a pseudodiverticulum following the myotomy necessary for the removal of the tumor.

Similarly, duplication cysts of the esophagus may simply be enucleated. The esophagus may return to a normal appearance postoperatively or may show pseudodiverticular formation similar to that
following removal of a leiomyoma (Fig. 2.11). One alternative to enucleation is opening the cyst and removing its lining; marsupialization
is another.

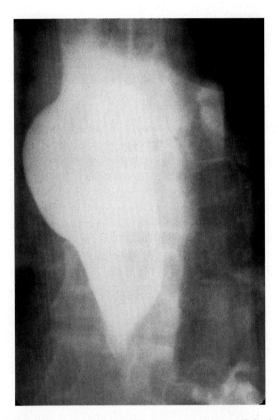

FIGURE 2.11. **Pseudodiverticulum following extramucosal lesion resection.**
Frontal film of the distal half of the thoracic esophagus demonstrates a broad-
based outpouching (pseudodiverticulum) of the right lateral wall of the esophagus following removal of an esophageal duplication cyst.

Esophageal Stents

Many different therapies have been proposed for the treatment or palliation of esophageal carcinoma. These include resection, bypass, radiation therapy, laser ablation (neodymium/yttrium–aluminum–garnet),
bougienage, chemotherapy, photodynamic therapy, bicap tumor
probes, and feeding tube placement. Another palliative option consists
of esophageal stents; previously rigid plastic stents were used, but now
expandable metal stents are available.

Leroy d'Etoiles, a French surgeon of the 1840s, utilized a decalcified
ivory tube as a stent. In 1885 Sir Charles Symonds placed a tube made
of boxwood and German silver. He eventually utilized ivory as
well [36–38]. This tube was held in place by strings that passed through
the patient's nostrils and either looped behind the ears, or were
attached to a mustache. In 1902 Gootskin modified the straight tube
with a proximal inverted funnel and distal rim to mitigate against
migration [39].

Traction placement, necessitating a laparotomy and gastrostomy to
deliver the stent has now been replaced by pulsion techniques. A
Celestin tube became the stent of choice before the advent of expandable metallic stents. This tube was modified by the placement of a
wider proximal end to direct food and secretions into the tube lumen
away from the native esophagus, especially in cases of local perforation or esophageal–airway fistulization. The proximal flare might also
limit proximal migration of the stent. Various modifications included
a collar (Souttar tube), funnel (Palmer tube), cup (Mousseau–Barbin
tube), or tulip tip (Celestin tube) [36]. The placement of all non-
expandable metal stents had to be preceded by bougienage to a diameter 3F to 6F greater than the stent to be placed [39]. Procedure-related
complication rates approached 20%, with a mortality of almost 9% following placement of rigid endoprostheses. In comparison, expandable
metal stents have fewer complications, decreased hospitalization time,
and comparable results of palliation [40]. One very unusual complication related to Celestin stents is fragmentation, with subsequent migration of the pieces, which have been known to cause obstruction or even
bowel perforation [41,42]. These problems have not been associated
with expandable metal stents.

The Nitinol mesh stent is made of knitted single strands of Nitinol
elastic alloy wire, a heat-sensitive metal alloy that expands at body
temperature. It is delivered in a gelatin mold and may take as long as
a week to reach its maximum diameter [43]. Because it is an open wire
mesh, it is not suited for covering esophageal–airway fistulas. Its chief
advantage is that of longitudinal flexibility [40,43].

The Wallstent is made of stainless steel that is intertwined in a double
layer. Both coated and uncoated varieties have been manufactured,
although only the coated kind is presently made [39]. The coated
variety is very effective in sealing esophageal–airway fistulas [40]. The
presence of flared ends (funnel shaped) makes this endoprosthesis a
good choice in tumors that do not present a good proximal shelf to
anchor a stent. These ends are not coated, even when the stent itself is

[36]. The stent is mounted in a delivery tube and self expands within 24 h [39]. Alternatively, balloon dilatation may speed the attainment of the maximal diameter of the stent [43]. Like all expandable stents, the prosthesis shortens considerably upon deployment. The presence of fixation hooks makes repositioning or removal difficult.

Gianturco Z stents are made of a stainless steel cage with wires in a zigzag pattern [36,39,40]. They may be covered with either silicone or urethane. Funnel-shaped ends are present at both proximal and distal ends. The deployment system is complex, consisting of a pusher tube and compression catheter. Prior to deployment, the esophagus must be dilated to at least 30F diameter. Although the stent is self-expanding, balloon dilatation may be needed to reach a satisfactory luminal diameter [43]. Similar to the Wallstent, the coated Z stent is a good choice for covering esophageal–airway fistulas [40].

The Esophacoil is made of a flat wire coiled-spring arrangement of a superelastic nickel–titanium alloy [36,43]. It is wrapped over an insertion catheter. Pulling of restraining threads releases the stent. The Slinkylike configuration leads to marked shortening upon deployment (50%) [40]. The device expands spontaneously in just a few seconds. The Esophacoil is particularly valuable in crossing tight and/or angulated strictures [43] because the radial force developed during its deployment is the greatest of all the stents. However, this very advantage may also lead to erosion of the esophageal wall, with resultant fatal hemorrhage.

The complications of esophageal stents are summarized in Table 2.1. Prior radiation and/or chemotherapy may lead to an increased rate of complications [40]. There are many reasons for esophageal perforation to occur during or after stent deployment. Many stents require predeployment dilatation of the esophagus. This itself may cause a perforation. Angulated lesions cause eccentric mechanical forces to be placed upon the esophageal wall, especially with noncompliant stents [36]. The considerable radial force developed by the Esophacoil may cause disruption of the wall.

Over the longer term, pressure necrosis may lead to perforation. The rate of perforation may reach as high as 14% for patients treated with rigid stents, although the numbers appear to be lower for the newer expandable stents [36,44–46]. The wire struts on some stents may lead to chronic esophageal ulceration or frank perforation [40].

TABLE 2.1. **Complications of esophageal stents.**

1. **Perforation**
2. **Malposition**
3. **Migration (including fragmentation of Celestin tube)**
4. **Tumor ingrowth**
5. **Tumor overgrowth**
6. **Obstruction by food bolus**
7. **Tracheal compression**
8. **Stent infolding**
9. **Stent motion during MR imaging**

The radiographic findings are often marked and easy to recognize. They include local extravasation of contrast agent or the presence of contrast in the mediastinum, pleural space, or subphrenic collections (Fig. 2.12). Pneumomediastinum or pneumothoraces may also be present. When perforations occur, they may be treated conservatively by leaving the covered stent in place or placing an overlapping stent to cover the perforation [47].

Malposition of a stent is usually the result of migration during or shortly after insertion. Other causes may include a discrepancy between the stent outer diameter and the maximum luminal diameter of the esophagus, inadequate anchoring of the prosthesis, too short a stent length, or deployment at the wrong level (seen in cases of inadequate predeployment localization of the stricture) [36]. At radiography, there is lack of coverage of the stricture by the stent or continued filling of a perforation or fistula. Stents placed near the gastroesophageal (GE) junction or across angulated lesions are more prone to malposition, as are those placed in cases of abrupt change in luminal caliber or lacking

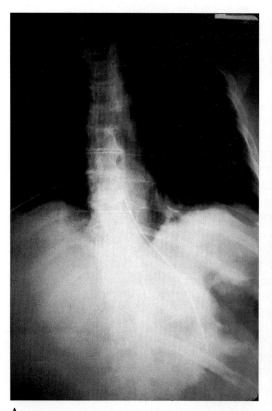
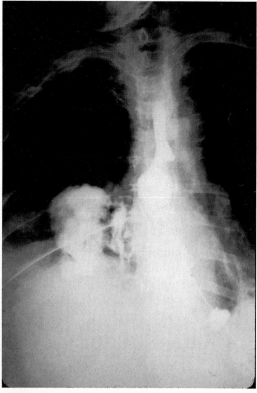

A

B

FIGURE 2.12. **Esophageal stents.** (A) Frontal film of the lower chest and upper abdomen reveals an esophageal endoprosthesis bridging the gastroesophageal junction with most of the tube in the stomach. (B) Perforated esophageal stent. Contrast outlines a large mediastinal collection of contrast as well as a right lower lobe abscess secondary to perforation of the proximal end of the esophageal endoprosthesis.

a distal anchoring point for the prosthesis [36] (Fig. 2.13). Very proximal lesions, such as those near the cricopharyngeus muscle (upper esophageal sphincter), are also prone to malpositioning [47].

Stent migration may be detected by serial examinations showing progressive or abrupt changes in the position of a previously placed stent. Stents have been noted to pass through the entire length of the GI tract until they are expelled through the rectum [48]. Migration may be secondary to inadequate anchoring, especially at the proximal edge of the stricture, or the lack of sufficient radial force exerted by an expandable stent.

Even though coating is not applied to the anchoring ends of coated metal stents, plastic and coated Wallstents have migration rates reported to be as high as 25% [45,49]. Z stents are prone to migration, especially when placed across the GE junction [40,50]. When this occurs, the stent may have to be removed via a gastrostomy, or it may be necessary to insert a second, overlapping stent [47].

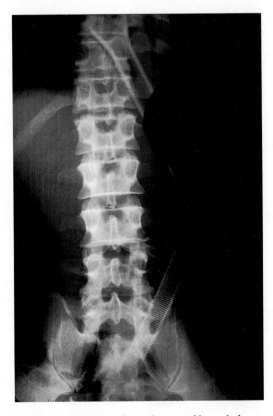

FIGURE 2.13. Migrated Celestin tubes. Supine film of the upper abdomen revealing two Celestin tubes that have migrated from the more proximal esophagus. Note the pneumomediastinum just lateral to the flange of the proximal tube, which lies partially dislodged in the distal esophagus.

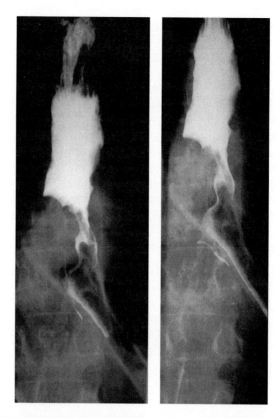

FIGURE 2.14. **Tumor ingrowth inside a stent.** Two films from a barium esophagogram revealing an irregular filling defect at the proximal end of an endoprosthesis. This represents tumor ingrowth from a carcinoma.

Tumor ingrowth may occur only in uncoated stents, or in cases of covered stents damaged during deployment [46]. The Ultraflex and uncovered Wallstents are most prone to tumor ingrowth [40]. Rates of tumor ingrowth may be as high as 36% for uncovered Nitinol stents [36]. Tumor ingrowth is usually detected approximately 3 months after stent insertion [51]. It may be detected by progressive narrowing of the inner diameter of the stent with irregularity of the stent lumen.

Tumor overgrowth of the stent may occur at the proximal or distal end of the stent, or at both ends (Fig. 2.14). Overgrowth may result in obstruction, or it may leave the patient prone to obstruction from an impacted food bolus. To prevent this complication, the stent should be long enough to extend 1- to 3 cm both proximal and distal to the gross tumor margins [36]. Occasionally, a marked inflammatory response to the presence of the stent may mimic neoplastic overgrowth [40]. The use of coated stents helps to decrease the rate of this hyperplastic tissue response. When tumor overgrowth occurs, it may be treated with an additional, interlocked stent, or laser ablation [47].

Multiple factors may lead to the impaction of a food bolus. These include inadequate chewing and food processing and improper selection of food, as well as an inadequate lumen within the stent (Fig. 2.15).

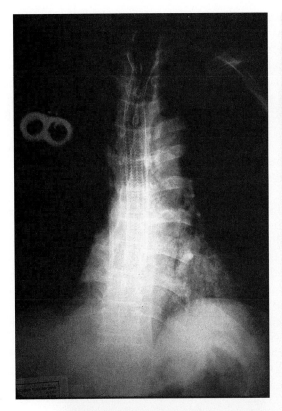

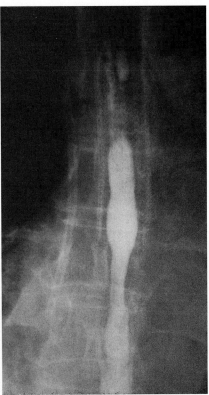

A

B

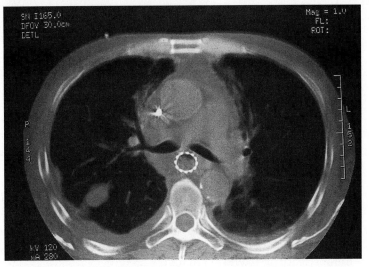

C

FIGURE 2.15. Obstructed endoprosthesis. (A) Frontal film of the chest reveals an esophageal metallic endoprosthesis in situ. (B) Frontal film from a contrast esophagogram on the same patient reveals marked narrowing and irregu- larity to the lumen of the endoprosthesis. This represents clogging from food in debris. (C) CT image of the same patient at the level of the carina reveals almost complete obliteration of the endoprosthesis lumen.

Food impaction has been noted more frequently in rigid stents [52]. It is less common in self-expanding metal stents, reflecting their larger internal diameters. The finding of one or more lobulated filling defects at the proximal end, or within a stent, should suggest an impacted food bolus. The differential diagnosis includes tumor in- or overgrowth, as well as stent migration uncovering the primary lesion. Endoscopic removal of the offending material is the usual treatment [47].

A more immediate, and potentially fatal complication is tracheal compression, which may necessitate stent retrieval, intubation, or placement of a tracheal stent [40]. The sudden onset usually precludes imaging.

Esophageal–airway fistulas are a common indication for esophageal stent placement. When left untreated, most patients expire within a month of diagnosis [53]. Esophageal stenting can result in a 90% closure rate for these fistulas [47]. However, continued filling of an airway fistula can be considered to be a complication (or failure) of stent placement. This lack of closure may be due to passage of contrast through the stent lumen, around the distal end of the prosthesis, and then, in a retrograde fashion, along the external wall of the stent until the fistula is reached [47]. Alternatively, if the esophagus proximal to the lesion is dilated to a diameter that exceeds the largest stent external diameter (28F), contrast will leak around the proximal end, leading to filling of the fistula [47]. Stent malpositioning or migration may also uncover a previously occluded fistula.

Infolding of the stent lumen is another possible complication. It is more commonly seen in patients with Ultraflex stents, and to a lesser extent, the Z stent [40]. It may be secondary to tumor growth exceeding the radial strength of the stent or to defective expansion during deployment [36]. Balloon dilatation may correct the problem, although in at least one case, the passage of the endoscope itself dilated the stent [36].

As MR imaging of the thorax increases in usage, caution must be used when a patient has an esophageal stent in situ. The European version of the Wallstent is made with titanium and does not pose a problem during imaging [54]. However, the U.S. version of the same stent is made with stainless steel and is ferromagnetic. Therefore it is theoretically susceptible to both attractive forces and torque while in the bore of a magnet. The Z stent is similarly affected. A useful guideline, similar to that used for patients with endovascular stents, is to wait 6 weeks after deployment before imaging. This allows sufficient fibrotic reaction to relatively fix the stent in place.

Another factor to be considered is the type of magnet to be used for imaging. In most closed-bore systems, the static field is aligned with the long axis of the patient. Because an esophageal stent generally is also aligned along the same axis, there should be relatively little torque applied to the stent. However, some open-air magnets have their static magnetic field aligned perpendicular to the patient's long axis. In these units, a ferromagnetic stent may be subject to considerable torque and possible dislodgment. Studies performed in both types of unit may be subject to image degradation secondary to ferromagnetic artifact due to stainless steel, but not titanium-based stents [40].

Esophageal Replacement

Patients with either benign or malignant disease are often treated by esophageal resection. Reestablishment of the continuity of the gastrointestinal tract must then be performed. This can be done by a variety of methods involving the stomach, jejunum, or colon.

The technique of "blind" or "blunt" esophagectomy was first performed by Denk in 1913, revised by Turner in 1931, and further updated by Orringer and Sloan in 1978 [55]. This technique, described in more detail shortly, allowed the surgeon, and the patient, to avoid an open thoracotomy. In addition, Orringer and Sloan placed the esophagogastric anastomosis in the neck. Ivor Lewis, in 1946, described the technique of transthoracic esophagectomy, followed by esophagogastrostomy via a right thoracotomy and laparotomy [55]. Among the many factors that determine the technique that will be used are the preference of the surgeon, the patient's general medical condition including prior surgical history, the location of the tumor, the choice and suitability for use of the esophageal substitute, and a history of prior radiation [55]. The two most important criteria in determining the actual surgery are the location of the tumor and the surgeon's preference.

Orringer and his colleagues popularized the transhiatal esophagectomy with an esophagogastric anastamosis in the neck [56]. This surgery avoids a thoracotomy and is usually performed for lesions in the lower third of the esophagus and/or the gastric cardia. An upper midline abdominal incision allows access to the stomach, which is then mobilized. The esophageal hiatus is opened. Some surgeons perform a pyloromyotomy to enhance emptying of the transposed stomach, once it is in the chest. After reaching into the mediastinum from below, the surgeon bluntly dissects the esophagus. A neck incision, usually on the left is then made, freeing up the esophagus, whereupon a short portion is delivered into the neck and out the incision. Care is taken to avoid injuring the left recurrent laryngeal nerve in the process. The remainder of the esophagus, including the tumor, is delivered through the esophageal hiatus into the abdomen. The stomach is then delivered through the mediastinal canal into the neck, where the primary anastomosis is performed. Besides avoiding a thoracotomy, the major advantage of this technique is that the cervical location of the anastomosis avoids the possibility of mediastinal soilage and mediastinitis in the case of leakage.

The Ivor Lewis technique is radically different [57]. It is the most frequently used technique for managing carcinomas of the middle to distal third of the esophagus. Initially performed as a two-stage procedure, it is now performed via simultaneous right thoracotomy and laparotomy. The abdomen is opened first, and in the absence of gross metastatic disease, the stomach is mobilized. A pyloromyotomy, or preferentially, a pyloroplasty, is performed. The esophageal hiatus is widened to allow delivery of the stomach into the chest. Following collapse of the left lung, the chest is opened, the esophagus mobilized, and the tumor-containing portion resected. The stomach is delivered into the chest and the proximal portion resected with wide margins if possible. The lesser curvature is resected to help form a tubular stomach that is then anastomosed to the esophageal remnant. This anastomosis is always performed above the level of the azygos vein, to help achieve adequate tumor margins and to aid in the reduction of gastroesophageal reflux.

The choices for benign disease are greatly influenced by the period of time during which the conduit must function. Unlike esophageal carcinoma, where patient survival is measured in months, or a few years, many patients with benign disease face decades of life with an esophageal substitute. Therefore, the colon has been advocated as the conduit of choice. Although the gastric pull-through is technically easier, many patients suffer from symptoms related to duodenogastric reflux and rapid gastric emptying, especially in the upright position [58]. As opposed to the stomach, the colon functions as a reservoir for the retained gastric antrum. The distal stomach, which remains in its normal subdiaphragmatic location, aids in a more normal and physiological emptying pattern [58]. This subdiaphragmatic location avoids the pressure gradient encountered when the stomach is placed in the thoracic compartment, where the pressure is relatively lower. This pressure gradient contributes to the development of duodenogastric reflux. The intra-abdominal portion of the colon is relatively collapsed by the positive pressure of the abdomen, further decreasing the possibility of reflux of contents into the native esophagus. Therefore, the development of a Barrett's esophagus is much less likely in patients with a colonic bypass [59,60]. Few if any long-term histological changes are encountered in the colon that has been used as an esophageal replacement [61].

Preoperative evaluation of the colon is required. The presence of diverticula does not preclude the use of the left colon for the construction of a conduit. Frank diverticulitis with pericolonic inflammation does limit the ability to transpose the colon into the chest. Vascular anatomy of the colon is also important in assessing the viability of the segment that is to be relocated.

The colon may be placed in the posterior mediastinum (Fig. 2.16A,B), or substernally (Fig. 2.17). The former placement allows better emptying of the cervical esophagus [58]. However, when adhesions prevent freeing up of the esophagus, the substernal route provides a viable alternative route. This procedure may require resection of portions of the manubrium, clavicle, and first rib to enlarge the thoracic inlet and avoid unnecessary compression of the colonic graft. Some authors prefer this route [62]. If a colonic segment is used in cases of esophageal carcinoma, the substernal route may avoid the complication of mediastinal recurrence involving the bypass graft [62]. However, higher rates of complications are associated with the substernal or even subcutaneous route. For examples, there may be anastomotic leaks and poorer function [63,64]. The former may be secondary to lack of adequate support from the surrounding structures.

Another decision to be made is whether the colonic graft should be iso- or antiperistaltic (i.e., utilizing the right or left colon, respectively).

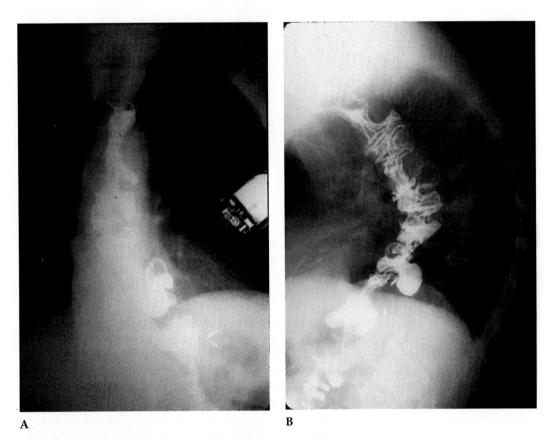

A   B

FIGURE 2.16. **Mediastinal colonic interposition.** Posteroanterior (A) and lateral (B) films of the chest show a barium-filled colon interposed between the esophagus and stomach traversing the posterior mediastinum.

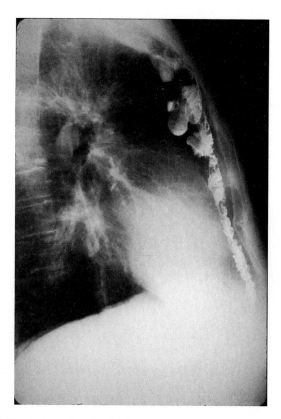

FIGURE 2.17. Retrosternal colonic interposition. Lateral film of the chest reveals the retro- or substernal course of a colonic interposition.

This choice is usually predicated on vascular anatomy, but the isoperistaltic alternative is preferred. Antiperistaltically placed colons may actually transport a barium bolus in a retrograde manner, leading to choking and possible aspiration [58]. The left colon's thicker wall and closer approximation in diameter to the esophageal remnant are additional reasons for its preferential use [60].

In the immediate postoperative period, single-contrast barium is used. Double-contrast studies with their need for effervescent granules are to be avoided to prevent excessively rapid overdistention of the lumen. An upright, delayed film is used to assess intrathoracic emptying. If a leak is suspected, water-soluble contrast should be used initially, and then barium if no leak is identified. The patient should be in the right posterior position on the fluoroscopy table with reverse Trendelenberg table tilt to help prevent possible aspiration [65]. The examination should be extended to include the proximal small bowel, since many problems may be encountered distal to the esophagogastric anastomosis [5].

Esophagogastric anastomoses have an angular appearance because the type usually used is end (esophagus) to side (gastric pull-through) (Fig. 2.18). There may be slight narrowing at the level of the anasto-

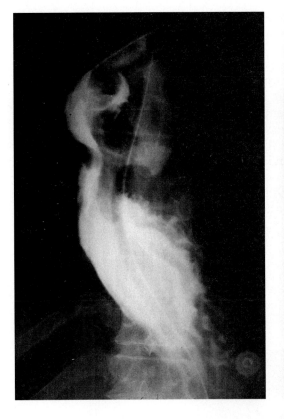

A

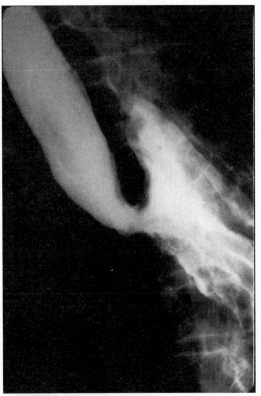

B

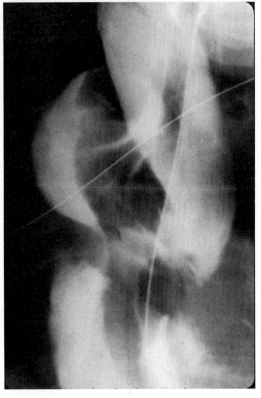

C

FIGURE 2.18. **Blind-ending gastric pouches.** (A)–(C) These three separate examples of blind-ending gastric pouches alongside and proximal to the esophagogastric anastomosis are the result of an end- (esophagus) to-side (stomach) anastomosis.

mosis, and gastric folds can be seen radiating up to the suture line [66]. A blind pouch of stomach extends above and behind the anastomosis, since the gastric remnant is often sutured to the prevertebral fascia (if the anastomosis is made in the neck) [67]. The closure of the gastric remnant, near the old cardia, leads to mucosal irregularity that can mimic ulceration or even recurrent disease [67]. The stapled closure is usually seen along the anterior wall when the patient is imaged in the left posterior oblique position [66]. It extends to the level of the esophagogastric anastomosis (Fig. 2.19). Surgical clips and sutures usually mark the closure line and may make its recognition easier. The closed stapler insertion site is marked by a row of staples along the anterior gastric wall. These do not reach as high as the gastric resection closure line, which lies more posteriorly and to the right when viewed in the

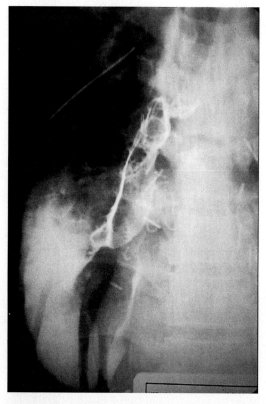

FIGURE 2.19. Gastric pull-through staple line. Upper GI series reveals the linear filling defect of the staple line that closes the gastric remnant.

frontal projection [66] (Fig. 2.20). Emptying of the stomach is often delayed in the immediate postoperative period. Gastric emptying takes four times as long in patients without a pyloroplasty than in those who have undergone the procedure [68]. This delay is usually alleviated in 3 to 4 weeks [67].

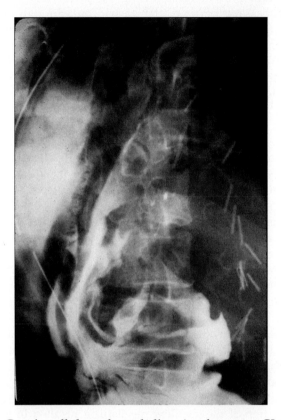

FIGURE 2.20. **Gastric pull-through staple line.** Another upper GI series shows the linear filling defect from the gastric stapler insertion site closure.

The pylorus usually straddles the diaphragm, with the duodenal bulb lying intra-abdominally. Because the stomach is placed in the right paravertebral region, contrast has to flow from right to left to transit the diaphragmatic hiatus to reach the abdomen [69]. Therefore, placing the patient semiupright and left posterior oblique aids in the process and evaluation of gastric emptying. The pylorus may be deformed secondary to pyloromyotomy or pyloroplasty [66]. There may be pancreatitis, related to the mobilization of the stomach and/or the duodenum [70].

Examinations performed weeks after the surgery reveal a fully distensible anastomosis without evidence of nodularity. The gastric pull-through appears to be tubular in configuration, with parallel folds. At this time it should empty more promptly [67].

Imaging by CT has a limited role to play in the immediate postoperative course. Anastomotic leaks, swallowing difficulties including aspiration, stricture, and emptying problems are all best evaluated by routine contrast studies. Evaluation of the neck and mediastinum for abscess and other fluid collections following esophagography is the best indication for CT imaging during this period [69].

With the passage of time, the gastric pull-through undergoes a change in appearance. The mucosal folds are said to become more parallel, and the overall width of the lumen decreases, approximating the appearance of the esophagus [67]. Others have described similar changes in the transplanted colon (see later).

Early postoperative complications are usually related to the esophagogastric anastomosis. Leaks at this site are the most commonly encountered problem and are probably underreported [71]. While rates vary considerably from one series to another, Agha et al. reported that pharyngoesophageal anastomoses leaked at a rate almost six times that of cervical esophagogastric ones [67]. Thoracic anastosmoses are even less frequently affected by leaks, perhaps because of tension on the suture line or ischemic changes [71]. Other authors consider all anastomotic leaks to be secondary to faulty technique [70]. Other leaks may develop from underlying diseases, at the other gastric suture or staple lines (closure of the cardia, gastrostomy site for insertion of the stapling device, or staple line for creation of a gastric tube of restricted diameter), or at the point of fixation to the prevertebral fascia [67]. The propensity to leak may be exacerbated by previous gastric surgery and its effect on that organ's vascular supply. Such leaks may be made worse by the bellows effect, associated with the negative intrathoracic pressure and respiratory motion, which sucks luminal contents into the mediastinum. The resultant mediastinitis may cause reflex bronchorrhea and copious mucus secretions within the lungs [70]. The morbidity of this extravasation is also increased by gastroesophageal reflux.

Incoordination of the swallow mechanism resulted in aspiration in approximately 5% of patients [67]. This is an important factor to consider in choosing the contrast agent to be used, even if an anastomotic leak is not suspected. This aspiration may be related to failure of the cricopharyngeus to properly relax prior to the arrival of a contrast bolus or, following its passage, to close to protect the airway [71,72].

Plain film examination of the chest may be misleading in cases of anastomotic or other suture line disruptions as a chest tube is placed alongside the gastric pull-through and may prevent the accumulation of fluid in the pleural space [66]. Once the chest tube has been removed, any significant reaccumulation of fluid, especially if rapid, may be suspect. If leaks are discovered, follow-up examinations until the leaks are closed are recommended [66,73,74]. Pleural effusions may also be chylous, and secondary to disruption of the thoracic duct, in slightly less than 1% of patients [71]. A disrupted thoracic duct may be difficult to diagnose in the immediate postoperative period. This may occur because the patient is not allowed to eat or drink or is not ingesting a

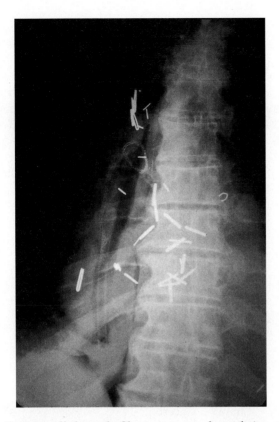

FIGURE 2.21. **Gastric pull-through.** Chest x-ray reveals a soft tissue density, surgical clips, and a linear collection of air in the right hemithorax in the classic appearance of a gastric pull-through.

diet containing fats or lipids. As the diet is advanced, the chylous nature of the pleural fluid may then become apparent. A chylothorax may carry a mortality as high as 50% [70,75,76].

In approximately 75% of patients, the gastric pull-through lies in the midline or to the right of midline in the mediastinum [69,77] (Fig. 2.21). Thus any air seen to the left, especially in the retrocardiac region, is suspect for inadvertent herniation of some abdominal contents into the chest [77] (Fig. 2.22). The differential diagnosis for air in the left

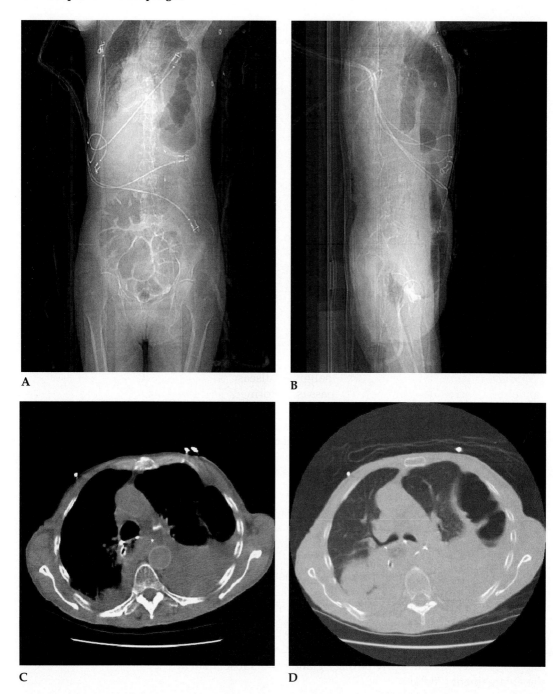

FIGURE 2.22. **Colon herniation following gastric pull-through.** Frontal (A) and lateral (B) scanograms of a patient who had recently undergone a gastric pull-through reveal a large and abnormal collection of air in the left hemithorax. A CT section at the level of the aortic arch (C) reveals a nasogastric tube in the distal esophagus and a large left-sided air and fluid collection. Another section, more caudal and viewed at lung windows (D), reveals that the air lies inside the herniated colon. (Courtesy of Marc Gollub, MD, New York, NY)

side of the mediastinum includes a left-sided gastric pull-through (Fig. 2.23), a mucocele [78], and a pneumo- or hydropneumothorax [77]. Occasionally, this differentiation is made easier by the presence of haustrations or the continuity of the air into subdiaphragmatic bowel [77]. The herniation is usually that of colon, but small-bowel herniation has also been reported [77,79–81]. The incidence of herniation is estimated to be no more than 4% [79,80]. A retrospective review of nine cases of herniation found the most significant risk factor to be that of an extended enlargement of the diaphragmatic hiatus during the gastric pull-through [81].

These herniations are usually noted during the acute postoperative phase on routine chest films. They can be confirmed by CT imaging and/or by routine contrast studies of the bowel. Some patients are asymptomatic; some have cough, dyspnea, or other signs of respiratory distress; others present with signs and symptoms of bowel obstruction [79,81] or strangulation [77]. A rare instance of extrapericardial tamponade by herniated omentum has also been reported [82]. Therefore it has been recommended to electively close (narrow) the esophageal diaphragmatic hiatus after the stomach has been delivered into the chest and before closure of the abdomen [80,82]. Others recommend performing an omentectomy to remove the possible leading edge for the herniation [79].

Occasionally, in both benign and malignant disease, the esophagus cannot be resected before surgical bypass is performed. This restriction might be secondary to unresectable malignancy or periesophageal inflammatory changes in cases of trauma or caustic ingestion [83,84]. In these instances, the thoracic esophagus is isolated (excluded) from the remainder both proximally and distally, by ligation or stapling the esophagus and then dividing it. Gastrointestinal continuity is then restored with either the stomach or colon. This procedure is fraught with difficulty, and complication rates of up to 60% have been reported [84]. The complications include anastomotic leaks, disruption of the distal portion of the isolated esophagus, fistula formation, and infection.

A well-described complication of leaving the esophagus in situ is that of an esophageal mucocele. This is defined as a closed, cystic space containing secretions high in protein [84]. This is secondary to continuing production of mucus by the submucosal glands and not secondary to adenomatous metaplasia, as might be suspected [78]. Mucoceles may occur in as many as 40% of patients in whom the esophagus cannot be resected [84]. Eventual increases in the esophageal remnant intraluminal pressure result in atrophy of these glands and subsequent arrest of the enlargement [78,84].

The onset of an esophageal mucocele usually occurs in the first two postoperative months, and most often the cyst remains stable in size [84]. Although rare, continued enlargement due to continued mucus production has been reported [84]. Esophageal mucoceles are usually small (mean 4 × 6.5 cm) and more often related to either the proximal or distal end of the excluded esophagus [84]. However, they may involve its entire length [78,84]. Obviously, routine contrast

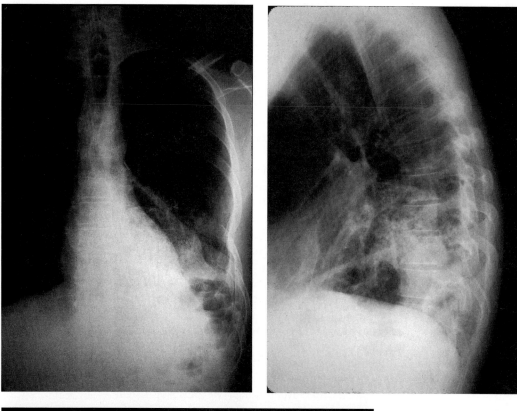

A

B

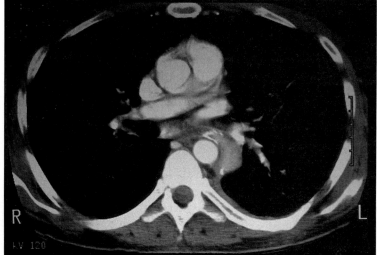

C

FIGURE 2.23. **Left-sided gastric pull-through.** Antero-posterior (A) and lateral (B) films of the chest reveal a large air and soft tissue density within the left hemithorax. A CT section just below the level of the left main stem bronchus (C) reveals surgical staples marking the esophagogastric anastamosis of a left-sided gastric pull-through. A film from an upper GI series (D) confirms the presence of the pull-through and better demonstrates the anastamotic integrity. Another CT section (E), more caudal than that in (C), reveals the fluid-filled intrathoracic stomach. The extent of the pull-through is further demonstrated on another film from the upper GI series (F).

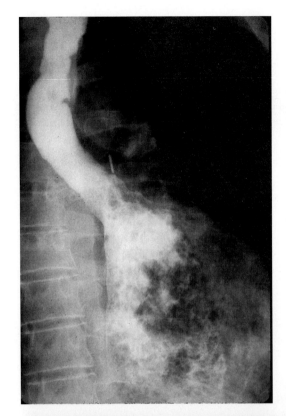

D

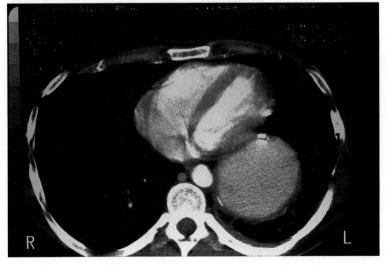

R   L

E

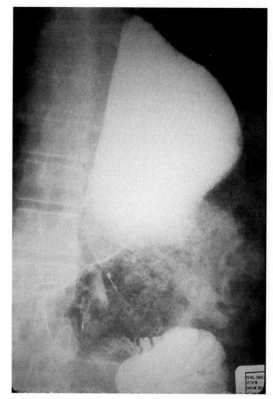

F

FIGURE 2.23. **Left-sided gastric pull-through.** (*Continued*)

examinations do not fill a mucocele. Instead, either CT or MR (with its multiplanar capabilities) imaging can reveal the presence, help identify its cystic nature, and confirm the proteinaceous contents of the mucocele [78,83,84].

Mucoceles are usually asymptomatic [83]. However, in one series of six patients, five were symptomatic [78]. Three patients suffered from respiratory distress, while two others had pain and nausea. In the former group, the mucoceles were of long-standing duration but were actually the smallest of the mucoceles encountered [78]. One reason for the failure of mucoceles to become symptomatic is masking of symptoms by the underlying disease, which may even lead to the patient's demise before symptoms can develop [83].

If a mucocele is thought to be infected, then CT- or ultrasound-guided aspiration may be performed [78,85,86]. Internal drainage can be performed in patients in whom the isolated esophagus cannot be resected [78]. Rupture of a mucocele leading to a subphrenic abscess has also been reported [87].

Dysphagia is often the symptom that prompts examination of the patient after the acute postoperative phase has passed. Oftentimes that examination reveals an anastomotic stricture. Classically smooth, symmetric, and tapered ending at the level of the esophagogastric anastomosis [66], these strictures are most likely secondary to previous leaks, even undetected, at the level of the anastomosis [67,88]. The type of suture material used for the anastomosis was once thought to be an etiology for stricture formation, but this is no longer thought to be true [89].

In one series, no surrounding mass was noted in cases of benign strictures, but 25% had associated ulcerations, either at or just proximal to the narrowing [66]. These authors reported that in no case was any abnormality found on the gastric side of the anastomosis. As the degree of narrowing increases, a "jet phenomenon" may be observed during esophagography [67]. This may be used to actually measure the degree of anastomotic narrowing. As a rule, CT imaging is not of benefit in following patients with benign strictures [69]. When a stricture is found less than 3 months postoperatively, it usually is benign [71].

The delayed onset of anastomotic leaks can be found in up to 16% of postoperative patients [90]. Half these patients with delayed onset of leaks were asymptomatic with no evidence of fever, chest pain, or other sign of a leak at the time of their examination. Eventually one of these patients developed signs and symptoms of infection. Reexamination showed that the leak had progressed to a gastropleural fistula. Patients who were symptomatic at the time of examination had much more extensive leaks, including gastropleural and gastrobronchial fistulas [90]. Another patient had an esophagogastric fistula paralleling the esophagogastric anastomosis, resulting in a double channel at that level.

When dysphagia occurs more than 3 months postoperatively, tumor recurrence must strongly be considered [71]. When tumor recurs, it may appear locally at the anastomotic site, or it may involve other portions of the gastric pull-through, from contiguous spread from the mediastinum, or even at the site of the pyloroplasty or myotomy [67,69]. Anastomotic recurrence is almost never found at a cervical anastomosis, perhaps because the shorter cervical esophageal remnant affords wider margins of resection [67,91,92]. Yet superior mediastinal adenopathy was much more common in the patients [92]. Recurrent left laryngeal nerve palsy, with its associated vocal changes and possible aspiration, was much more common as well in these patients with high anastomoses [92].

When recurrences are detected at barium studies, the narrowings are often associated with masses at or near the anastomoses [66]. In almost half these patients, the mass effect extends inferior to the level of the anastomosis, unlike benign strictures, in which there is no mass effect. In slightly greater than half these patients, ulceration may occur. The presence of ulceration (Fig. 2.24) is not adequate to differentiate benign from anastomotic recurrence [66]. More important differential features include narrowing below the anastomosis, eccentric narrowing of the lumen, and formation of fistulas [66]. Esophageal–airway fistulas have also been described, and these are often due to necrotic tumor mass and/or radiation therapy administered to treat the recurrence [66].

Most recurrences originate extramucosally [66,69,91] and therefore computed tomography is of significant value in its detection. The CT appearance of recurrence is varied and may include a perianastomotic soft tissue mass (most common), mediastinal soft tissue masses at the level of the original tumor, mediastinal masses above or below that level, or nodular thickening of the gastric wall [91]. Masses at the pyloromyotomy site have also been described [69]. Apparent gastric wall thickening without mass should not be considered to be a sign of recurrence [69].

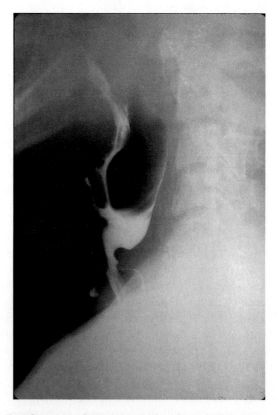

FIGURE 2.24. Esophagogastric anastomotic ulcer. Following a gastric pull-through, a film from an upper GI series shows a benign anastomotic ulcer (along with leakage alongside the relocated stomach).

Caveats in the interpretation of CT images include a blind gastric pouch associated with the closure of the cardia, or other gastric outpouchings, which may present as a soft tissue mass that simulates recurrence on CT imaging unless properly distended by air and/or oral contrast [91]. Wall thickness is also difficult to properly evaluate because the interposed stomach is underdistended. Especially on older generation CT images, artifacts from metal clips in the mediastinum may add to the difficulties encountered [91]. Infiltration of the mediastinal fat may be secondary to inflammation and scar tissue, rather than indicating neoplastic spread [91].

Other areas of recurrent tumor that can be detected by CT imaging include liver metastases, abdominal lymphadenopathy, pleural masses, peritoneal and omental carcinomatosis, and skin and adrenal involvement [69,91]. In a 1987 study, CT imaging served to diagnose distant spread in half of all patients who presented with local recurrence [91].

Vomiting and retrosternal fullness may suggest pyloric narrowing and resultant outlet obstruction of the pull-through. Pyloric stenosis is usually evidenced by a dilated interposed stomach on plain film or CT images (Fig. 2.25A). There is delayed gastric emptying, even with the

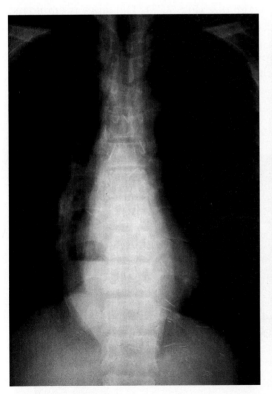 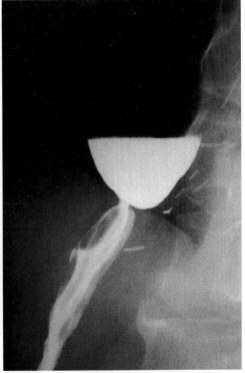

A   B

FIGURE 2.25. Delayed emptying of gastric pull-through. Upright chest film (A) reveals an air–fluid level above the right hemidiaphragm in a patient with a previous gastric pull-through. This represents delayed gastric emptying, presumably at the level of the pylorus. Upright film of the pyloric region (B) shows delayed emptying through a narrowed pylorus, located just at the level of the diaphragm.

patient in the upright position (Fig. 2.25B). Postoperative pyloric stenosis can readily be treated by dilatation [67].

Reflux into the esophageal remnant may be secondary to gastric atony and/or loss of the lower esophageal sphincter [71]. Duodenogastric bile reflux into the interposed stomach may lead to the development of adenocarcinorna in that organ [93]. Barrett's esophagus with ulceration may also be seen. In at least one patient, this led to an esophagopericardial fistula with severe mediastinitis [94]. Reflux may also affect the colon when that organ is used as an esophageal substitute (see later).

The problems following colonic interposition are similar to those encountered with gastric pull-through procedures. Because the gastric antrum is preserved and maintained in its normal position, its contractions three times per minute aid in prompt emptying of the colonic reservoir [58]. The subdiaphragmatic portion of interposed colon is partially compressed by the relatively high (vs the chest) intra-abdominal pressure (Fig. 2.26). This leads to a decreased rate of duodenogastroesophageal reflux and subsequent decreased rates of esophagitis; also possible are stenoses or even Barrett's esophagus [58].

A finding similar to that seen in gastric pull-through is that of a pseudodiverticulum at the proximal esophagocolonic anastomosis secondary to an end-to-side technique (Fig. 2.27). The latter is employed because of a mismatch in size between the esophageal remnant and the interposed colon [95].

The colon often develops a peculiar mucosal pattern with redundant folds during the postoperative period. This can be seen in 20 to 50% of

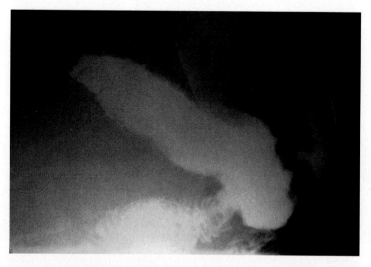

FIGURE 2.26. Cologastric anastomosis following colonic interposition. Lateral film from an upper GI series shows the collapsed intra-abdominal segment of colon anastomosed to the anterior wall of the colon. This type of anastomosis is used in retro- or substernal placement of the interposed colon.

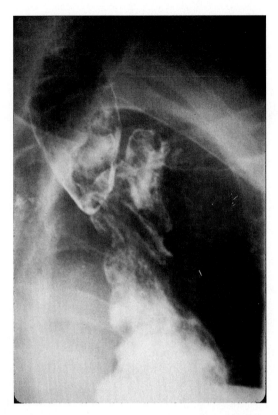

FIGURE 2.27. **Esophagocolic blind pouch.** Oblique film from an upper GI series shows a dilated esophageal remnant and a large blind-ending pouch or pseudodiverticulum, resulting from an end- (esophagus) to-side (interposed colon) anastomosis.

patients and has variably been called esophagization or jejunization [60,65,96]. In the colon the folds become longitudinally aligned and are slightly thicker than those seen in the native esophagus. Visible in the proximal portion of the transplanted colon, these folds become more marked with time from the original surgery. Tuszewski concluded that such changes are an adaption of the colonic mucosa to its new function, that primarily of transport, and not storage and water resorption [96]. The changes have been ascribed to postoperative edema or to an adaptation of the colonic mucosa due to its new function [65,96].

In the early postoperative period, the abnormality most commonly encountered is anastomotic narrowing [60]. Such changes may occur either proximally or distally and most often are related to postprocedure edema (Fig. 2.28). Anastomatic stricture is usually self-limited, but when persistent is remediable by dilatation. A transient nodular appearance to the perianastomotic site is also most likely secondary to edema [60]. Stasis within the interposed segment was also seen, although less frequently. Slightly more than half the patients with stasis had narrowing of the distal colonic esophageal anastomosis.

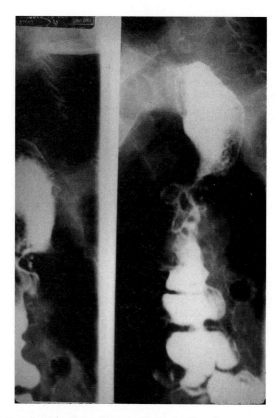

FIGURE 2.28. Esophagocolic stricture. Oblique film from an upper GI series shows marked smooth narrowing at an esophagocolic anastomosis. This is the typical appearance for a benign stricture.

Leaks from the anastomoses are five times more frequently encountered at the proximal esophageal colon anastomosis than the distal one [60]. Only half these leaks seal spontaneously. Perforations of the colon have also been reported, as well as other cases of ischemic necrosis [60]. Aspiration was noted during the acute postoperative phase in slightly less than 10% of patients. A rare case of obstruction of the interposed colon due to an intrathoracic axial volvulus has also been reported [60].

During the late phase, aspiration and anastomotic strictures were equally observed (~15% of patients) [60]. The strictures were evenly distributed between the proximal and distal esophageal colonic anastomoses [60]. Gastric stasis has also been observed, but not as frequently as aspiration or strictures. Gastrocolic and gastrocoloesophageal reflux is observed in slightly less than 10% of patients. This reflux may lead to ulceration. In one case, the ulcer penetrated into the aorta, resulting in an aortocolonic fistula [97].

Colonic stasis is occasionally secondary to a long, redundant intraabdominal portion of the colon, which may be acutely angulated just proximal to the cologastric anastomosis [60,95]. Diverticular disease

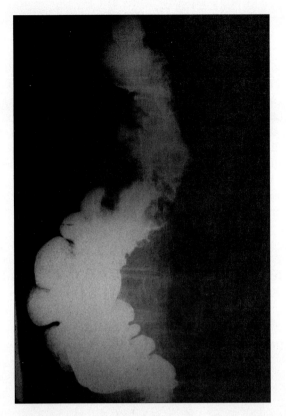

FIGURE 2.29. **Carcinoma that developed in interposed colon.** Film from a barium study reveals a colonic interposition. Annular constricting lesion in the midportion of the interposed colon represents a carcinoma.

[98] has been known to develop in the interposed colonic segment, as well as adenocarcinoma (Fig. 2.29) [55,93,99–101].

Varices

Esophageal varices are most often the result of portal hypertension. Patients with esophageal varices are often prone to gastrointestinal bleeding that may be life threatening. In trying to control varices and variceal bleeding, both local and systemic therapies may be employed. Medications that result in the lowering of portal venous hypertension (nonselective β-adrenergic blockers or oral nitrates) may be used, especially for long-term control [102]. More recently, transjugular intrahepatic portosystemic shunts (TIPS) have been of considerable help in lowering portal venous pressures, often replacing operative shunts. However, elevated serum ammonia levels with resultant hepatic encephalopathy and/or reduced flow through the shunts reduce the overall efficacy and clinical usefulness of these procedures.

Alternatively, local therapies are of value, especially in the short-term management of variceal bleeding. The oldest therapy is that of balloon tamponade via a Sengstaken–Blakemore tube. This tube has multiple components. First is a long proximal balloon that lies within the esophagus. A second balloon, rounder and larger in diameter, is located distally. The longitudinal balloon is used to compress esophageal varices, while the distal round balloon compresses gastric fundal varices. Care must be taken to insufflate the distal balloon in the capacious stomach, not in the limited diameter of the esophagus (Figs. 2.30 and 2.31). Improper inflation can lead to esophageal disruption with dire consequences for the patient (Fig. 2.32).

Other, more permanent methods of control include esophageal variceal sclerotherapy or variceal banding. Less likely to be used, especially in the United States is esophageal devascularization (Sugiura–Futagawa procedure). In sclerotherapy, small amounts of sclerosant are injected directly into, or immediately adjacent to the esophageal varices [102–106]. Sodium morrhuate (5%) [104,105], ethanolamine oleate [106], and tetradecyl sulfate have all been used to produce a local

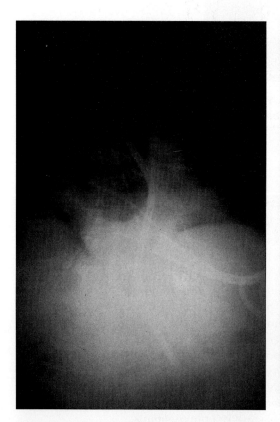

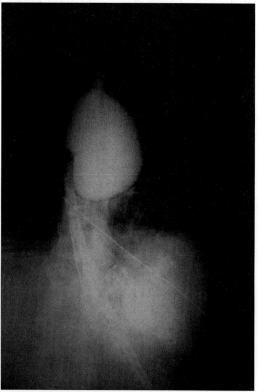

FIGURE 2.30. Malpositioned Sengstaken–Blakemore tube. Anteroposterior film of the chest following inadvertent inflation with air of the gastric balloon of a Sengstaken–Blakemore tube in the esophagus.

FIGURE 2.31. Malpositioned Sengstaken–Blakemore tube. Anteroposterior film of the chest shows a large gastric balloon of a Sengstaken–Blakemore tube filled with contrast medium while still in the patient's esophagus.

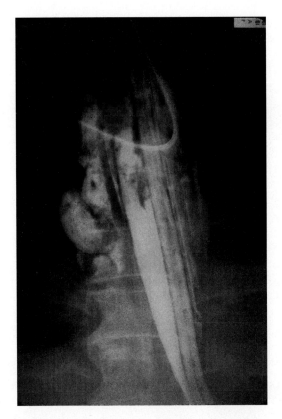

FIGURE 2.32. Esophageal perforation secondary to malpostioned Sengstaken–Blakemore tube. Film from a water-soluble contrast esophagogram following attempted placement of a Sengstaken–Blakemore tube shows marked disruption of the esophagus with multiple mediastinal tracts.

inflammatory reaction that obliterates the varices. Sodium morrhuate, a mixture of unsaturated fatty acids found in cod liver oil [105], includes oleic and linoleic acids. Early on in the postinjection period, the overlying mucosa may ulcerate. These ulcers are usually focal and related to the injection site [104]. Following extensive injection therapy, the ulceration may become more diffuse and confluent, even leading to sinus tract and fistula formation. A double-barreled appearance may result from extensive intramural tracking [104]. When the ulcerations are deep, perforation may ensue [104].

The local inflammatory response may lead to esophageal luminal narrowing. If the region of injection therapy was circumferential, the resultant narrowing may also be circumferential, mimicking an annular carcinoma [104]. When less extensive, the perivariceal inflammatory and hemorrhagic response produces mucosal or extramucosal defects that may vary in size and shape [104]. These local defects secondary to edema usually regress in a few days.

In patients in whom the inflammatory response was more marked, or deeper in extent, esophageal strictures may develop over time (Fig. 2.33). Therefore, patients with deep ulcers or sinus tracts early on in

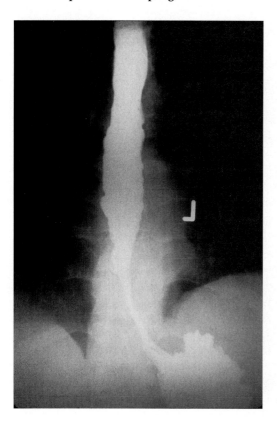

FIGURE 2.33. Sclerotherapy-induced esophageal changes. Postsclerotherapy esophagogram reveals multiple ulcerations in the proximal to middle thirds, and a long stricture distally.

their course are more prone to develop a stricture [104]. Most strictures are short and may be at the site of a previous ulceration. Contour defects noted in the early post-procedure period may persist as nodules or even plaques on later follow-up examinations. Stiffening of the injected portions of the esophageal wall may also result. Dysmotility in the area, perhaps secondary to neuromuscular damage, has been reported as well.

A new, and now widely used therapy for the control and prevention of variceal hemorrhage is that of endoscopic variceal ligation (or banding) [102,107,108]. Reportedly, this procedure has several advantages over sclerotherapy, including fewer complications, fewer treatments necessary, lower rebleeding rates, and an overall lower mortality [107]. In esophageal variceal ligation, the varix is snared with endoscopic suction and drawn into the ligator. A small O-ring ligature is then placed around the base of the varix and released. The placement of the rubber ligature results in strangulation of the varix, with eventual thrombosis, sloughing, and fibrosis [109].

When a varix sloughs, an ulceration of the mucosa may result. If deep enough, the ulcer may heal with stricturing [108]. When studied in the immediate postprocedure period, patients with esophageal variceal ligation show smooth rounded nodules that range in size from 5 to 10mm. Because blood does not flow into or out of the ligated varix, the vein does not change in size or shape as opposed to a nontreated varix. Ulcerations may also be seen in these patients, but these are usually healed within 2 weeks of the initial insult [108].

Esophageal devascularization is another, and more controversial method of controlling esophageal varices [110]. As the procedure is commonly performed, the esophagus is devascularized distal to the level of the inferior pulmonary vein. The greater and lesser curvatures of the stomach are also devascularized, with the ligation of the short gastric veins along the greater curvature and the left gastric veins along the high lesser curvature. The esophagus is then transected and reanastomosed by means of a stapling device. A splenectomy is performed along with the esophagogastric surgery. Truncal vagotomy and pyloroplasty are concomitantly performed in most patients. If a selective vagotomy is performed, there may not be a need for the pyloroplasty.

Initial results from Japan, in nonalcoholic cirrhotic patients, showed 66% 5-year survival and recurrent hemorrhage in less than 10% of patients [111]. A more recent study from France replicated these results [112]. In North America, the results have been significantly worse, and the procedure is usually reserved for emergencies.

There is little written about the radiographic appearance of the esophagus following the Sugiura procedure (Fig. 2.34). One series of 11 patients showed a significant number of complications including pleural effusions, ascites, ileus, and pneumonia [113]. Esophageal varices were either markedly reduced in size or absent altogether on

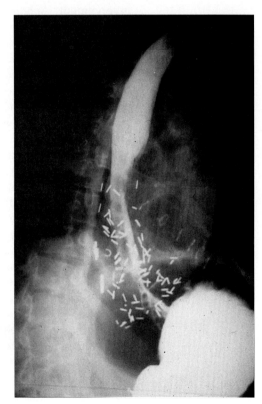

FIGURE 2.34. **Sugiura procedure.** Innumerable surgical clips outline the esophagus in this patient, who has undergone a devascularization procedure. A long segment of narrowing is noted distally.

postoperative studies. A less striking reduction in gastric varices was also seen. Two patients had dysphagia with stricture formation. One resolved spontaneously and the other required bougienage. One patient developed gastroesophageal reflux symptoms postoperatively, and esophagitis was noted on endoscopy. Some irregularity to the esophageal wall was noted, but it was difficult to differentiate esophagitis from postprocedure deformity. Two cases of anastomotic leakage were noted, one with fatal consequences. The surgical literature notes that fistulization or frank dehiscence of the anastomotic line is not unheard of [114,115]. A new modification of the procedure involves a submucosal interruption of the esophageal wall, leaving the mucosa intact. This measure reportedly has decreased the incidence of these two serious complications [116].

Esophageal Dilatation

Strictures of the esophagus are usually treated by dilatation. Passage of a 45F dilator usually signals the ability to eat most foods [117]. Tight strictures are usually dilated stepwise, with each session limited to passage of a dilator 6F to 10F larger than the first one that encounters resistance. Perforation may occur with too rapid a dilatation at one setting. Patients with previous corrosive ingestion are at higher risk for perforation than those with peptic strictures [118]. This is because of the extensive periesophageal fibrotic response as well as the length of involvement. Achalasia patients have a more serious clinical course than others owing to spillage of food, sometimes in copious amounts.

Although Willis attempted an esophageal dilatation during the mid-1600s, it was Hurst and his mercury-filled dilator that revolutionized the technique in 1915 [119]. The Hurst dilator was modified by Maloney, who replaced the blunt end with a tapered tip to allow easier passage through a stricture. During the 1950s, olive-shaped metal dilators, passed over a metal guide wire, were introduced (Eder–Puestow) [119]. Eventually, hollow-core polyvinyl dilators (Savary–Guillard, American), more rigid devices that are best for tight and/or long strictures, further increased the therapeutic armamentarium. Balloon dilators, a newer additional choice, have the advantage of developing a lower shear force than is possible with traditional bougienage [118].

Perforation is the most common and dreaded complication of esophageal dilatation, no matter what instrument is used. Rates following bougienage may be as high as 9%, while balloon dilatation may lead to rates between 1 and 2% [120]. However, the rate depends on what is actually defined as a perforation. Kang et al. proposed a grading system, with types 1 and 2 representing intramural and transmural tears, respectively, and type 3 being a complete disruption with mediastinal spill [118]. Types 1 and 2 differ radiographically with respect to whether the contrast is retained within the tear (type 2). Using these criteria, Kang's team found the rate of type I disruptions to be equal to that of types 2 and 3. If the mucosal flap that separates the lumen from the tear seals over, an extramucosal mass (hematoma) may develop. This may appear similar to a leiomyoma or other intramural mass. Preprocedure comparative films or follow-up examinations usually make this differentiation easy. Perforation may not only involve the thoracic esophagus but also the subdiaphragmatic portion. When the latter is involved, air may be present in the lesser sac [121].

Alternative Therapies

Other modalities available for the palliation of esophageal carcinoma include lasers, photodynamic therapy, bipolar electrocoagulation therapy (BICAP™), and local injection therapy, along with radiation therapy (including brachytherapy).

The neodymium/yttrium–aluminum–garnet laser (Nd/YAG) was introduced in 1982 [122]. The laser, which operates at a wavelength of 1060 nm, widens the lumen by locally heating and vaporizing the tumor. When feasible, the endoscope is passed through the tumor and the therapy performed during withdrawal. This allows better control and a lower perforation rate than can be obtained with antegrade therapy [123]. Following laser therapy, the esophageal lumen is increased in diameter but may show residual tumor mass. In other cases, the mucosal surface may be irregular and thickened, resembling an esophagitis. In still others, the residual lumen is narrowed with smooth margins, appearing as a benign stricture, though this is less commonly encountered [124]. Early complications include perforation, bleeding, and airway fistulization (Fig. 2.35). Complication rates range

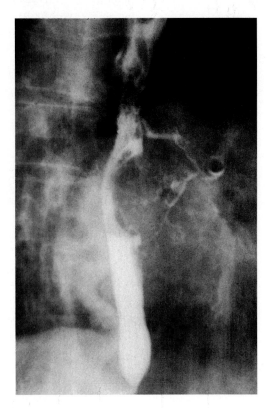

FIGURE 2.35. Esophageal changes following laser therapy. Esophagogram demonstrates an irregular margin to the esophagus consistent with a carcinoma. An esophageal–bronchial fistula has developed secondary to recent laser therapy of the obstructing lesion. Note that there is no longer any significant esophageal obstruction.

as high as 20% for those treated with laser therapy [122]. Both pneumomediastinum and pneumoperitoneum have been reported post-therapy [124]. Restenosis may occur over time.

Photodynamic therapy is based on the administration of a photo-sensitizing agent that is preferentially localized in neoplastic tissue. In Canada and Europe, 5-aminolevulenic acid is orally administered [122,125]. In the United States, porfirmen sodium is the only approved agent, and it is administered intravenously. On exposure to a properly tuned laser (wavelength of 630 nm) oxygen free radicals are formed [122,125]. These cause local cell death and subsequent tumor necrosis. The depth of affected tissue is less than that seen with conventional laser therapy, and therefore perforation is expected less often. Side effects include sunburn and are more commonly seen than in conventional laser treatments [122].

The BICAP™ technique is based on the direct application of heat generated by an electric current. An olive-shaped bipolar electrode is utilized, and no grounding plate is needed because the electrodes are situated close together on the probe. The electrocoagulation probe is placed distal to the malignant stricture following preliminary dilatation. An electric current, applied as the endoscope and electrode are withdrawn, circumferentially deposits the energy in the surrounding malignant tissue. This results in tissue desiccation during which the tissue resistance increases, thus limiting the depth of the destructive effect [125]. Inflatable balloon probes have also been developed [122].

Local injection therapy, which acts via tissue necrosis and subsequent sloughing, has also been utilized in palliating malignant strictures [122]. Substances injected have included dehydrated ethanol, sodium morrhuate, polidocanol, and chemotherapeutic agents [125]. Carbon-adsorbed peplomycin, a bleomycin derivative, has also shown promising results [126,127].

Fundoplication

The causation of lower esophageal sphincter incompetence that can lead to gastroesophageal reflux is multifactorial. The list may include transient lower esophageal sphincter (LES) relaxation not related to a swallow, decreased resting tone of the LES, gastric motility disturbances, and distortion of the gastroesophageal junction anatomy (lack of a flap valve mechanism) [128]. The relationship of reflux and the presence of a hiatal hernia is unclear.

The surgical management of gastroesophageal reflux is based on restoration of competency of the valve. To achieve this goal, six basic principles must be met [128]:

1. The distal esophagus must be wrapped by a fundoplication that is affixed to the esophagus to keep it in place.
2. No tension can be placed on the fundoplication.
3. The esophagus must allow the passage of a large bougie (~55–60F).

4a. The plication should be 2 cm long anteriorly, and slightly longer posteriorly if a complete wrap is performed.
4b. If a partial fundoplication is performed (as described shortly) it should be 3 to 4 cm long.
5. The wrapped portion of the esophagus must be subdiaphragmatic in position.
6. The diaphragmatic hiatus must be narrowed about the esophagus proximal to the level of the wrap.

Many variations of fundoplication have been proposed and utilized. They all try to balance adequate reflux control without excessive dysphagia [129]. As described by Stirling and Orringer [130], Nissen originally proposed a complete, 360° wrap with the gastric fundus wrapped posteriorly, to the right, and then anteriorly to encompass the entire circumference of the distal esophagus. Eventually, this wrap was shortened from 4 to 5 cm to approximately 2 cm, the wrap was performed over a large-bore dilator, and the short gastric vessels were divided to prevent traction on the fundoplication. These measures effectively loosened the fundoplication, and the procedure has been termed a floppy fundoplication (Fig. 2.36).

If there is insufficient length of esophagus to allow a subdiaphragmatic wrap to be performed without undue tension on the fundoplication, a Collis gastroplasty may be performed [70,128,131,132]. This procedure, which is often performed with the following techniques, effectively lengthens the abdominal portion of the esophagus. It is performed by dividing the stomach along the lesser curvature just lateral to the left border of the distal esophagus with a GI stapling device. A large bougie is placed in the esophagus as a guide and to prevent inadvertent narrowing of the tube created [128,131,132].

Toupet, Dor, Skinner and Belsey, and Hill have made further modifications to the original technique. Toupet modified the Nissen wrap by making it incomplete, only encompassing the posterior wall of the esophagus and attaching the fundoplication to the anterior wall

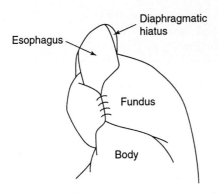

FIGURE 2.36. Nissen fundoplication. Schematic drawing of a Nissen fundoplication.

of the esophagus and the diaphragmatic hiatus, which is not closed [128,131].

Dor reversed the Toupet procedure, encompassing the anterior wall of the distal esophagus [128,131] (Fig. 2.37). This approach may be used following a lower esophageal myotomy, in which the wrap covers the myotomy site [128].

The Belsey Mark IV differs from the preceding wraps by invaginating the distal esophagus into the fundus, rather than wrapping the fundus transversely about the distal esophagus. Only 270° of the esophagus is wrapped, leaving the posterior wall uncovered [131].

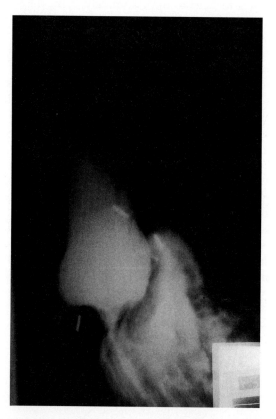

FIGURE 2.37. **Incomplete fundal wrap around esophagus.** Film from an upper GI series showing an incomplete fundoplication, perhaps of the Dor type.

Hill advocated attaching portions of the lesser curvature to the median arcuate ligaments of the diaphragm, rather than to the esophagus. Although not strictly speaking a fundoplication, it acts as one, and it is aimed at restoring the normal flap valve anatomy at the gastroesophageal junction [128].

Many variations of these techniques have been introduced. In addition, the traditional open surgical technique is rapidly being supplanted by laparoscopic surgery. All aim at providing symptomatic relief for heartburn and regurgitation. However, if the fundoplication is too tight, either dysphagia or "gas bloat" syndrome may occur.

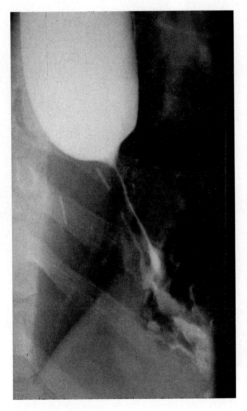

FIGURE 2.38. **Tight fundoplication.** Long narrowing of the distal esophagus due to an overly tight fundoplication.

Dysphagia is the most common symptom and is seen in 30 to 40% of patients in the immediate postoperative period. Over time this decreases to 5% of patients. Some of the dysphagia is initially due to perioperative edema. If persistent, esophageal narrowing may be secondary to a wrap that is too tight. An upper GI series performed with barium may help to identify the narrowing in symptomatic patients (Fig. 2.38). However, the use of a barium tablet (12.5 mm diameter) aids in the diagnosis of significant lesions, especially in patients who experience dysphagia only for solid foods (Figs. 2.39 and 2.40). When encountered, narrowings can be successfully dilated. Less than 1% of patients end up requiring reoperation [132].

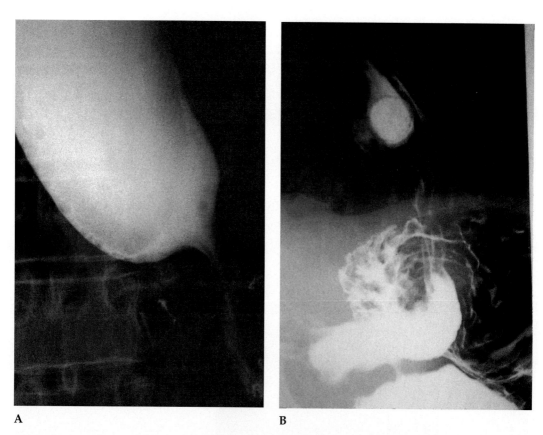

A   B

FIGURE 2.39. **Tight wrap with entrapped barium tablet.** Upper GI series (A) demonstrates a dilated esophagus with a short, smooth, symmetrical narrowing secondary to a tight wrap. Use of a barium tablet reveals obstruction to a swallowed solid (B). The tablet dissolved a few minutes afterward.

"Gas bloat" syndrome, the inability to eructate, causes abdominal discomfort [128,132]. For reasons that remain unclear, it occurs less frequently following laparoscopic surgery [133]. Some authors comparing partial and Nissen fundoplications have reported no significant difference in esophageal motility [134]. Others, however, have reported better overall motility in patients with partial fundoplications [135].

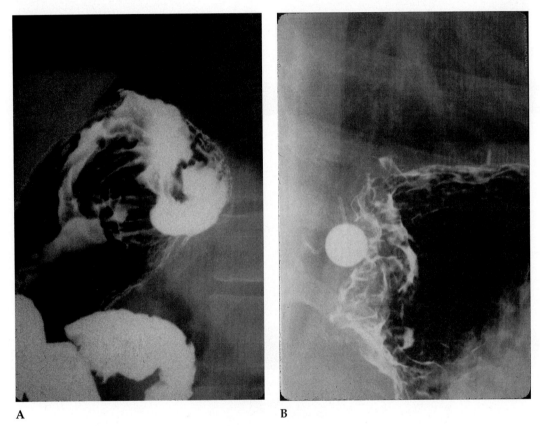

A   B

FIGURE 2.40. Whirled appearance in a tight fundoplication. Double-contrast upper GI series (A) reveals the whirled appearance of the fundus following fundoplication. A second film from this exam (B) shows the obstructed barium tablet in a deformed fundus.

Some deformity of the stomach may be observed in patients who have undergone a fundoplication. There may be a mass indentation at the level of the fundus where the esophagus enters the stomach (Fig. 2.41), or the submerged portion of the esophagus may be narrowed as it passes through the wrap itself (Fig. 2.42). Sometimes, especially on

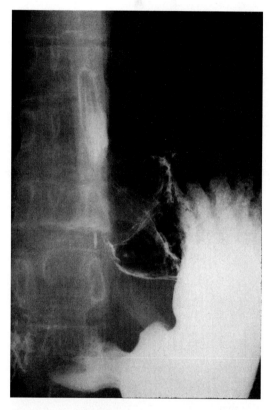

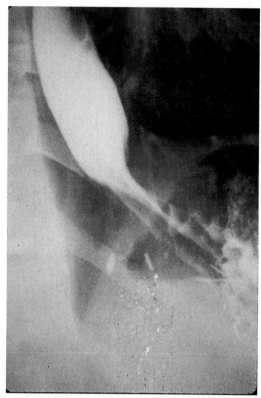

FIGURE 2.41. Fundoplication defect. A deformed fundus with a large filling defect is noted following fundoplication.

FIGURE 2.42. Fundoplication defect. The submerged segment of the esophagus is narrowed as it passes through a plication defect.

double-contrast examinations, the soft tissues of the wrap may sur-
round the enwrapped esophagus (Figs. 2.43 and 2.44). On CT scans,
the fundal gastric mucosa has a whirled appearance as it wraps around
the esophagus (Fig. 2.45).

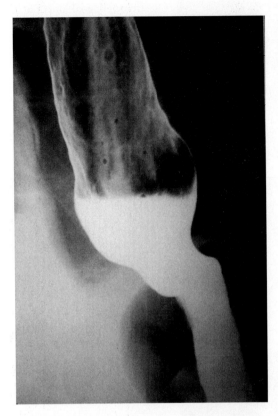

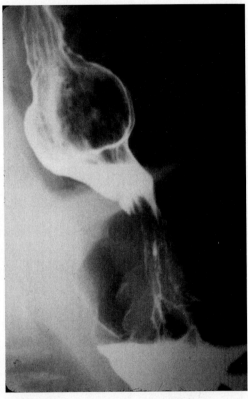

FIGURE 2.43. Fundal mass secondary to wrap.
Double-contrast esophagogram reveals part of a
fundoplication as a soft tissue mass about the
intragastric portion of the esophagus.

FIGURE 2.44. Fundal mass secondary to wrap.
Excellent demonstration of a fundal wrap
with its soft tissues surrounding the distal
esophagus.

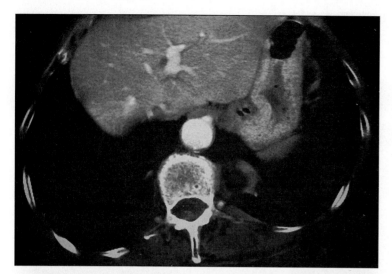

A

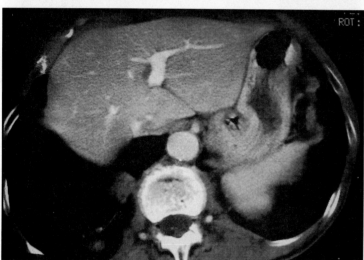

B

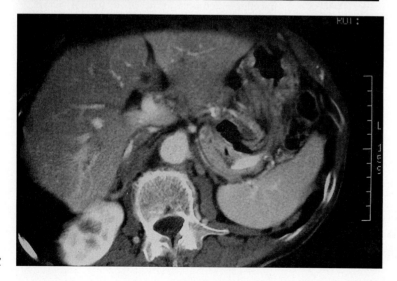

C

FIGURE 2.45. Whirled CT appearance of fundoplication. Three CT sections demonstrating the whirled appearance of a fundoplication from the level of the gastroesophageal junction (A) to the fundus (B) to the proximal body of the stomach (C).

FIGURE 2.46. Type I failed fundoplication. Schematic diagram of a type I failed fundoplication.

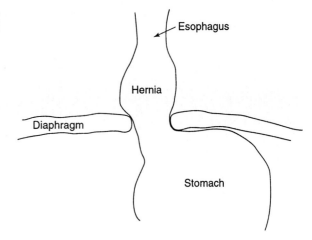

Four different patterns of fundoplication failure have been described [131]. In type I, the fundal wrap becomes undone and the hiatal hernia recurs, with the stomach slipping back into the chest (Figs. 2.46 and 2.47). In type II, the wrap is maintained and remains infradiaphragmatic in location. However, part of the stomach reenters the chest. The diaphragm pinches the herniated stomach, causing an "hourglass"

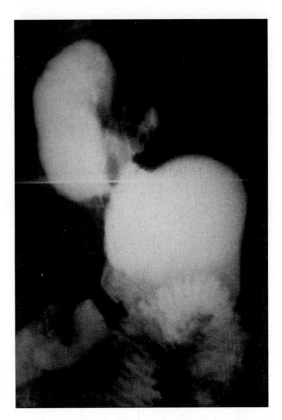

FIGURE 2.47. Type I failed fundoplication. Film from an upper GI series showing a type I failure with undoing of the plication and herniation of the stomach above the diaphragm.

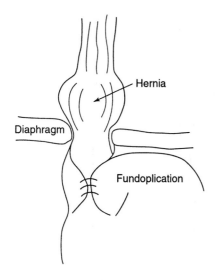

FIGURE 2.48. Type II failed fundoplication. Schematic diagram of a type II failed fundoplication.

deformity (Figs. 2.48 and 2.49). In type III, part of the stomach lies above the fundal wrap but still is infradiaphragmatic in location. This also gives rise to an "hourglass" deformity (Figs. 2.50–2.52). This is the so-called slipped Nissen repair. In a type IV failure, the wrap remains intact, but the distal esophagus and its wrap herniate through the esophageal hiatus into the chest (Fig. 2.53).

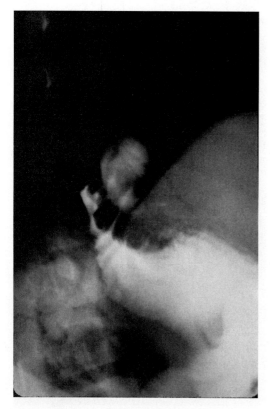

FIGURE 2.49. Type II failed fundoplication. Film from an upper GI series showing a type II failure with an intact wrap below the diaphragm, but herniation of the stomach into the chest.

FIGURE 2.50. Type III failed fundoplication. Schematic diagram of a type III failed fundoplication.

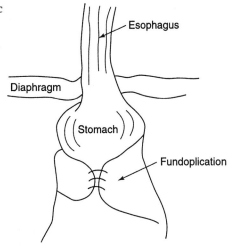

FIGURE 2.51. Type III failed fundoplication. Single-contrast upper GI series showing a small portion of stomach proximal to the fundoplication defect, but still infradiaphragmatic in location.

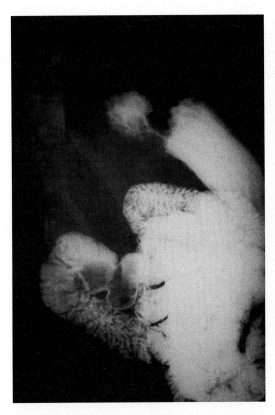

FIGURE 2.52. Type III failed fundoplication. Double-contrast upper GI series showing a large portion of the stomach proximal to the plication defect, but below the diaphragm.

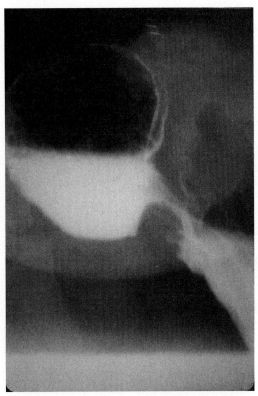

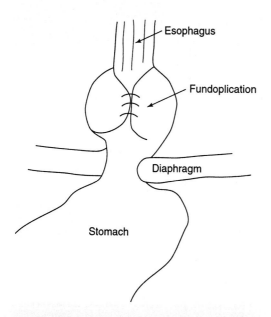

Esophagus

Fundoplication

Diaphragm

Stomach

FIGURE 2.53. Type IV failed fundoplication. Schematic diagram of a type IV failed fundoplication.

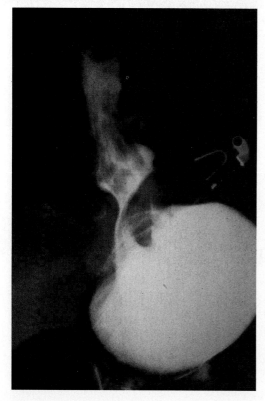

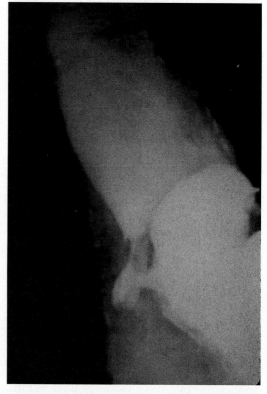

FIGURE 2.54. Gastroesophageal reflux following failed fundoplication. Upper GI series demonstrating a type II failure, with marked gastroesophageal reflux.

FIGURE 2.55. Peptic stricture following fundoplication. Upper GI series showing a short peptic stricture in a patient with a prior fundoplication.

When reflux symptoms recur postoperatively, they are usually less intense than before the surgery [132]. Up to 8% of patients are symptomatic 10 years after open surgery. It is expected that laparoscopic surgery will yield similar long-term results. Medical therapy is usually sufficient to control the symptoms as long as the fundoplication is intact. Leaks may occur that are silent clinically. These are often due to improper (too deep) placement of a suture plicating the fundus to the esophagus. These small leaks may be observed and treated expectantly [70]. When reflux is severe (Fig. 2.54), the patient is subject to the development of reflux esophagitis, peptic stricture formation (Figs. 2.55 and 2.56), Barrett's metaplasia, and even carcinoma formation (Fig. 2.57).

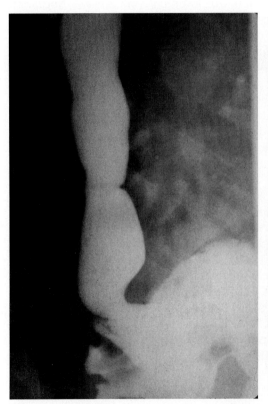

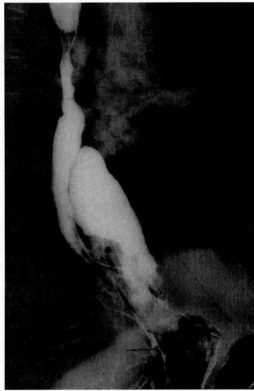

FIGURE 2.56. Peptic stricture following failed fundoplication. Upper GI series demonstrating an annular peptic stricture in a patient whose fundoplication has become almost completely undone.

FIGURE 2.57. Failed fundoplication with Barrett's carcinoma. Single-contrast esophagram of a patient with a type IV failure. Note the irregular narrowing of the midesophagus from an adenocarcinoma.

Angelchik Prosthesis

In 1979 Angelchik and Cohen described a new and novel approach for the prevention of gastroesophageal reflux [136]. They designed a C-shaped prosthesis made out of silicone and filled with a silicone gel. The inner diameter was 2.5 × 3.1 cm with an outer diameter of 6 × 7 cm². The device was anchored in place by a Dacron fiber strap and had a tantalum-filled marker for radiographic localization. Originally the device had a 1 cm gap in the radiopaque marker that sometimes led to the diagnosis of a nonexistent fracture in the device. The gap was closed in 1982. The device was inserted via an abdominal incision in which the collar of the prosthesis is wrapped around the distal esophagus and held in place anteriorly by the Dacron straps [137,138].

The Angelchik prosthesis has had a checkered history and has generally fallen out of favor [137–146]. Many complications have been described, including migration, displacement, and erosion. Migration due to breaks in the Dacron tapes was eliminated by the change in design in 1982. Displacement occurred either into the mediastinum through a widened esophageal hiatus [139,140] or into the abdomen because of an excessive mobilization of the cardia at the time of surgery [139]. Even a fatal case of suppurative pericarditis was reported [141]. Erosion may be due to placement near a preexisting suture line in the stomach, or accidental entry into the gastric lumen may occur during surgery. In the absence of development of an acute abdomen, however, the slow and insidious movement of the prosthesis may also suggest a chronic form of migration, with the formation of surrounding adhesions [142,143].

The prosthesis appears as a doughnut encircled by an opaque tantalum band 2 mm wide [138]. When properly positioned, it should be at the gastroesophageal junction [137]. It may cause a nipplelike protrusion in the center of the gastric fundus [137]. On CT images the ring has attenuation similar to the liver or spleen [144]. It may be obliquely oriented and not completely imaged on any single section through the gastroesophageal junction. The tantalum strap is easily visible, and the prosthesis should not be difficult to recognize. When either intra- or extraluminal dislodgment has occurred, the radiopaque marker should make the CT or even plain film diagnosis of the complication easy.

The Angelchik prosthesis may cause dysmotility, and many patients will have prolonged esophageal transit times as measured by a marshmallow swallow [145]. However, the absence of abnormal motility does not mean that a complication is not present [146]. Gas bloat, usually indicative of an overly tight gastroesophageal junction, has also been reported in patients with this prosthesis.

Achalasia

Achalasia, a failure of the lower esophageal sphincter to relax, has an estimated incidence, in the United States, of 1 per 100,000 population per year [147]. Males and females are equally affected. The characteristic plain film findings include a widened mediastinum with an air–fluid level in the upright position. The increased mediastinal density may wander from the right in the upper chest to the left in the retrocardiac region. On barium studies, a beaklike deformity of the submerged segment (subdiaphragmatic) is a classic finding. Although the more proximal esophagus is classically atonic, a significant percentage of patients show esophageal contractions, so-called vigorous achalasia.

Various therapies have been used over time to treat achalasia. Surgery, systemic medications, and various endoscopic techniques all have their advantages and disadvantages. Nitrates and calcium channel blockers work as smooth muscle relaxants with some relief of symptoms [especially isosorbide dinitrate (Isordil)]. These are of use early in the course of the disease [147].

More recently, direct injection of botulinum toxin (botox) has been proposed as a therapeutic measure. However, the treatment's effect is not permanent, and multiple procedures are necessary to ensure long-standing relief. Botox still plays a role in the frail and elderly, who are not good candidates for surgery and/or pneumatic dilatation.

Surgical therapy, initially through a laparotomy, but also performed via thoracotomy is a long-standing therapeutic option. More recently, it has become possible to perform the procedure laparoscopically. Heller, in 1914, first described the performance of two longitudinal myotomies on opposite sides of the distal esophagus [148]. As a consequence of the myotomy, many patients have gastroesophageal reflux, and therefore many surgeons perform an antireflux procedure at the same time. A Nissen fundoplication may close the gastroesophageal junction too tightly, and therefore an anterior (Dor) or a posterior (Toupet) fundoplication is used to control the reflux. The former is used in elderly patients and those with a megaesophagus (>7 cm diameter), while the latter is reserved for less severe dilatation, especially in younger patients [148].

The last treatment option is that of pneumatic dilatation. The esophagus must reach a diameter of at least 3 cm to partially disrupt the circular muscle fibers of the lower esophageal sphincter [147]. Endoscopes and standard bougies do not reach this size, and therefore balloon dilatation is necessary. Many different dilators have been used over the years, but only two are currently available in the United States. These are the Rigiflex and Witzel dilators. Both utilize polyethylene balloons, with the former positioned fluoroscopically over a guide wire and the latter mounted on an endoscope [147].

The efficacy of all these therapies is difficult to determine. Relief of symptoms is a subjective criterion, while completeness of esophageal emptying is objective [149]. However the correlation between the two criteria is not always good [150–152]. Therefore, de Oliveira and colleagues proposed a timed barium swallow to evaluate the patient's response to therapy [149]. In this procedure, the patient drinks medium density barium in the upright position until satiated. Films of the esophagus are then taken at 0, 2, and 5 minutes postingestion, being careful to maintain the same magnification factors for all views.

Measurements yield the percentage of emptying over time. This exam can be repeated to measure the response post-therapy.

Following myotomy, the herniation of the mucosa through the incised circular muscle fibers of the lower esophageal sphincter may cause the formation of pseudodiverticula [153] (Fig. 2.58). This condition has been reported to progress to a giant epiphrenic diverticulum measuring 8 cm in greatest diameter [154]. A similar deformity may be seen following pneumatic dilatation as well [155]. Because of the decreased effectiveness of the lower esophageal sphincter, it is not surprising that gastroesophageal reflux is a complication of both myotomy and pneumatic dilatation. Barrett's metaplasia and even carcinoma have been reported [156].

Immediately following pneumatic dilatation, there may be improved emptying of the esophagus. However, edema and hemorrhage in the wall as well as spasm of the lower esophageal sphincter may actually lead to decreased emptying. Therefore the immediate post-procedure study is a poor predictor of the patient's ultimate response [157]. Imme-

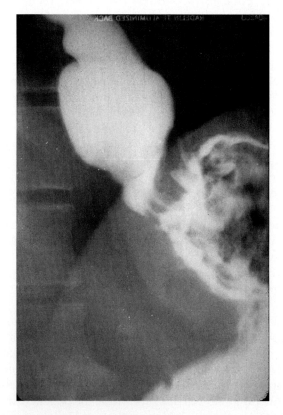

FIGURE 2.58. **Heller myotomy.** Single-contrast esophagram of a patient who had undergone a Heller myotomy. Paired bulges from the distal esophagus represent pseudodiverticula through the operative muscle defects.

diate post-procedure studies should be performed only to exclude an esophageal tear (which may be clinically silent).

Patients at highest risk for having a perforation are those with blood on the dilator, tachycardia, and chest pain more than 4 hours after the procedure [158]. The Rigiflex dilator is associated with a significantly lower rate of perforation than the Witzel dilator [159].

The radiographic findings of esophageal injury vary with the depth of the mural disruption. More limited injuries, confined to the mucosa, may present as a linear extraluminal collection of contrast paralleling the esophageal lumen [160] (Fig. 2.59). A somewhat deeper injury may present as a double-barreled appearance to the esophagus similar to that seen in an aortic dissection, or communicating hematoma [160] or thermal injury of the esophagus [161]. The mucosal stripe separating the two lumina is readily evident as a thin lucency between the two contrast collections. Alternatively, if the intramural hematoma is non-communicating (the mucosal flap has sealed over), a smooth filling defect in the esophageal wall is noted [162]. A through-and-through

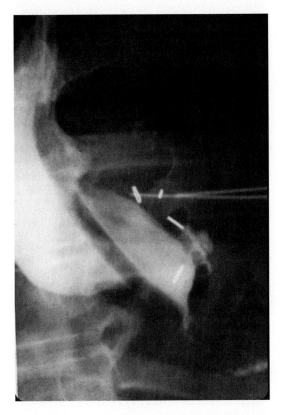

FIGURE 2.59. **Achalasia pneumatic dilatation tear.** Immediate post–pneumatic dilatation esophagogram shows a well-contained extraluminal collection of contrast representing a mucosal tear.

disruption would present with one or more of the following: pneumo-mediastinum, subcutaneous air, pleural fluid, and extravasation of air beyond the normal confines of the esophagus. The latter may include air in the lesser sac from perforation of the "submerged" subdia-phragmatic portion of the esophagus [163]. Perforation of the segment can be confirmed on conventional contrast studies and/or CT imaging. Incomplete tears are usually managed conservatively with operative intervention needed for full-thickness disruption [164].

These complications, including frank perforation, resolve with no serious long-term sequelae [158] (Fig. 2.60). However, as many as half of all patients studied over a 5-year period continue to have symptoms [155].

Another unusual complication is an intradiaphragmatic abscess. One such abscess was noted following a 3-week relatively asymptomatic period following pneumatic dilation. Both conventional and CT pre-operative studies failed to identify the exact site of this abscess, which had to be drained operatively [165].

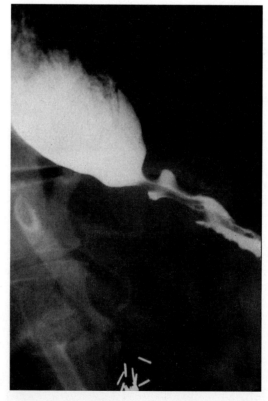

FIGURE 2.60. **Post–pneumatic dilatation esophageal deformity.** Repeat study of the same patient in Figure 2.59, many months later, reveals a bilobed out-pouching of contrast at the distal esophagus, similar to, but smaller than that seen following a Heller myotomy.

References

1. Moore KL. The Developing Human. Philadelphia: WB Saunders; 1988; 207–245.
2. Brookes M, Zietman AL. Clinical Embryology: A Color Atlas and Text. Boca Raton, FL: CRC Press; 1998;78–82.
3. Patti MG, Gantert W, Way LW. Surgery of the esophagus. Anatomy and physiology. Surg Clin North Am 1997;77:959–970.
4. Ekberg O, Besjakov J, Lindgren S. Radiographic findings after cricopharyngeal myotomy. Acta Radiol 1987;28:555–558.
5. Rubesin SE, Beatty SM. The postoperative esophagus. Semin Roentgenol 1994;29:401–410.
6. Olsen KD, DeSanto LW. Resection of the larynx and the pharynx for cancer. In: Nyhus LM, Baker RJ, Fischer JE, eds. Mastery of Surgery, 3rd ed. Boston: Little, Brown; 1996:411–437.
7. Tomkinson A, Shone GR, Kingle A, Roblin DG, Quine S. Pharyngocutaneous fistula following total laryngectomy and post-operative vomiting. Clin Otolaryngol 1996;21:369–370.
8. Seikaly H, Park P. Gastroesophageal reflux prophylaxis decreases the incidence of pharyngocutaneous fistula after total laryngectomy. Laryngoscope 1995;105:1220–1222.
9. Smit CT, Tan J, Mathus-Vliegen LM, et al. High incidence of gastropharyngeal and gastroesophageal reflux after total laryngectomy. Head Neck 1998;20:619–622.
10. Fradis M, Podoshin L, Ben David J. Post-laryngectomy pharyngocutaneous fistula—A still unresolved problem. J Laryngol Otol 1995; 109:221–224.
11. Muller-Miny H, Eisele DW, Jones B. Dynamic radiographic imaging following total laryngectomy. Head Neck 1993;15:342–347.
12. Oursin C, Pitzer G, Fournier P, Bongartz G, Steinbrich W. Anterior neopharyngeal pseudodiverticulum. A possible cause of dysphagia in laryngectomized patients. Clin Imaging 1999;23:15–18.
13. Woisard V, Serrano E, Yardeni E, Puech M, Pessey JJ. Deglutition after supra-glottic laryngectomy. J Otolaryngol 1993;22:278–283.
14. Jung TTK, Adams GL. Dysphagia in laryngectomized patients. Otolaryngol Head Neck Surg 1980;88:25–33.
15. Torres WE, Fibus TF, Coleman III JJ, Clements Jr JL, Bernandino ME. Radiographic evaluation of the free jejunal graft. Gastrointest Radiol 1987;12:226–230.
16. Neifeld JP, Merritt WA, Theogaraj SD, Parker GA. Tubed pectoralis major musculocutaneous flaps for cervical esophageal replacement. Ann Plast Surg 1983;11:24–30.
17. Williford ME, Rice RP, Kelvin FM, Fisher SR, Meyers WC, Thompson WM. Revascularized jejunal graft replacing the cervical esophagus: Radiographic evaluation. AJR Am J Roentgenol 1985;145:533–536.
18. Cordeiro PG, Shah K, Santamaria E, Gollub MJ, Singh B, Shah JP. Barium swallows after free jejunal transfer: Should they be performed routinely? Plast Reconstr Surg 1999;103:1167–1175.
19. Kerlin P, McCafferty GJ, Robinson DW, Theile D. Function of a free jejunal "conduit" graft in the cervical esophagus. Gastroenterology 1986;90: 1956–1963.
20. Wilson JA, Maran AG, Pryde A, Walker WE, Heading RC. The function of free jejunal autografts in the pharyngo-oesophageal segment. J R Coll Surg Edinb 1995;40:363–366.

21. Gluckman JL, McDonough J, Donegan JO. The role of free jejunal graft in reconstruction of the pharynx and cervical esophagus. Head Neck Surg 1982;4:360–369.

22. Duranceau A, Jamieson G, Hurwitz AL, Jones RS, Postlethwait RW. Alteration in esophageal motility after laryngectomy. Am J Surg 1976;131:30–35.

23. Little AG. Motility disorders of the esophagus. In: Bell Jr RH, Rikkers LF, Mulholland MW, eds. Digestive Tract Surgery. A Text and Atlas. Philadelphia: Lippincott-Raven; 1996:27–42.

24. Collard JM, Otte JB, Kestens PJ. Endoscopic stapling technique of esophago-diverticulostomy for Zenker's diverticulum. Ann Thorac Surg 1993;56:573–576.

25. Baldwin DL, Toma AG. Endoscopic stapled diverticulotomy: A real advance in the treatment of hypopharyngeal diverticulum. Clin Otolaryngol 1998;23:244–247.

26. Zeitoun H, Widdowson D, Hammad Z, Osborne J. A video-fluoroscopic study of patients treated by diverticulectomy and cricopharyngeal myotomy. Clin Otolaryngol 1994;19:301–305.

27. Tsai JY, Berkery L, Wesson DE, Redo SF, Spigland NA. Esophageal atresia and tracheoesophageal fistula: Surgical experience over two decades. Ann Thorac Surg 1997;64:778–783.

28. McKinnon LJ, Kosloske AM. Prediction and prevention of anastomotic complications of esophageal atresia and the tracheoesophageal fistula. J Pediatr Surg 1990;25:778–781.

29. Ashcraft KW, Goodwin C, Amoury RA, Holder TM. Early recognition and aggressive treatment of gastroesophageal reflux following repair of esophageal atresia. J Pediatr Surg 1977;12:317–321.

30. Spitz L, Kiely E, Brereton RJ. Esophageal atresia: Five-year experience with 148 cases. J Pediatr Surg 1987;22:103–108.

31. Chittmittrapap S, Spitz L, Kiely EM, Brereton RJ. Anastomotic leakage following surgery for esophageal atresia. J Pediatr Surg 1992;27:29–32.

32. Solomon MP, Rosenblum H, Rosato FE. Leiomyoma of the esophagus. Ann Surg 1993;199:246–248.

33. Rendina EA, Venuta F, Pescarmona EO, et al. Leiomyoma of the esophagus. Scand J Thorac Cardiovasc Surg 1990;24:79–82.

34. Bardini R, Segalin A, Ruol A, Pavanello M, Peracchia A. Videothorascopic enucleation of esophageal leiomyoma. Ann Thor Surg 1992;54:576–577.

35. Postlethwait RW, Lowe JE. Benign tumors and cysts of the esophagus. In: Zuidema GD, ed. Shackelford's Surgery of the Alimentary Tract, 4th ed. Philadelphia: WB Saunders; 1996;369–385.

36. Gollub MJ, Gerdes H, Bains MS. Radiographic appearances of esophageal stents. RadioGraphics 1997;17:1169–1182.

37. Girardet RE, Ransdell Jr HT, Wheat Jr MW. Collective review: Palliative intubation in the management of esophageal carcinoma. Ann Thorac Surg 1974;18:417–427.

38. Angorn IB, Haffeje AA. Endoesophageal intubation for palliation in obstructing esophageal carcinoma. In: Delarue CW, Wilkins Jr EW, Wong J, eds. International Trends in General Thoracic Surgery. St. Louis, MO: Mosby; 1998:410–419.

39. Kozarek RA. Expandable endoprostheses for gastrointestinal stenoses. Gastrointest Endosc Clin North Am 1994;4:279–295.

40. Nevitt AW, Kozarek RA, Conti N, Hauptmann E, Cummings F. Complications encountered with use of expandable esophageal prostheses. Appl Radiogr May 1999;27–35.

41. Laughlin EH, Walker WY. Fragmentation of Celestin tube: A cause of fatal intestinal perforation. J Thorac Cardiovasc Surg 1980;80:17–20.

42. Palafox BA, Lifschutz H, Juler G, Stemmer E, Mason GR. Fragmentation of a Celestin tube causing intestinal obstruction. Case report and review of the literature. J Thorac Cardiovasc Surg 1984;87:698–701.

43. Nevitt AW, Kozarek RA, Kidd R. Expandable esophageal prostheses: Recognition, insertion techniques, and positioning. AJR Am J Roentgenol 1996;167:1009–1013.

44. Earlem C, Cunha-Melo K. Malignant oesophageal strictures: A review of techniques for palliative intubation. Br J Surg 1982;69:61–68.

45. Knyrim K, Wagner HJ, Bethge N, et al. A controlled trial of an expansile metal stent for palliation of esophageal obstruction due to inoperable cancer. N Engl J Med 1993;329:1302–1307.

46. Schaer J, Katon RM, Ivancev K, et al. Treatment of malignant esophageal obstruction with silicone-coated metallic self-expanding stents. Gastrointest Endosc 1992;38:7–11.

47. Morgan RA, Ellul JPM, Denton ERE, Glynos M, Mason RC, Adam A. Malignant esophageal fistulas and perforations: Management with plastic-covered metallic endoprostheses. Radiology 1997;204:527–532.

48. Cwikiel W, Stridbeck H, Transberg KG, et al. Malignant esophageal strictures: Treatment with a self-expanding Nitinol stent. Radiology 1993;187:661–665.

49. Watkinson AF, Ellul J, Entwisle K, et al. Esophageal carcinoma: Initial results of palliative treatment with coated self-expanding endoprostheses. Radiology 1995;195:821–827.

50. Kozarek RA, Raltz S, Brugge WR, et al. Prospective multicenter trial of esophageal Z-stent placement for malignant dysphagia and TE fistula. Gastrointest Endosc 1996;44:562–567.

51. Acunas B, Rozanes I, Akpinar S, et al. Palliation of malignant esophageal strictures with self-expanding Nitinol stents: Drawbacks and complications. Radiology 1996;648–652.

52. Han YM, Song HY, Lee JM, et al. Esophagorespiratory fistulae due to esophageal carcinoma: Palliation with a covered Gianturco stent. Radiology 1996;199:65–70.

53. Do YS, Song HY, Lee BH, et al. Esophagorespiratory fistula associated with esophageal cancer: Treatment with a Gianturco stent tube. Radiology 1993;187:673–677.

54. Taal BG, Muller SH, Boot H, Koops W. Potential risks and artifacts of magnetic resonance imaging of self-expandable stents. Gastrointest Endosc 1997;46:424–429.

55. Lee RB, Miller JI. Esophagectomy for cancer. Surg Clin North Am 1997; 77:1169–1196.

56. Orringer MB. Transhiatal esophagectomy without thoracotomy. In: Orringer MB, Zuidema GD, eds. Shackelford's Surgery of the Alimentary Tract, 4th ed; vol I: The Esophagus. Philadelphia: WB Saunders; 1996: 414–445.

57. Lewis I. The surgical treatment of carcinoma of the oesophagus with special reference to the new operation for growths in the middle third. Br J Surg 1946;34:18–31.

58. Watson TJ, Peters JH, DeMeester TR. Esophageal replacement for end-stage benign esophageal disease. Surg Clin North Am 1997;77:1099–1114.

59. Belsey R. Reconstruction of the oesophagus. Ann R Coll Surg Engl 1983; 65:360–364.

60. Christensen LR, Shapir J. Radiology of colonic interposition and its associated complications. Gastrointest Radiol 1986;11:233–240.
61. Isolauri J, Helin H, Markkula H. Colon interposition for esophageal disease: Histologic findings of colonic mucosa after a follow-up of 5 months to 15 years. Am J Gastroenterol 1991;86:277–280.
62. van Lanschot JJB, van Blankenstein M, Oei HY, Tilanus HW. Randomized comparison of prevertebral and retrosternal gastric tube reconstruction after resection of oesophageal carcinoma. Br J Surg 1999;86:102–108.
63. Bartels H, Thorban S, Siewert JR. Anterior versus posterior reconstruction after transhiatal oesophagectomy: A randomized controlled trial. Br J Surg 1993;80:1141–1144.
64. Bardini R, Bonavina L, Asolati M, Ruol A, Castoro C, Tiso E. Single-layered cervical esophageal anastomoses: A prospective study of two suturing techniques. Ann Thorac Surg 1994;58:1087–1090.
65. Agha F, Orringer MB. Colonic interposition: Radiographic evaluation. AJR Am J Roentgenol 1984;142:703–708.
66. Owen JW, Balfe DM, Koehler RE, Roper CL, Weyman PJ. Radiologic evaluation of complications after esophagogastrectomy. AJR Am J Roentgenol 1983;140:1163–1169.
67. Agha FP, Orringer MB, Amendola MA. Gastric interposition following transhiatal esophagectomy: Radiographic evaluation. Gastrointest Radiol 1985;10:17–24.
68. Fok M, Cheng WK, Wong J. Pyloroplasty versus no drainage in gastric replacement of the esophagus. Am J Surg 191;162:447–552.
69. Gross BH, Agha FP, Glazer GM, Orringer MB. Gastric interposition following transhiatal esophagectomy: CT evaluation. Radiology 1985;55:177–179.
70. Orringer MB. Complications of esophageal surgery. In: Zuidema GD, Orringer MB, eds. Shackelford's Surgery of the Alimentary Tract, 4th ed; vol I: The Esophagus. Philadelphia: WB Saunders; 1996:446–473.
71. Katariya K, Harvey JC, Pina E, Beattie EJ. Complications of transhiatal esophagectomy. J Surg Oncol 1994;57:157–163.
72. Heitmiller RF, Jones B. Transient diminished airway protection after transhiatal esophagectomy. Am J Surg 1991;162:442–446.
73. Chassin JL. Esophagogastrectomy data favoring end-to-side anastomosis. Ann Surg 1978;188:22–27.
74. Fekete F, Breil P, Ronsse H, Tossen JC, Langonnet F. EEA stapler and omental graft in esophagogastrectomy. Ann Surg 1981;193:825–830.
75. Ferguson MK, Little AG, Skinner DB. Current concepts in the management of postoperative chylothorax. Ann Thorac Surg 1985;40:542–545.
76. Lam KH, Lim STK, Wong J, Ong GB. Chylorthorax following resection of the esophagus. Br J Surg 1979;66:105–109.
77. Gollub MJ, Bains MS. Herniation of the transverse colon after esophagectomy: Is retrocardiac air a normal postoperative finding? AJR Am J Roentgenol 1997;169:481–483.
78. Kamath MV, Ellison RG, Rubin JW, Moore HV, Pai GP. Esophageal mucocele: A complication of blind loop esophagus. Ann Thorac Surg 1987;43:263–269.
79. Heitmiller RF, Gillinov AM, Jones B. Transhiatal herniation of colon after esophagectomy and gastric pull-up. Ann Thorac Surg 1997;63:554–556.
80. Orringer MB. Invited commentary. Ann Thorac Surg 1997;63:556.
81. van Sandick JW, Kneghens JL, van Lanschot JB, Obertop H. Diaphragmatic herniation following oesophagectomy. Br J Surg 1999;86:109–112.

82. Granke K, Hoshal VL Jr., Vanden Belt RJ. Extrapericardial tamponade with herniated omentum after transhiatal esophagectomy. J Surg Oncol 1990;44:273–275.

83. Erasmus JJ, McAdams HP, Goodman PC. Diagnosis please. Case 5: Esophageal mucocele after surgical bypass of the esophagus. Radiology 1998;209:757–760.

84. Glickstein MF, Gefter WB, Low D, Stephenson LW. Esophageal mucocele after surgical isolation of the esophagus. AJR Am J Roentgenol 1987; 149:729–730.

85. Olsen CO, Hopkins RA, Postlethwait RW. Management of an infected mucocele occurring in a bypassed excluded esophageal segment. Ann Thorac Surg 1985;40:73–75.

86. Jones GRM, Nicholson DM. Percutaneous ultrasound-guided esophagostomy. J Ultrasound Med 1988;7:643–645.

87. Orringer MB. Substernal gastric bypass of the excluded esophagus— Results of an ill-advised operation. Surgery 1984;96:467–470.

88. Barbier PA, Becker CD, Wagner HE. Esophageal carcinoma: Patient selection for transhiatal esophagectomy. A prospective analysis of 50 consecutive cases. World J Surg 1988;12:263–269.

89. Curran AJ, Gough DB, O'Muircheartaigh I, Keeling P. Transhiatal oesophagectomy in the management of advanced oesophageal carcinoma. J R Coll Surg Edinb 1992;37:225–228.

90. Anbari MM, Levine MS, Cohen RB, Rubesin SE, Laufer I, Rosato EF. Delayed leaks and fistulas after esophagogastrectomy: Radiologic evaluation. AJR Am J Roentgenol 1993;160:1217–1220.

91. Becker CD, Barbier PA, Terrier F, Porcelini B. Patterns of recurrence of esophageal carcinoma after transhiatal esophagectomy and gastric interposition. AJR Am J Roentgenol 1987;148:273–277.

92. Ribet M, Debrueres B, Lecomte-Houcke M. Resection for advanced cancer of the thoracic esophagus: Cervical or thoracic anastomosis? Late results of a prospective randomized study. J Thorac Cardiovasc Surg 1992; 103:784–789.

93. Akiyama H, Nakayama K. Carcinomas arising in the reconstructed oesophagus. Int Adv Surg Oncol 1982;5:145–161.

94. Salo JA, Heikkila L, Nemlander A, Lindahl H, Louhimo I, Mattila S. Barrett's oesophagus and perforation of gastric tube ulceration into the pericardium: A late complication after reconstruction of oesophageal atresia. Ann Chir Gynaecol 1995;84:92–94.

95. Kotsis, Krisar Z, Imre J, Csikos M. Complications of oesophagoplasty with isoperistaltic transverse colon. Scand J Thorac Cardiovasc Surg 1983; 17:317–321.

96. Tuszewski FK. The radiologic appearance of the reconstructed esophagus. Acta Radiol Diagn 1972;12:193–216.

97. Debras B, Kanane O, Enon B, Robert M. Aorto-colonic fistula as a late complication of colon interposition for oesophageal atresia. Eur J Pediatr Surg 1996;6:310–311.

98. Raia A, Gama AH, Pinotti HW, Rodriguews JJG. Diverticular disease in transposed colon used for esophagoplasty: Report of two cases. Ann Surg 1973;177:70–74.

99. Goldsmith H, Beattie Jr E. Malignant villous tumour in a colon bypass. Ann Surg 1968;167:98–100.

100. Houghton AD, Jourdan M, McColl I. Dukes A carcinoma after colonic interposition for oesophageal stricture. Gut 1989;30:880–881.

101. Licata AA, Fecanin P, Glowitz R. Metastatic adenocarcinoma from oesophageal colonic interposition graft for oesophageal stricture. Lancet 1978;1:285.
102. Wolf DC. The management of variceal bleeding: Past, present and future. Mt Sinai J Med 1999;66:1–13.
103. Memon MA, Jones WF. Injection therapy for variceal bleeding. Gastrointest Endosc Clin N Am 1999;9:231–252.
104. Agha FP. The esophagus after endoscopic injection sclerotherapy: Acute and chronic changes. Radiology 1984;153:37–42.
105. Monroe P, Morrow Jr CF, Millen JE, Fairman RP, Glauser FL. Acute respiratory failure after sodium morrhuate esophageal sclerotherapy. Gastroenterology 1983;85:693–699.
106. Zeller FA, Cannan CR, Prakash UBS. Thoracic manifestations after esophageal variceal sclerotherapy. Mayo Clin Proc 1991;66:727–732.
107. Woods KL, Qureshi WA. Long-term endoscopic management of variceal bleeding. Gastrointest Endosc Clin N Am 1999;9:253–270.
108. Low VHS, Levine MS. Endoscopic banding of esophageal varices: Radiographic findings. AJR Am J Roentgenol 1999;172:941–942.
109. Stiegmann GV, Goff JS, Sun JH, Davis G, Bozdech J. Endoscopic variceal ligation: An alternative to sclerotherapy. Gastrointest Endosc 1989;35:431–434.
110. Sugiura M, Futagawa S. A new technique for treating esophageal varices. J Thorac Cardiovasc Surg 1973;66:677–685.
111. Idezuki Y, Kokudo N, Sanjo K, Sandai Y. Sugiura procedure for management of variceal bleeding in Japan. World J Surg 1994;18:216–221.
112. Mariette D, Smadja C, Borgonovo G, Grange D, Franco D. The Sugiura procedure: A prospective experience. Surgery 1994;115:282–289.
113. Greenspan R, Kressel HY, Laufer I, Rosato EF. Radiographic findings in the esophagus following the Sugiura procedure. Radiology 1982;144:245–247.
114. Mercado MA, Orozco H, Vasquez M, et al. Comparative study of 2 variants of a modified esophageal transection in the Sugiura–Futagawa operation. Arch Surg 1998;133:1046–1049.
115. Orozco H, Mercado MA, Takahashi T, Hernandez-Ortiz J, Capellan JF, Garcia-Tsao G. Elective treatment of bleeding varices with the Sugiura operation over 10 years. Am J Surg 1992;163:585–589.
116. Mercado MA, Takahashi T, Orozco H. An alternate low risk technique for esophageal transection in the Sugiura–Futagawa procedure. Am Surg 1993;59:461–464.
117. Saeed ZA, Winchester CB, Ferro PS, et al. Prospective randomized comparison of polyvinyl bougies and through-the-scope balloons for dilation of peptic strictures of the esophagus. Gastrointest Endosc 1995;41:189–195.
118. Kang SG, Song H-Y, Lim M-K, Yoon HK, Goo D-E, Sung K-B. Esophageal rupture during balloon dilation of strictures of benign or malignant causes: Prevalence and clinical importance. Radiology 1998;209:741–746.
119. Koshy SS, Nostrant TT. Pathophysiology and endoscopic/balloon treatment of esophageal motility disorders. Surg Clin North Am 1997;77:971–992.
120. Michael GS, Peter HH, Michael GW, Kettlewell MC. Peroral pulsion intubation of malignant esophageal strictures using a fiberoptic technique. Am Surg 1984;50:437–440.
121. Han SY, Tishler JM. Perforation of the abdominal segment of the esophagus. AJR Am J Roentgenol 1984;143:751–754.

122. Ponec RJ, Kimmey MB. Endoscopic therapy of esophageal cancer. Surg Clin North Am 1997;77:1197–1218.

123. Vanmoerkerke I, Rutgeerts P, Vantrappen G. The role of laser therapy in the palliative treatment of esophageal cancer. J Belge Radiol 1991; 74:401–406.

124. Wolf EL, Frager J, Brandt LJ, Frager DH, Bernstein LH, Beneventano TC. Radiographic appearance of the esophagus and stomach after laser treatment of obstructing carcinoma. AJR Am J Roentgenol 1986;146:519–522.

125. Rahmani EY, Rex DK. Endoscopic therapy for polyps and tumors. In: Yamada T, ed. Textbook of Gastroenterology, 3rd ed. Philadelphia: Lippincott, Williams & Wilkins; 1999:2880–2898.

126. Hagiwara A, Takahashi T, Kojima O, et al. Endoscopic local injection of a new drug-delivery format of peplomycin for superficial esophageal cancer: A pilot study. Gastroenterology 1993;104:1037–1043.

127. Kitamura K, Hagiwara A, Sasabe T, et al. Significant clinical response of activated carbon-adsorbed peplomycin against esophageal cancer: A pilot study. J Surg Oncol 1993;52:56–60.

128. Horgan S, Pellegrini CA. Surgical treatment of gastroesophageal reflux disease. Surg Clin North Am 1997;77:1063–1082.

129. Watson DI, Jamieson GG, Pike GK, Davies N, Richardson M, Devitt PG. Prospective randomized double-blind trial between laparoscopic Nissen fundoplication and anterior partial fundoplication. Br J Surg 1999;86: 123–130.

130. Stirling MC, Orringer MB. Surgical treatment after failed antireflux opeation. J Thorac Cardiovasc Surg 1986;92:667–672.

131. Hinder RA. Gastroesophageal reflux disease. In: Bell Jr RH, Rikkers LF, Mulholland MW, eds. Digestive Tract Surgery. A Text and Atlas. Philadelphia: Lippincott-Raven; 1996:3–26.

132. Hinder RA, Klingler PJ, Perdikis G, Smith SL. Management of the failed antireflux operation. Surg Clin North Am 1997;77:1083–1098.

133. Hinder RA, Filipi CJ, Wetscher GJ, et al. Laparoscopic Nissen fundoplication is an effective treatment for gastroesophageal reflux disease. Ann Surg 1994;220:472–483.

134. Anderson JA, Myers JC, Watson DI, Gabb M, Mathew G, Jamieson GG. Concurrent fluoroscopy and manometry reveal differences in laparoscopic Nissen and anterior fundoplication. Dig Dis Sci 1998;43:847–853.

135. Skinner DB, Belsey RHR. Surgical management of esophageal reflux and hiatus hernia-long term results with 1030 patients. J Thorac Cardiovasc Surg 1967;53:33–54.

136. Angelchik JP, Cohen R. A new surgical procedure for the treatment of gastroesophageal reflux and hiatal hernia. Surg Gynecol Obstet 1979;148: 246–248.

137. Burhenne LJW, Fratkin LB, Flak B, Burhenne HJ. Radiology of the Angelchik prosthesis for gastroesophageal reflux. AJR Am J Roentgenol 1984;142:507–511.

138. Lewis RA, Angelchik J-P, Cohen R. A new surgical prosthesis for hiatal hernia repair. Radiographic appearance. Radiology 1980;135:630.

139. Crookes PF, DeMeester TR. The Angelchik prosthesis: What have we learned in fifteen years? Ann Thorac Surg 1994;57:1385–1386.

140. Albin J, Noel T, Allan K, Khalil KG. Intrathoracic esophageal perforation with the Angelchik antireflux prosthesis: Report of a new complication. Gastrointest Radiol 1985;10:330–332.

141. Hill IR, Limage SJ. Suppurative pericarditis due to Angelchik prosthesis. Am J Forensic Med Pathol 1989;10:71–72.

142. Haney PJ, Gunadi IK, Arnold J, Diaconis JN. Spontaneous penetration of an antireflux prosthesis into the stomach. Gastrointest Radiol 1983; 8:303–305.
143. Curtis DJ, Benjamin SB, Kerr R, Castell DO. Angelchik anti-reflux device: Radiographic appearance of complications. Radiology 1984;151:311–313.
144. Sussman SK, Illescas FF, Woodruff WW III, Cooper C. Angelchik antireflux device: Computed tomography appearance. J Comput Tomogr 1987; 11:212–215.
145. Maxwell-Armstrong CA, Steele RJ, Amar SS, et al. Long-term results of the Angelchik prosthesis for gastro-oesophageal reflux. Br J Surg 1997;84:862–864.
146. Demmy TL, Caron NR, Curtis JJ. Severe dysphagia from an Angelchik prosthesis: Futility of routine esophageal testing. Ann Thorac Surg 1994; 57:1660–1661.
147. Kahrilas PJ. Motility disorders of the esophagus. In: Yamada T, ed. Textbook of Gastroenterology, 3rd ed. Philadelphia: Lippincott, Williams & Wilkins; 1999:1199–1234.
148. Hunter JG, Richardson WS. Surgical management of achalasia. Surg Clin North Am 1997;77:993–1016.
149. de Oliveira JMA, Birgisson S, Doinoff C, et al. Timed barium swallow: A simple technique for evaluating esophageal emptying in patients with achalasia. AJR Am J Roentgenol 1997;169:473–479.
150. Birgisson S, Richter JE. Achalasia: What's new in diagnosis and treatment? Dig Dis 1997;15(suppl 1):1–27.
151. Eckardt VF, Aignherr C, Bernhard G. Predictors of outcome in patients with achalasia treated by pneumatic dilation. Gastroenterology 1992;103: 1732–1738.
152. Vantrappen G, Hellemans J, Deloof W, Valembois P, Vandembroucke J. Treatment of achalsia with pneumatic dilation. Gut 1971;12:268–275.
153. Rubesin SE, Kennedy M, Levine MS, et al. Distal esophageal ballooning following Heller myotomy. Radiology 1988;167:345–347.
154. Dobashi Y, Goseki N, Inutake Y, Kawano T, Endou M, Nemoto T. Giant epiphrenic diverticulum with achalasia occurring 20 years after Heller's operation. J Gastroenterol 1996;31:844–847.
155. Eckardt VF, Kanzler G, Westermeier T. Complications and their impact after pneumatic dilation for achalasia: Prospective long-term follow-up study. Gastrointest Endosc 1997;45:349–353.
156. Feczko PJ, Ma CK, Halpert RD, Batra SK. Barrett's metaplasia and dysplasia in postmyotomy achalasia patients. Am J Gastroenterol 1983;78: 265–268.
157. Ott DJ, Wu WC, Gelfand DW, Richter JE. Radiographic evaluation of the achalasic esophagus immediately following pneumatic dilatation. Gastrointest Radiol 1984;9:185–191.
158. Nair LA, Reynolds JC, Parkman HP, et al. Complications during pneumatic dilation for achalasia or diffuse esophageal spasm. Analysis of risk factors, early clinical characteristics, and outcome. Dig Dis Sci 1993;38: 1893–1904.
159. Borotto E, Gaudric M, Danel B, et al. Risk factors of oesophageal perforation during pneumatic dilatation for achalasia. Gut 1996;39:9–12.
160. Bradley JL, Hans SY. Intramural hematoma (incomplete perforation) of the esophagus associated with esophageal dilatation. Radiology 1979;130: 59–62.
161. Javors BR, Panzer DE, Goldman IS. Acute thermal injury of the esophagus. Dysphagia 1996;11:72–74.

162. Ott DJ, Donati D, Wu WC, Chen MY, Gelfand DW. Radiographic evaluation of achalasia immediately after pneumatic dilation with the Rigiflex dilator. Gastrointest Radiol 1991;16:279–282.
163. Healy ME, Mindelzun. Lesser sac pneumoperitoneum secondary to perforation of the intraabdominal esophagus. AJR Am J Roentgenol 1984; 142:325–326.
164. Molina EG, Stollman N, Grauer L, Reiner DK, Barkin JS. Conservative management of esophageal nontransmural tears after pneumatic dilation for achalasia. Am J Gastroenterol 1996;91:15–18.
165. Mercer CD, Hill LD. Intradiaphragmatic abscess. An extremely rare complication of pneumatic dilatation of the esophagus. Dig Dis Sci 1985; 30:891–895.

3

The Stomach

Operations of the stomach have evolved greatly since Billroth first described the partial gastrectomy in 1881. General indications for gastric surgery include resection of neoplasms, peptic ulcer disease (PUD), and obesity. Various factors, including decreased incidence of PUD and evolving medical therapy for it, have contributed to an overall decrease in the amount of gastric surgery being performed. Radiographic contrast examinations remain the most useful means of evaluating early and late complications of gastroduodenal surgery.

Radiographic Technique

The radiographic evaluation of the postoperative stomach can be challenging because normal anatomy is often disrupted. To avoid confusion, it is critical to know beforehand the type of surgery that has been performed, although unfortunately this information may be difficult to obtain. A careful review of the scout film is often helpful, since the pattern of staples and clips can provide clues to the procedure performed. The plain film may also be helpful in assessing for obstruction, gastric distention, bezoars, and abscesses. Previous films, if available, should always be reviewed before contrast agent is administered. It is strongly recommended that a baseline contrast study be obtained several weeks after surgery. This is helpful in increasing the accuracy of assessing for postoperative complications and sequelae. As with any procedure, it is important to obtain a history from the patient.

The choice of contrast and type of study will depend on several factors. In the early postoperative period when leaks are suspected, water-soluble contrast is the agent of choice. The choice between single and double contrast depends on physician preference and clinical circumstances. Single-contrast examinations are more useful in delineating fistulas, assessing for obstruction, and determining the direction of flow of barium (i.e., preferential filling of the afferent or efferent limb); also, they are easier to perform in debilitated patients who are unable to change position rapidly. Initial studies comparing the accuracy of the single-contrast upper gastrointestinal (UGI) series with endoscopy and surgery reported fairly poor results for the UGI, with the accuracy ranging from 20 to 70% [1,2]. Reasons for this include the presence of a small gastric pouch, positioned under the ribs and inaccessible to palpation and compression, limited distensibility of the gastric remnant with rapid emptying, postoperative changes misinterpreted as pathology, and conversely, pathology mistaken as postoperative change. In the late 1970s double contrast became widely used for routine upper GI studies. Owing to its superiority in assessing mucosal detail, the double-contrast study became recognized for its usefulness in the postoperative patient [3–5]. The superiority of double contrast over single contrast has been challenged in a study by Ott et al., however [6]. In their series double contrast failed to perform better than single contrast, and overall sensitivity was fairly poor for both methods.

The radiographic assessment of the postoperative stomach requires attention to detail and modification of the routine standard technique. Initially a small amount of contrast should be given slowly (especially if the type of surgery performed is not known). This avoids flooding the pouch (if a gastric resection has been performed) and the small bowel with contrast. Glucagon is generally but not universally advocated with double-contrast technique to relieve spasm, permit bowel distention, decrease postoperative artifacts, and provide a longer period of time for the performance of the study. In patients with antecolic Billroth II anastomoses and/or gastric stasis, upright and/or prone films may be necessary because gastric outlet obstruction may be simulated in the supine position as barium pools in the dependent fundus. It may be difficult to fill the afferent limb (A limb); prone, right-side-down films and/or compression of the efferent loop may help direct barium into the A limb. Delayed films may be helpful in filling the A limb in patients with gastric stasis or poor filling of the A limb on initial films. In the postoperative weight reduction surgery patient, additional challenges exist as will be discussed later.

Historical Perspective and Rationale for Surgery in Peptic Ulcer Disease

Various operations for ulcer disease have been in vogue and have waxed and waned in popularity over the years. The objectives of surgery for duodenal ulcer disease are to eradicate the disease, leave the gastrointestinal tract as normal as possible, and achieve these goals with the lowest possible mortality and morbidity rate [7]. As medical therapy has become more effective, and the role that *Helicobacter pylori* plays in the etiology of PUD has been established, most surgery is now performed for complications of the condition: bleeding, perforation, and obstruction.

To understand the rational for surgery in PUD, a basic understanding of the physiology of gastrin and acid production, and the role of the vagus nerve is necessary. Gastrin stimulates gastric acid secretion.

Gastrin is produced primarily by the parietal cells in the gastric antrum. Stimuli for the antral release of gastrin are vagal activity, antral distention, and contact with an alkaline pH. The vagus nerve (tenth cranial nerve) has two main divisions: the anterior, or left, and the posterior, or right. The anterior or left division divides above the cardia and gives off small branches to the body and fundus, including the gastrohepatic nerve and the main anterior nerve of the lesser curvature (Latarjet's nerve). Latarjet's nerve innervates approximately two thirds of the anterior wall of the stomach and ends 5 to 7 cm from the pylorus. The gastrohepatic nerve divides into the hepatic nerve and the pyloric nerve. The pyloric nerve innervates the distal antrum, pylorus, and proximal duodenum. Antropyloric emptying is controlled by the pyloric nerve and distal twigs of Latarjet's nerve. The posterior, or right, vagus nerve has a pattern similar to that of the left, but instead of a gastrohepatic branch it gives off a branch to the celiac plexus.

Operations attempt to alter physiology so that ulcers heal and do not recur. The surgical procedure will vary with respect to the amount of the gastric resection performed, the type of anastomosis, and the presence and type of vagotomy: truncal, selective, or superselective. In the 1950s and 1960s a distal partial gastrectomy without vagotomy was widely performed. Antral resection removes the gastrin-producing cells present in the antrum. The high incidence of recurrent ulcer with this type of surgery, however, led to the adoption of a truncal vagotomy (Dragstedt operation) along with an antrectomy, or vagotomy and drainage procedure as the operations of choice. Vagotomy decreases acid production and parietal cell response to gastrin. An emptying procedure, a gastroenterostomy or pyloroplasty, must accompany a truncal vagotomy or a selective vagotomy because these types of vagotomy induce gastric stasis. More recently, superselective vagotomy (parietal cell vagotomy) alone has become a common operation for PUD. The branches of the vagus nerve that innervate the acid-producing parietal cells are sectioned (the pericardial gastric branches and the twigs of the nerves of Latarjet that innervate the fundus), but the remaining hepatic, celiac, and distal antral and pyloric branches are left intact, and a drainage procedure is therefore not required.

Terminology and Normal Appearances

Billroth I and Billroth II

To perform a technically adequate study and to obtain all the pertinent information required, the radiologist must be familiar with the many types of gastric surgical procedure that may be performed. There are multiple eponyms and descriptive terminology used in gastric surgery. "Billroth I" is loosely used to refer to any partial gastric resection with an anastomosis to the duodenal stump (Fig. 3.1). "Billroth II" loosely refers to any partial gastric resection with a gastrojejunostomy: the duo-

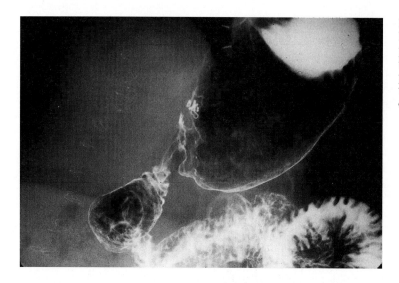

FIGURE 3.1. Billroth I. Double-contrast left posterior oblique view of the stomach following partial gastric resection with anastomosis to the duodenal bulb.

denal bulb is closed off and becomes part of the afferent limb with the efferent limb leading away from the stomach distally (Fig. 3.2). In fact, however, there are multiple modifications and variations, primarily in the nature of the anastomosis, of the standard "Billroth I and II" operations (Fig. 3.3). In 1939, Polya described 49 different methods for

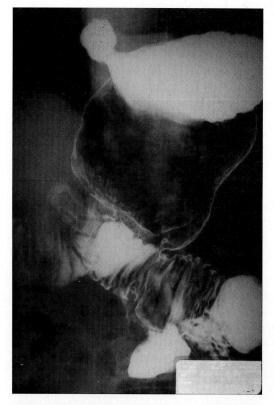

FIGURE 3.2. Billroth II. Double-contrast supine view of the stomach following partial gastric resection with a gastrojejunostomy. There is filling of the efferent limb and a small portion of the afferent limb.

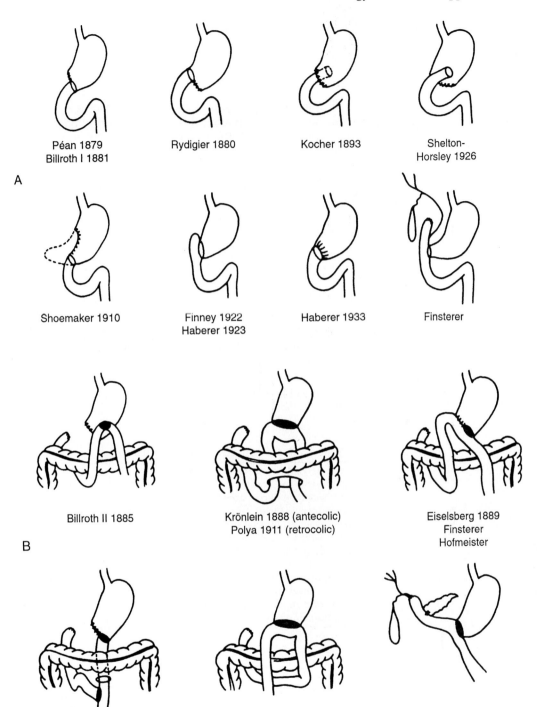

A

B

FIGURE 3.3. Modifications of the Billroth operations. (A) Varieties of gastroduodenostomy. (B) Varieties of gastrojejunostomy. (From Burhenne, HJ. Am J Roentgenol 91:732, 1964. © 1964. American Roentgen Ray Society. Reprinted with permission.)

establishing gastrointestinal continuity after gastric resection, many with eponyms attached. To highlight the confusion in terminology, he brought attention to the fact that the "Polya" procedure had been performed earlier by 11 different surgeons, including Hofmeister, and the "Hofmeister procedure" was first performed by Eiselsberg. The Billroth I was in fact first performed by Péan and bears his name in some countries. To avoid confusion, descriptive terminology, rather than eponyms should be used. Burhenne has outlined 11 basic components of gastric surgery [8] (Table 3.1). The extent of gastric resection will depend on the indication for surgery (i.e., malignancy, benign tumor, or PUD) and the surgical objective (e.g., removal of the gastrin-producing portion of the stomach). The anastomosis may be end to end, end to side, side to side, or side to end. It is now customary to perform an end-to-side anastomosis with a Billroth II.

In relation to gastrojejunostomy, the terms "anterior" and "posterior" refer to the position of the jejunal anastomosis with respect to the anterior and posterior walls of the stomach. The anastomosis is not always made to the cut end of the stomach; indeed, it may be at a separate area distinct from that site.

The jejunal anastomosis may also be either antecolic or retrocolic. With the antecolic anastomosis, the jejunum is anastomosed to the stomach anterior to the transverse colon, whereas the retrocolic anastomosis is performed posterior to the transverse colon through an incision in the transverse mesocolon.

TABLE 3.1. Basic components of gastric surgery.

Extent of gastric resection
End of side anastomosis
Anterior or posterior anastomosis
Superior or inferior anastomosis
Large or small stomal diameter
Slow or rapid gastric emptying
Antecolic or retrocolic gastrojejunostomy
Right-to-left or left-to-right direction of
    anastomosis
Short or long proximal jejunal limb
Horizontal or oblique plane of anastomosis
Direction of gastric emptying

Source: Ref. 8.

Variations also exist in the method of performing the gastrojejunal anastomosis itself, which in turn affects stomach size. The entire gastric pouch can be left patent and sutured to the jejunum, or a portion of the lesser curvature can be oversewn to create a restricted stoma. The terminology has evolved to refer to an unrestricted gastric pouch as a Polya and a partially restricted pouch as a Hofmeister. A characteristic postsurgical change called the Hofmeister defect is observed in a small proportion of cases with this procedure (Fig. 3.4). The Hofmeister

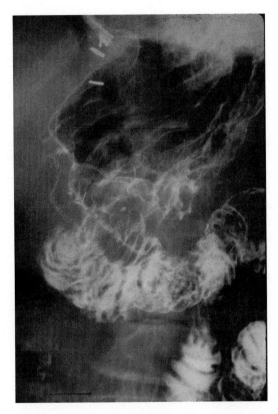

FIGURE 3.4. **Hofmeister defect.** Supine film from an upper GI series demonstrating a defect along the lesser curvature of the gastric remnant corresponding to the closure line of the invaginated cut surface of the stomach.

defect corresponds to the closure line of the invaginated cut surface of the stomach. Six out of 100 cases with this repair demonstrated this defect in one study [9]. It is important to recognize this as a postsurgical deformity, not to be confused with pathology, such as neoplasm. The defect is generally best seen in the early postoperative period and often decreases in size or disappears on subsequent examinations. It may appear as an ovoid, spherical, smooth, or lobulated defect up to 5 cm in diameter on the lesser curvature of the gastric remnant just above the anastomosis. Postoperative baseline studies are helpful in this regard, because this defect would not develop at a time distant from surgery, and in fact may decrease in size or disappear with time.

The terms "isoperistaltic" and "antiperistaltic" have been generally discarded because they have acquired different meanings, producing confusion and controversy. The terms "right to left" and "left to right" have replaced "iso-" and "antiperistaltic," and indicate that the A loop is located on the greater curvature (right to left) or the lesser curvature (left to right). This decision will be based on the patient's body habitus and the surgeon's preference.

A complete interpretation of the radiographic appearance of the postoperative stomach should include, where appropriate, estimation of the extent of the gastric resection, the type, position, direction, and orientation of any anastomosis, evaluation of the stoma or channel diameter, contour and location, and an assessment of the speed, direction, and completeness of gastric emptying [8,10].

Pyloroplasty

The various types of pyloroplasty include Heineke–Mikulicz, Finney, and Jaboulay, with the former being the most commonly performed. Pyloroplasty is a drainage procedure intended to widen the pyloric channel and therefore facilitate gastric emptying. In the Heineke–Mikulicz procedure a longitudinal incision of 2 to 5 cm is made across the pylorus, which is then sutured transversely (Fig. 3.5).

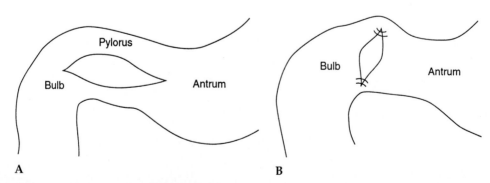

A   B

FIGURE 3.5. **Heineke–Mikulicz pyloroplasty.** (A) A longitudinal incision is made across the pylorus, which is then sutured transversely (B).

The postoperative appearance is variable, especially if the normal anatomy of the pyloroduodenal region is deformed from fibrosis and/or edema, and it is often difficult to distinguish postoperative deformity from recurrent ulcer. It has been noted that peristatic activity in the pouches can be observed fluoroscopically, and therefore pouches can be differentiated from ulcers on this basis [11]. A characteristic pseudodiverticulum appearance on both sides of the pyloric channel, which has been called a "beagle ear sign," may be identified (Fig. 3.6) [8,12]. The effect of the Heineke–Mikulicz pyloroplasty was studied theoretically and confirmed by cadaver and clinical studies by Toye et al. [13]. These authors hypothesized that the effect of the suturing would be to produce a pouch at the site of the suture line and traction on the longitudinal muscle fibers at either end of the incision. The traction produces a "sling" proximal and distal to the pouch. A ridge is formed by the pyloric muscle in the middle of the pouch. The longer the incision, the greater the size of the pouch and constrictions.

The Finney pyloroplasty, an incision followed by suturing in the form of an inverted U extending from the antrum across the pylorus into the duodenum, produces a characteristic ridgelike deformity with a wide pyloric channel. The Jaboulay pyloroplasty is a gastroduodenostomy with an anastomosis created between the antrum and second portion of the duodenum. This type of procedure is considered when severe scarring and deformity of the bulb renders the other procedures technically difficult.

In some cases, gastric and duodenal ulcers may be treated with simple closure or local excision. Plication defects may be identified in such circumstances, although often no radiological abnormality can be detected. Minor irregularities or deformity of the gastric or duodenal wall may be identified in some cases, and these may disappear with time [14]. Wedge and sleeve resection of the gastric wall leaves a permanent deformity that can be identified on barium studies.

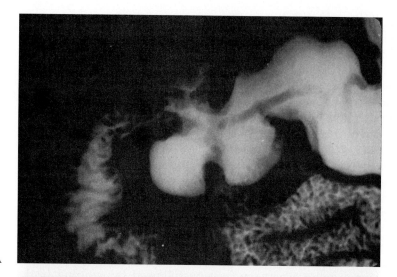

A

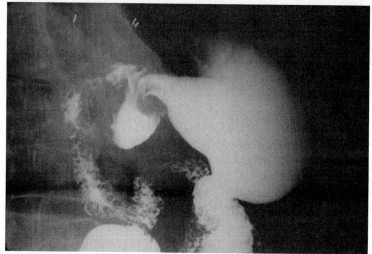

B

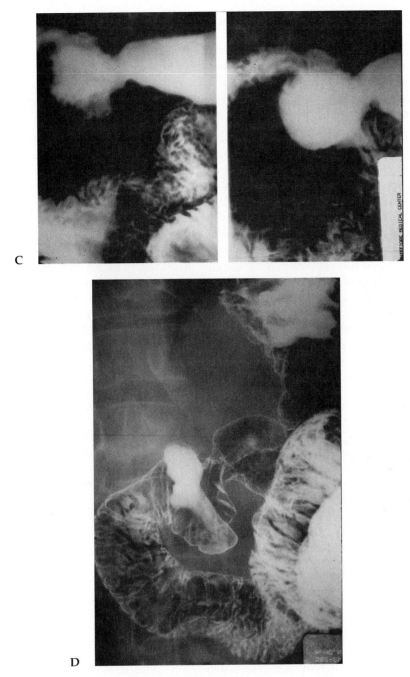

FIGURE 3.6. Pyloroplasty deformities. (A) Coned-down view of the pyloro-duodenal region showing characteristic pseudodiverticular outpouchings ("beagle ear sign") after Heineke–Mikulicz pyloroplasty. (B) Another patient with pseudodiverticular deformity following pyloroplasty. (C) Coned-down view of the pyloroduodenal region following pyloroplasty with a widened, deformed pyloric region. (D) Double-contrast view of the pyloroduodenal region after pyloroplasty with loss of the normal anatomy.

Complications of Billroth Surgery

Although most patients will not develop sequelae after surgery, there are unfortunately a large number of early and late postoperative complications that may ensue (Table 3.2).

Leaks

In the early postoperative period after Billroth surgery, anastomotic leaks may develop. Leaks are generally readily detected by water-soluble contrast administration or CT imaging. Subsequent subphrenic abscesses, usually left sided, may ensue. Leaks are the most common cause of mortality after gastric surgery [12].

Rupture of the duodenal stump ("duodenal stump blowout") after Billroth II is one of the most serious complications of gastric surgery. This may occur as early as the first or as late as the nineteenth postoperative day, although it is usually identified between the third to seventh postoperative day [15]. Contrast examination may be diagnostic, although complete filling of the A limb is necessary for diagnosis, and this may be difficult to achieve (Fig. 3.7). CT imaging may reveal extraluminal contrast, collections, and/or abscess adjacent to the duodenal stump or in the right subphrenic space (Fig. 3.8).

TABLE 3.2. Complications of gastroduodenal surgery.

Early
Duodenal stump blowout
Anastomotic leak
Anastomotic edema and gastric outlet obstruction
Intussusception (antegrade or retrograde)
Gastroileostomy
Late
Obstruction secondary to anastomotic stricture
Bezoars (food or yeast)
Intussusception (antegrade or retrograde)
Recurrent (marginal) ulcer
Gastric stump carcinoma
Dumping
Afferent limb syndromes (acute or chronic)
Alkaline reflux gastritis
Postgastroenterostomy contraction of gastric antrum
Efferent loop dysfunction
Fistula

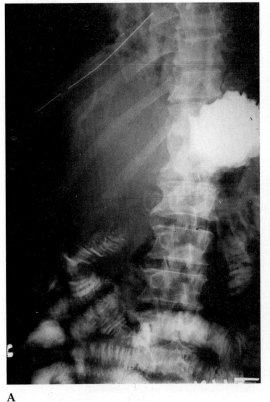

A

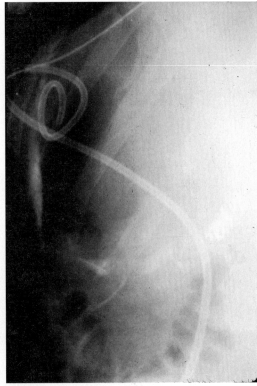

B

FIGURE 3.7. **Duodenal stump blowout.** (A) Upper GI series performed with water-soluble contrast agent demonstrates extraluminal contrast and air extending from the duodenal bulb to the peri- hepatic space. Drainage catheter was placed per-cutaneously. (B) Coned-down view of the same patient.

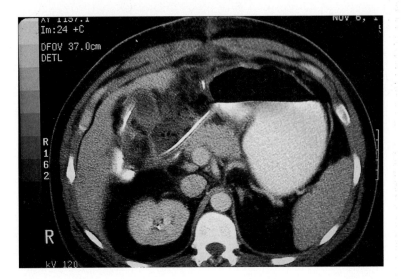

FIGURE 3.8. **Duodenal stump blowout.** CT scan of the upper abdomen shows a collection with extraluminal contrast medium in the right upper quadrant arising from the duodenal bulb. A drain is also present.

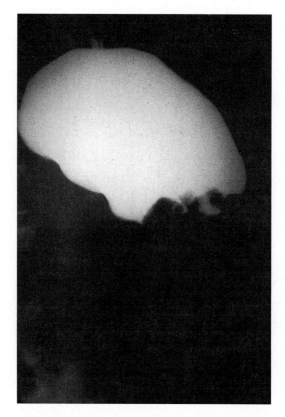

FIGURE 3.9. **Gastric outlet obstruction secondary to edema at the anastomotic site.** Supine view from an upper GI series 5 days after Billroth II shows that the stomach fails to empty secondary to edema at the anastomotic site. This condition resolved several days later.

Gastric Outlet Obstruction

Edema at the anastomotic site may lead to gastric outlet obstruction in the early postoperative period, but is usually self-limiting (Fig. 3.9). Obstruction may also be due to hematoma or an iatrogenic tight stoma.

Marginal Ulcer

Marginal ulcer (recurrent ulcer, stomal ulcer) may occur as soon as one week postoperatively. The incidence varies with the type of operation and the underlying condition for which the surgery was performed. The ulcer recurrence rate is highest with gastroenterostomy alone or antral exclusion procedures, and for this reason these techniques have been abandoned as therapy for PUD. The lowest recurrence rate (<1%), is for vagotomy and partial gastrectomy, with vagotomy and drainage about 5%. Traditionally, after Billroth II, marginal ulcers have been described as most commonly present in the efferent limb within the first 2 cm of the anastomosis, although they may develop in the gastric remnant as well (Figs. 3.10–3.12) [15]. In studies comparing the sensitivity of upper GI series with endoscopy for the detection of marginal ulcer, the UGI series performed poorly, identifying ulcers in only about 50% of cases [6]. Marginal ulcers may develop secondary to retained gastric antrum, incomplete vagotomy, or Zollinger–Ellison syndrome. Incomplete vagotomy is the major cause of recurrent ulcer at the present time.

Retained gastric antrum, an uncommon cause of marginal ulcer, occurs when portions of the antrum are unintentionally left behind after partial gastrectomy. Without acid bathing of the retained antrum, there is no inhibitory effect for the production of gastrin, and thus the parietal cells in the fundus and body of the stomach produce high levels of acid, with a resultant high incidence of ulcer recurrence. High blood levels of circulating gastrin are found. The diagnosis can be made on barium studies when there is filling of a portion of the antrum adjacent to the duodenal bulb [16,17]. Good opacification of the A limb is required for this to be seen. The retained gastric antrum may change position after surgery and instead of occupying its normal position to the left of the pylorus, it may be superimposed on the duodenum or to the right of it [16]. Retained gastric antrum can be simulated by the Bancroft procedure, in which the gastrin-producing mucosa is stripped, but the remaining antrum is left intact (Fig. 3.13). The Bancroft proce-

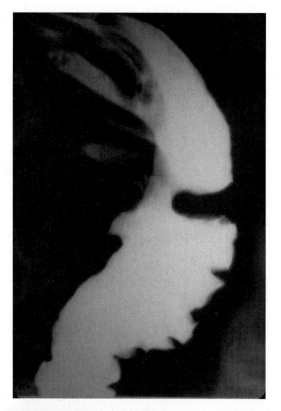

A

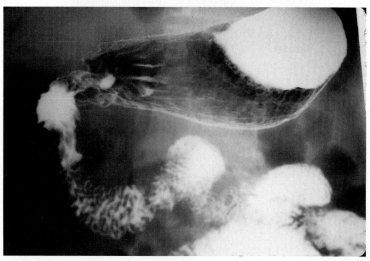

B

FIGURE **3.10. Marginal ulcer after Billroth I.** (A) Single-contrast UGI series demonstrating a marginal ulcer in the duodenum adjacent to the anastomosis. (B) Double-contrast study in a different patient showing an ulcer near the anastomosis in the gastric remnant.

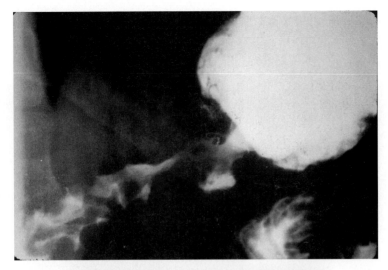

A

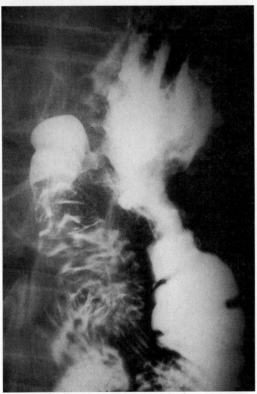

B

FIGURE 3.11. Marginal ulcer. (A) Marginal ulcer developed after Billroth I. Surgical conversion to a Billroth II was then performed. (B) Another marginal ulcer developed in the same patient years later.

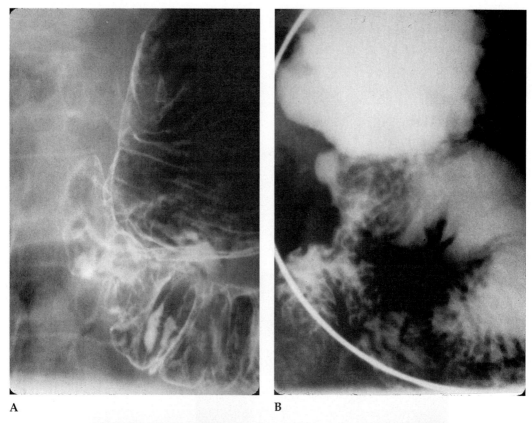

A   B

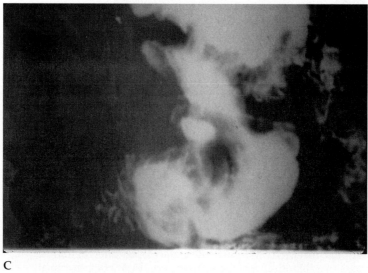

C

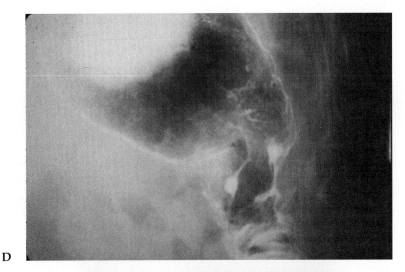

D

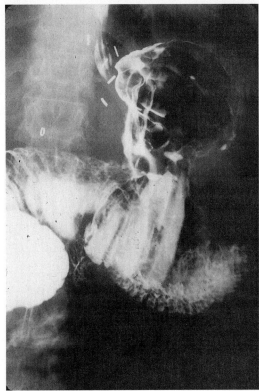

E

FIGURE 3.12. Marginal ulcers. (A–C) Three different patients with marginal ulcers in the jejunum adjacent to the gastrojejunal anastomosis. (D) Double-contrast UGI series showing multiple marginal ulcers in the jejunum. (E) Double-contrast UGI series revealing multiple ulcers in the gastric remnant.

dure may be performed when resection of the antrum is technically difficult. Retained gastric antrum can also be diagnosed by nuclear scintigraphy using pertechnetate scanning [18]. The method used is the same as that used in the search for ectopic gastric mucosa in Meckel's diverticulum. Radioactive technetium-99^m (^{99m}Tc) is handled in a biologically similar fashion to halogens and is excreted by normal gastric mucosa.

Now that simple gastroenterostomy has been abandoned as a primary operation for peptic disease and vagotomy has become routine, the complication of gastrojejunocolic fistula in marginal ulcers has declined in incidence (Fig. 3.14). In patients with a retrocolic anastomosis, the incidence of gastrojejuncolic fistula is increased. Barium enema has been shown to be the most reliable examination in making this diagnosis [12].

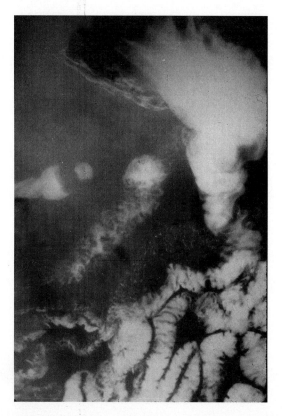

FIGURE 3.13. **Bancroft procedure.** Right anterior oblique view from an upper GI series shows contrast medium extending beyond the duodenal bulb into the distal antrum, simulating retained gastric antrum. The antral mucosa was stripped at the time of surgery.

FIGURE 3.14. Gastrojejunocolic fistula secondary to marginal ulcer after Billroth II. (A)
Upper GI series showing filling of the stomach, jejunum, and colon due to fistula formation from a marginal ulcer. (B) Barium enema
demonstrating the same. (C) Upper GI series
in another patient demonstrating a marginal
ulcer and gastrojejunocolic fistula.

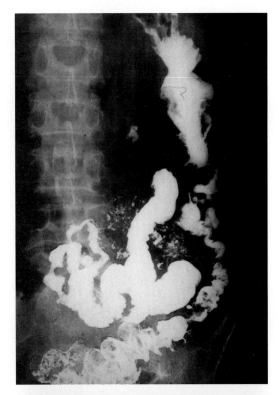

A

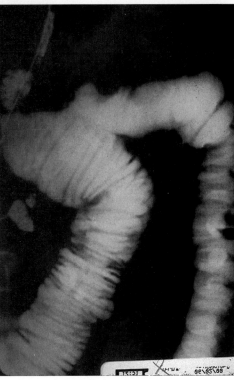

B

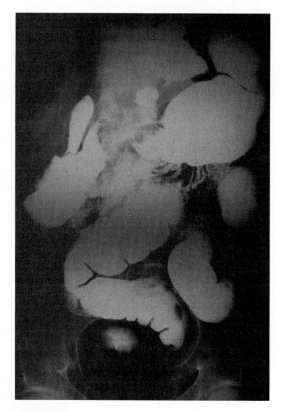

C

FIGURE 3.14. (*Continued*)

Gastric Stump Carcinoma

There is an increased incidence of carcinoma developing in the gastric remnant after the Billroth I and procedures II and after gastroenterostomy for benign disease [19,20]. The average interval for carcinoma to develop is about 20 years after surgery. The incidence is higher in patients who have undergone surgery for gastric ulcer than for duodenal ulcer [20]. The radiographic findings of carcinoma in the gastric remnant are similar to those in the unoperated stomach, including polypoid mass, diffuse infiltration, enlarged folds, and gastric outlet obstruction (Figs. 3.15–3.18). The tumor tends to occur at or near the anastomotic site. Errors in diagnosis may result from suboptimal technique and/or interpretive mistakes, such as attributing pathology to postoperative change. The value of having a baseline study for comparison is particularly apparent in this setting. Suture granulomas due to a foreign body reaction, which can develop after gastric surgery with nonabsorbable suture material, can be misinterpreted as neoplasm [21].

FIGURE 3.15. **Gastric stump carcinoma.** Plain film of the abdomen showing an abnormal gastric air bubble due to gastric carcinoma developing many years after Billroth II surgery for benign disease.

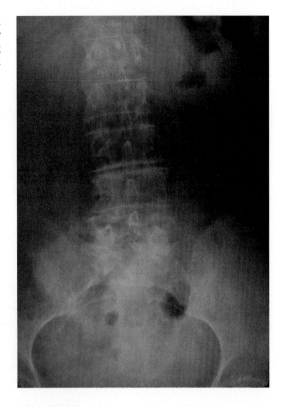

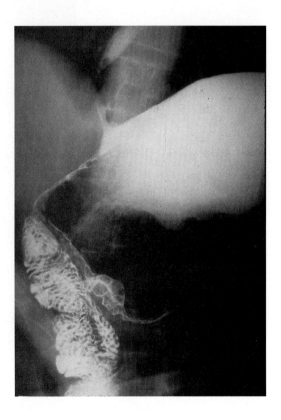

FIGURE 3.16. **Gastric stump carcinoma.** Double-contrast upper GI series showing a small polypoid lesion in the gastric remnant adjacent to the anastomosis due to carcinoma.

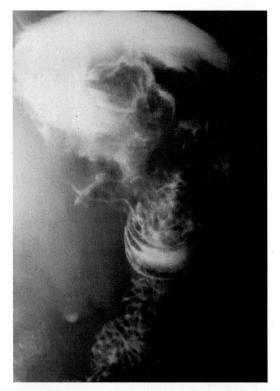

A

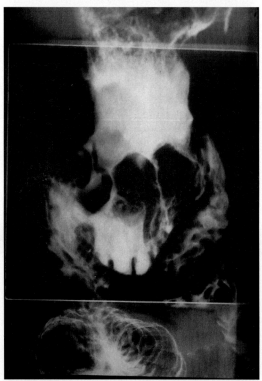

B

FIGURE 3.17. Gastric stump carcinoma. (A) Upper GI series showing a large fungating polypoid mass due to carcinoma after Billroth II. (B) Another patient with an infiltrating carcinoma with a non-distensible gastric remnant and markedly thickened folds at the anastomosis due to carcinoma.

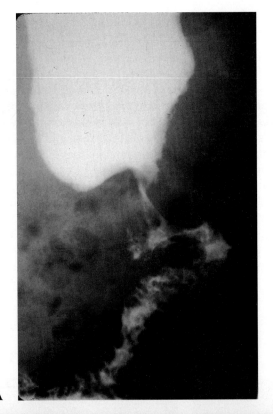

A

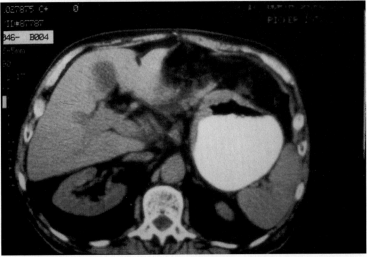

B

FIGURE 3.18. **Gastric stump carcinoma.** (A) Upper GI series demonstrating narrowing of the anastomosis with partial obstruction due to infiltrating carcinoma. (B) CT scan on the same patient showing irregular thickening of the anterior gastric wall.

Bezoars

Gastric and small-bowel bezoars are a well-recognized complication of Billroth I and II surgery, especially when a vagotomy has been performed [22,23]. Gastric bezoars are seen with both Billroth I and II, whereas small-bowel bezoars are generally seen after Billroth II. Phytobezoars, with the nidus usually composed of fruit and vegetable skins, seeds, and fibrous matter are most commonly found. Rarely fungus balls, generally composed of *Candida*, and less commonly *Torylopsis glabrata*, and concretions of antacids have been reported [24,25]. Bezoars may form shortly after surgery or many years later. Predisposing factors include loss of gastric enzymes and acid, gastric atony, decreased drainage, and improper mastication. Symptoms include early satiety, epigastric fullness, or symptoms related to gastric outlet obstruction. The diagnosis can be made on plain films, upper GI series, and CT images when mottled air collections trapped within the bezoar are identified (Figs. 3.19 and 3.20). A gastric bezoar will be freely

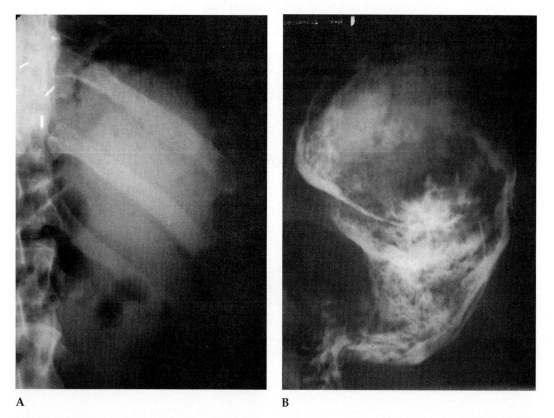

A   B

FIGURE 3.19. **Bezoar after Billroth II.** (A) Coned-down view of the left upper quadrant showing a mottled mass containing air in the stomach due to a bezoar. (B) Upper GI series in the same patient.

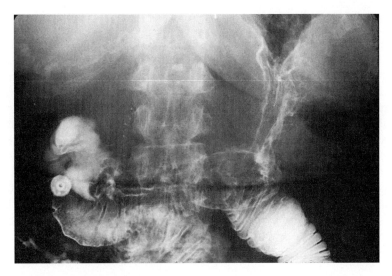

FIGURE 3.20. **Bezoar after vagotomy.** Upper GI series showing a bezoar in the stomach after vagotomy alone.

movable, changing position with patient motion. Recently, an obstructing small-bowel bezoar after Billroth II was diagnosed on CT imaging [26]. Esophageal atony may develop after vagotomy, and subsequent esophageal foreign bodies may ensue (Fig. 3.21).

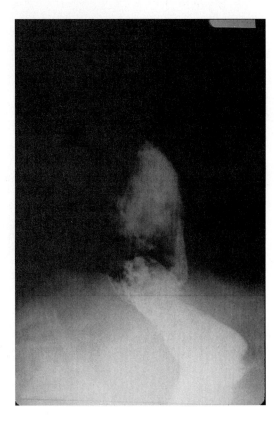

FIGURE 3.21. **Esophageal foreign body after vagotomy.** Upper GI series demonstrating a foreign body in the distal esophagus due to esophageal atony after vagotomy.

Intussusception and Prolapse

Intussusception after Billroth II surgery may be gastrojejunal or jejuno-gastric, with the jejunogastric form being more common. Acute and chronic forms exist. In the acute setting, which may be as soon as 4 days postoperatively, obstruction develops and surgery is required. The chronic form is usually intermittent and self-reducing.

In the jejunogastric form a characteristic striated filling defect or "coiled-spring pattern" is identified within the gastric remnant (Fig. 3.22). Both the efferent and afferent loops may intussuscept, with intussusception of the efferent limb accounting for approximately 75% of cases [27]. The gastrojejunal form typically shows gastric folds crossing the anastomosis into the proximal small bowel (Figs. 3.23 and 3.24). A degree of gastric outlet obstruction may be present. Incarceration may rarely develop, which would require immediate surgery.

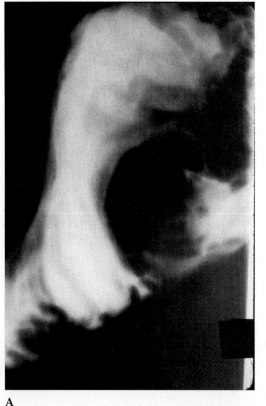
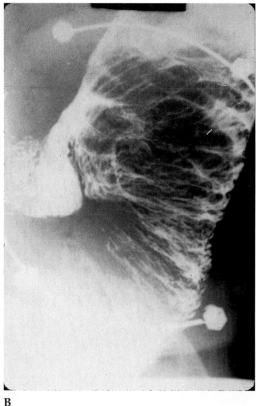

A   B

FIGURE 3.22. **Jejunogastric intussusception.** (A) Upper GI series showing a smooth defect in the gastric remnant adjacent to the anastomosis due to jejunogastric intussusception. (B) Upper GI series in another patient showing the characteristic "coiled-spring" appearance in the gastric remnant.

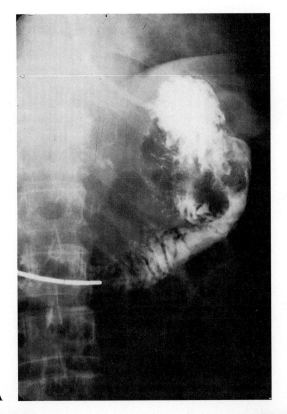

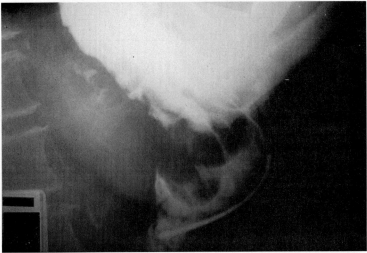

FIGURE 3.23. **Gastrojejunal intussusception.** (A) Upper GI series showing a smooth lobulated defect in the proximal jejunum due to gastrojejunal intussusception after Billroth II. (B) Coned-down view of the same patient.

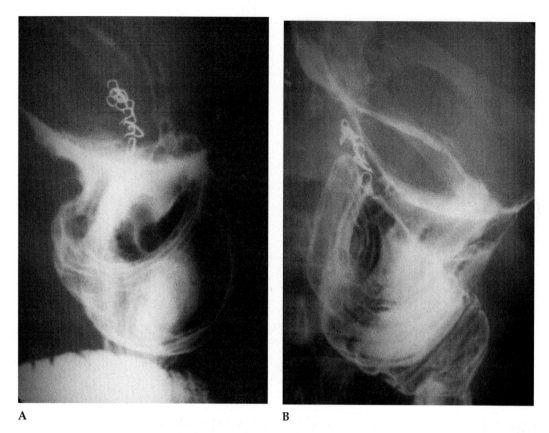

A   B

FIGURE **3.24. Gastrojejunal intussusception.** (A, B) Two views from an upper GI series showing a large smooth defect in the proximal jejunum due to intussusception.

Gastrojejunal or jejunogastric prolapse may be detected radiographically as well [28]. Prolapse involves mucosa alone, whereas intussusception indicates full-thickness invagination. Prolapse may be asymptomatic or may be responsible for obstruction and possibly bleeding. A well-defined, usually lobulated defect is typically identified in the stomach or small bowel adjacent to the anastomosis (Fig. 3.25).

Dumping Syndrome

There are two types of dumping syndrome: early and late with respect to the time interval following a meal. The early dumping syndrome consists of postprandial sweating, flushing, palpitation, vomiting, diarrhea, weakness, and dizziness, often relieved by assuming a recumbent position. It is in part due to rapid emptying of the gastric remnant and can be seen with all types of gastric surgery that cause disruption or bypass of the normal pyloric sphincter mechanism and subsequent loss of the gastric reservoir function. Stomach size may also contribute to the development of the dumping syndrome. It is thought that symp-

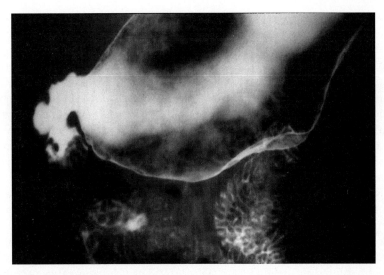

FIGURE **3.25. Jejunogastric prolapse.** Upper GI series shows a well-defined defect in the gastric remnant due to prolapse.

toms result from premature passage of hyperosmolar chyme into the small bowel with subsequent increased extracellular fluid and distention of the bowel leading to autonomic and adrenal medullary corrective mechanisms. It has been suggested that a better term for this condition is "jejunal hyperosmolarity syndrome." About 5 to 10% of postgastrectomy patients develop clinical symptoms of this condition [29].

The radiographic diagnosis of the dumping syndrome is unreliable. Some studies have used physiological contrast material or barium glucose rather then barium alone in an attempt to identify rapid transit fluoroscopically; however, consistent results have not been obtained with this technique [12].

The late dumping syndrome refers to the occurrence of the early dumping symptoms 2 to 3 hours after a meal. The etiology is thought to be hypoglycemia secondary to postprandial hyperglycemia.

Afferent Loop Dysfunction

Afferent loop dysfunction may be acute or chronic. The term "acute afferent limb obstruction" has been used to refer to mechanical obstruction of the afferent limb, which may occur at any time following surgery. Herniation of the afferent loop through a surgical defect is the most common etiology [15]. On barium studies, the A limb fails to fill, although failure to fill the A limb does not necessarily indicate obstruction. CT images may be more reliable in establishing the diagnosis by showing the dilated afferent loop.

"Chronic afferent limb obstruction," or the afferent limb syndrome, refers to incomplete obstruction of the A limb, which may be due to stricture, tumor, adhesions, kinking at the anastomosis, internal hernia, intussusception, or recurrent ulcer in the A limb near the anastomosis. Preferential filling of the A limb may also lead to dilation of the A limb and is due to technical factors, such as restriction of the efferent (E) limb, especially with a left-to-right anastomosis accompanied by the Hofmeister procedure (restricted stoma), or inferior placement of the A limb on the greater curvature of the gastric remnant [12]. An unusually long A limb may predispose a patient to this condition as well. Partial obstruction of the A limb leads to stasis with accumulation of secretions and/or food, which may result in bacterial overgrowth and malabsorption. Postprandial fullness relieved by bilious vomiting is a characteristic frequent presentation.

Radiographic findings on barium study include dilatation of the A limb with retained secretions, and retention of barium on delayed films (Fig. 3.26). In some cases, preferential filling of the A limb may be observed, and examination in the upright position may accentuate this finding. CT imaging may also be diagnostic, demonstrating a characteristic dilated fluid-filled loop (Fig. 3.27). The CT appearance is somewhat variable, depending on the length of the A limb [30]. Confusion with cystic masses in the upper abdomen is possible if the surgical history is not appreciated and/or if contrast medium has not entered the A limb. Sonography may also show a similar pattern of cystic masses. Hepatobiliary imaging studies can also be used to make this diagnosis, by demonstrating persistent activity in the afferent loop [31]. An advantage of this technique over barium studies is the ability to fill the A limb via the liver.

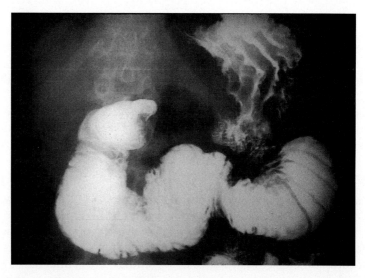

FIGURE 3.26. **Afferent limb syndrome.** Supine view from an upper GI series after Billroth II shows marked dilatation of the afferent limb, which failed to empty well on delayed films owing to afferent limb syndrome from recurrent carcinoma.

FIGURE 3.27. **Afferent limb syndrome.** (A–C) Three films from a CT scan of the upper abdomen with oral and intravenous contrast media showing a markedly dilated fluid-filled af-ferent limb after Billroth II.

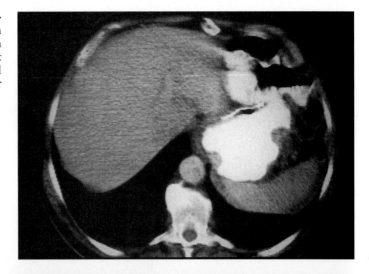

A

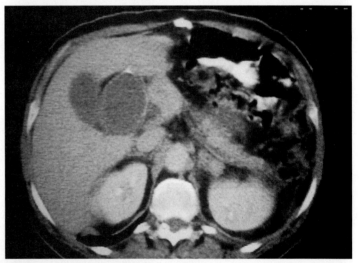

B

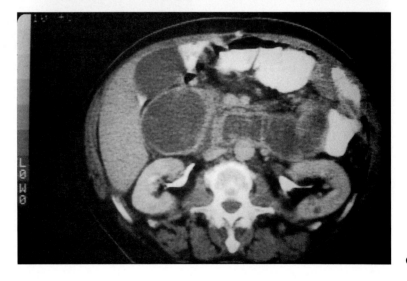

C

Efferent Loop Dysfunction

Acute and chronic forms of efferent loop dysfunction may occur. An upper GI series may show poor filling of the E limb, with preferential filling of the A limb (Fig. 3.28). The acute form is usually identified in the early postoperative period and is generally self-limiting. The postulated etiologies include spasm, inflammation, and neosphincters. Symptoms are typically abdominal pain and bilious vomiting.

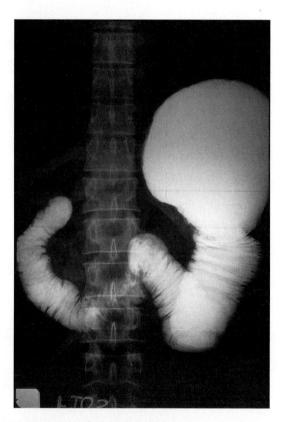

FIGURE **3.28. Efferent limb dysfunction.** Supine view from an upper GI series showing nonfilling of the efferent limb with preferential filling of the afferent limb.

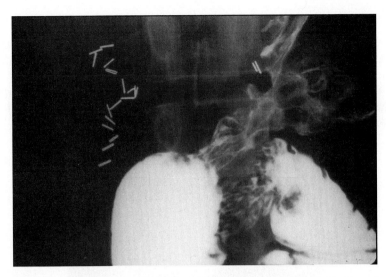

FIGURE 3.29. Postoperative alkaline reflux gastritis (bile gastritis). View from an upper GI series showing thickened folds in the gastric remnant after Billroth II.

Postoperative Alkaline Reflux Gastritis

A form of gastritis may develop beginning immediately after gastric surgery or years later. Although it has been termed bile gastritis, it has not been definitely established that bile reflux is the etiology. Characteristic symptoms are constant epigastric burning pain made worse by eating. Large gastric folds may be identified on upper GI series (Fig. 3.29). Bile reflux esophagitis may develop as a further consequence (Fig. 3.30).

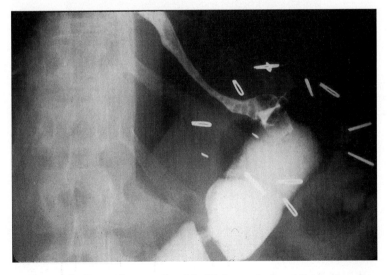

FIGURE 3.30. Alkaline reflux esophagitis. Right posterior oblique view from an upper GI series demonstrates a distal esophageal stricture from bile reflux after Billroth I.

Suture Granulomas

Suture granulomas, due to a foreign body reaction, may occur after gastric surgery with nonabsorbable suture material. Well-defined, rounded filling defects at the level of the anastomosis, identified radiographically may simulate tumor (Fig. 3.31) [21]. Endoscopically, smooth indentations with intact mucosa are identified at the level of the anastomosis.

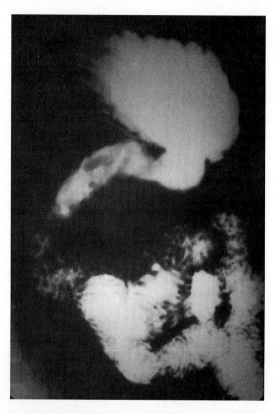

FIGURE 3.31. Suture granuloma. A small smooth defect is identified on an upper GI series in the region of the anastomosis after Billroth I.

Small-Bowel Changes After Vagotomy and Pyloroplasty

It has been observed that after vagotomy and pyloroplasty the diameter of the small bowel increases, the transit time becomes prolonged, and barium tends to precipitate [32]. These findings are attributed to the interruption of the parasympathetic nerve supply to the intestine which produces altered small-bowel motility with resultant bowel dilatation and prolongation of transit. In addition, disruption of the pyloric barrier may affect gastric digestion and interfere with the admixture of food with biliary and pancreatic secretions. The altered composition of the intestinal contents may lead to the observed small-bowel changes as well. The current routine use of selective and super-selective vagotomy avoids some of these problems.

Gastric Stasis

Gastric stasis may be an early or late complication of gastric surgery. In the early postoperative period it is more frequently observed in patients with diabetes, malnutrition, or gastric or pancreatic cancer and is usually self-limited [33]. In the later postoperative period, symptoms of gastric stasis, including postprandial vomiting, pain, and weight loss, develop in 1 to 25% of patients [34]. Although the etiology of postoperative gastric stasis is unclear, ineffective gastric emptying, impaired bowel motility, and alkaline reflux gastritis have been implicated. Nuclear medicine emptying studies are indicated to quantitate gastric emptying. Reoperation with reconfiguration of the anastomosis or a total gastrectomy may be required in severe cases.

Total Gastrectomy

Total gastrectomy may be necessary in some patients with primary or recurrent gastric carcinoma. In such cases, an esophagojejunostomy generally will be performed. This can be performed with a Roux-en-Y anastomosis, which can be either end to side or "J shaped"; alternatively, a jejunal loop can be brought up with an afferent and efferent limb (Figs. 3.32–3.34).

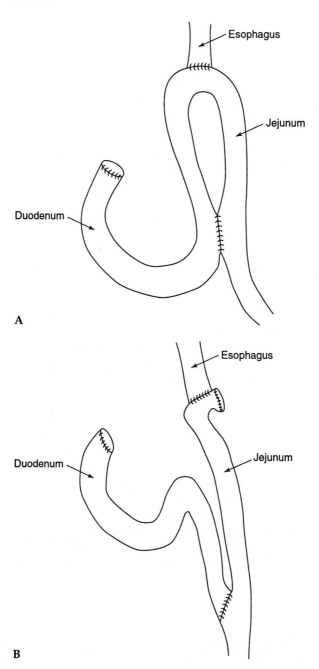

A

B

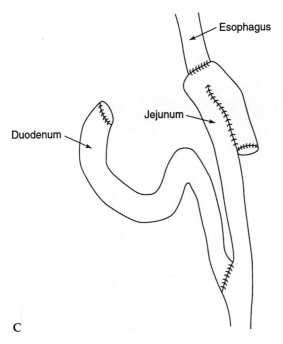

C

FIGURE 3.32. Various forms of esophagojejunal anastomoses after total gastrectomy. (A) Loop esophagojejunostomy with distal jejunojejunostomy. (B) With Roux-En-Y. (C) J shaped anastomosis with Roux-En-Y.

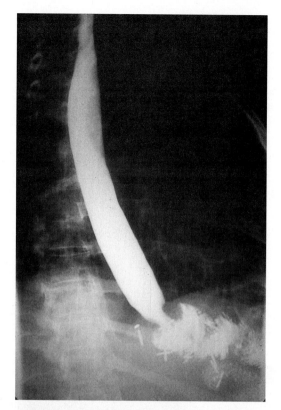

A

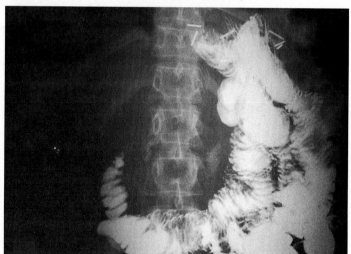

B

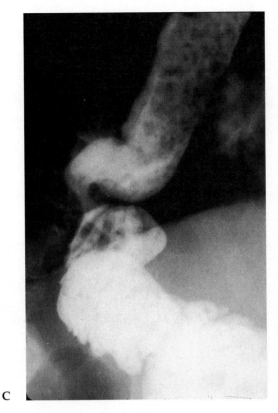

C

FIGURE 3.33. **Total gastrectomy.** (A, B) Film from an upper GI series following total gastrectomy with an end-to-side anastomosis. (C) Another patient with the same type of anastomosis.

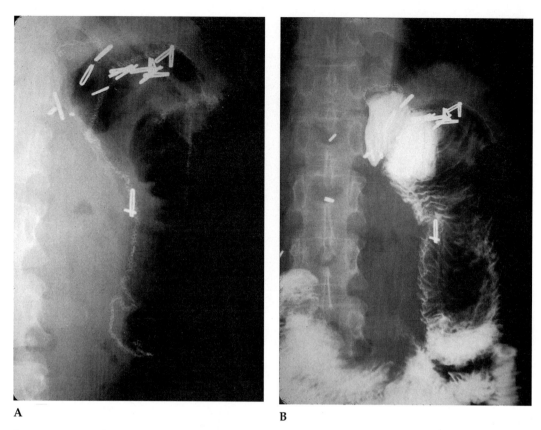

A   B

FIGURE 3.34. **Total gastrectomy with J pouch.** (A) Plain film of the abdomen. (B) Upper GI series after total gastrectomy for gastric carcinoma with a J-pouch esophagojejunostomy.

A variety of early and late complications may occur after total gastrectomy [35]. In the early postoperative period, anastomotic leaks may occur, usually from the esophagojejunal anastomosis, but also from the duodenal stump or jejunojejunal anastomosis if a Roux-en-Y procedure has been performed. Breakdown of the anastomosis with anatomic disruption will generally require surgery, while small leaks may be managed conservatively in some cases. Rarely, leaks may be identified in the later postoperative period, either from delayed recognition or delayed breakdown of the anastomosis. Edema at the anastomotic site may lead to obstruction in the early postoperative period as well. In the late postoperative period, recurrent tumor or fibrosis may lead to anastomotic narrowing and obstruction. Alkaline reflux esophagitis is common after esophagojejunostomy since there is no sphincter to prevent reflux. To prevent reflux of duodenal contents into the esophagus, it is recommended that a Roux-en-Y anastomosis be performed with the jejunojejunostomy placed about 40 cm distal to the esophagojejunal anastomosis.

Gastroenterostomy

A gastroenterostomy, usually gastrojejunostomy, may be performed as a drainage procedure with vagotomy for peptic ulcer disease and in patients with unresectable antral carcinomas and other conditions that may lead to antral narrowing, such as Crohn's disease. In the past, simple gastroenterostomy was a commonly performed procedure for PUD, although it was abandoned owing to the high ulcer recurrence rate. An anastomosis is generally made between the jejunum and the greater curvature of the stomach, as far as possible from the pylorus, in a side-to-side fashion, although other configurations are sometimes used (Figs. 3.35 and 3.36). The jejunum may be brought either to the anterior wall of the stomach superior to the omentum or to the

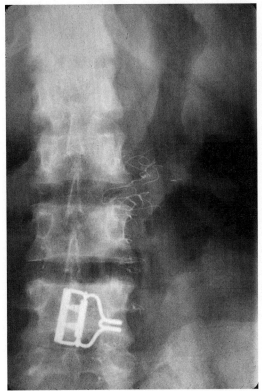 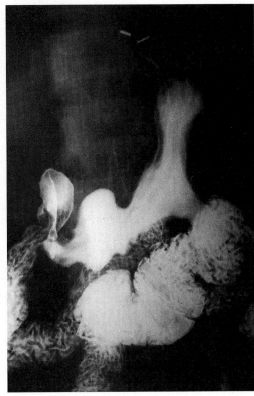

A   B

FIGURE 3.35. **Gastroenterostomy.** (A) Plain film. (B) Upper GI series demonstrating the gastrojejunal anastomoses along the greater curvature of the body of the stomach. Note contrast flows via the anatomic route and the gastrojejunostomy.

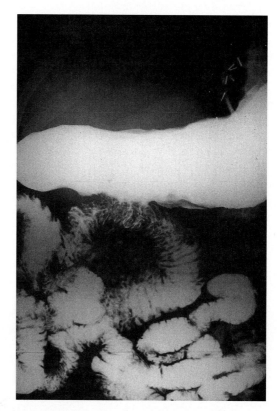

FIGURE 3.36. Gastrojejunostomy. Right anterior oblique view from an upper
GI series showing the gastroenterostomy at the distal body of the stomach.

posterior wall through an opening made in the transverse mesocolon.
When one is performing a contrast study, it is important to document
the direction of the flow of barium out of the stomach, with the preferable route being from the stomach to the efferent limb.

Complications of Gastroenterostomy

Antral Narrowing

Narrowing of the antrum may develop many years after gastroenterostomy, with or without vagotomy (Fig. 3.37). The etiology is
unclear. Narrowing may be due to disuse secondary to exclusion of the
antrum, as is known to occur in other portions of the bowel following
diversion procedures; or it may be related to antral gastritis with fibrosis or to postoperative adhesions. The entire antrum or only a portion
of the antrum may be affected. The narrowing is typically smooth and
concentric. The appearance may be confused with infiltrating carcinoma, which is increased in incidence following gastroenterostomy
over the general population [19]. Biopsy may be necessary to establish
a definitive diagnosis.

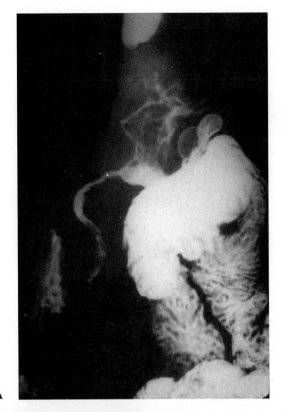

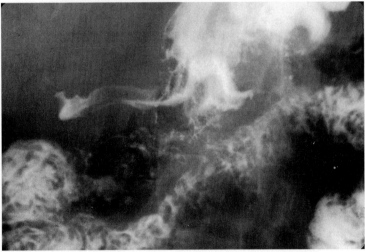

FIGURE 3.37. **Antral narrowing after gastroenterostomy.** (A) Single view from an upper GI series showing smooth antral narrowing after gastroenterostomy. (B) View of a different patient with similar findings.

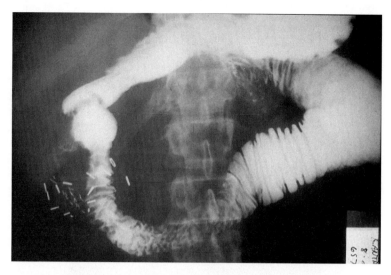

Figure 3.38. "Viscious circle" after gastroenterostomy. Supine view from an upper GI series shows filling of the afferent limb only. On fluoroscopy, barium was seen entering the A limb, then flowing retrograde into the stomach and back into the afferent limb.

"Viscious Circle"

Another complication of gastroenterostomy is the so-called viscious circle, when partial obstruction of the efferent limb causes food or contrast medium to be directed through the anastomosis into the A limb and retrograde through the pylorus back into the stomach. This sequence may be observed fluoroscopically and documented radiographically (Fig. 3.38). Revision of the anastomosis is required to correct the condition.

Gastroileostomy

Gastroileostomy is a possible iatrogenic complication of gastroenterostomy that is readily diagnosed in upper GI series by identifying direct communication between the stomach and the ileum.

Postsplenectomy Gastric Deformity

Gastric deformities may be observed following splenectomy. Ansel and Wasserman found mass- or polyplike deformities, most commonly in the posterolateral wall of the gastric fundus in 7% of postsplenectomy patients [36]. They ranged from 1.5 to 4.5 cm in diameter, and from small submucosal-appearing defects to larger polypoid masses simulating neoplasms (Fig. 3.39). These defects may vary in etiology but are postulated to be related to ligation of the short gastric vessels between the spleen and greater curvature of the gastric fundus, with resulting infolding of the stomach wall. Other postulated causes are local trauma with edema and/or hematoma, and foreign body suture granuloma.

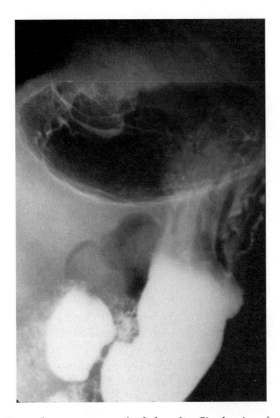

FIGURE 3.39. **Postsplenectomy gastric deformity.** Single view from a double-contrast upper GI series shows a smooth lobulated filling defect in the gastric fundus after splenectomy for lymphoma. Biopsy showed no tumor.

Whipple Procedure

The first successful pancreaticoduodenectomy was performed in 1912. Whipple popularized the procedure for periampullary tumors, reporting three cases in 1935. The original operation was performed in two stages. The morbidity and mortality rates after pancreaticoduodenectomy were high for several decades, and long-term survival was extremely poor. Since that time, numerous modifications and technical refinements have been made, and perioperative mortality rates have dropped from approximately 20% to less than 4% [37,38]. The "standard" Whipple procedure now consists of resection of the head and uncinate process of the pancreas, the common bile duct and gallbladder, and the duodenum, with formation of three anastomoses: a choledochojejunostomy, a gastrojejunostomy, and a pancreaticojejunostomy (Fig. 3.40).

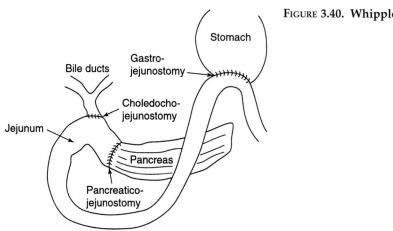

FIGURE 3.40. Whipple procedure.

Variations in the type and placement of the anastomoses are common. The jejunal loop may be placed in an antecolic or retrocolic position. Stents are sometimes left in the pancreatic duct and the chole-dochojejunal anastomosis temporarily after surgery. In the pylorus-preserving Whipple, which has become an alternative to the standard procedure, the pylorus and first portion of the duodenum are preserved (Fig. 3.41). This modification results in better postoperative weight gain due to the increased gastric reservoir, decreased bile reflux, and decreased jejunal ulceration (since gastrointestinal physiology is more normal). The operative time is also shortened. There may

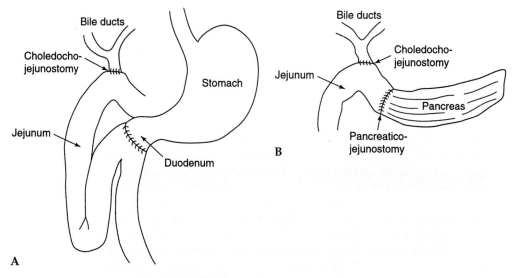

FIGURE 3.41. Pylorus-preserving Whipple procedure. (A) Gastrogejunel and biliary enteric anastamoses. (B) Pancreaticojejunal anastomosis.

however be a temporary delay in gastric emptying. Indications for the Whipple procedure include neoplasms of the periampullary region, symptomatic chronic pancreatitis, and trauma.

The evaluation of the postoperative Whipple patient is challenging because of the complexity of the surgery and the multiple anastomoses to be investigated. In the early postoperative period UGI series and CT are the most useful tools available, with CT imaging being preferable in the later postoperative period (Figs. 3.42 and 3.43). The CT features of the normal postoperative appearance and complications have been described by multiple authors [39–44]. Attempts should be made to identify the three anastomoses. The pancreaticojejunostomy and chole-dochojejunostomy may be difficult to identify because they are often not opacified with oral contrast medium, although if stents are placed across these anastomoses, they can generally readily be identified. Pneumobilia is seen in about 80% of patients; thus its absence does not imply obstruction of the choledochojejunal anastomosis [42]. Transient fluid collections in the surgical bed, in Morrison's pouch, in the right paracolic gutter, and in the region of the anastomoses are common findings but may be difficult to differentiate from leaks and abscesses [40]. When fluid collections are seen on CT scans, an UGI series with water-soluble contrast may be necessary to exclude a leak, and ultrasound- or CT-guided aspiration may be necessary to differentiate abscess from noninfected fluid. Reactive lymphadenopathy may be a normal inflammatory response to recent surgery and may be confused with metastatic disease. Serial scans are helpful in this regard, since reactive nodes

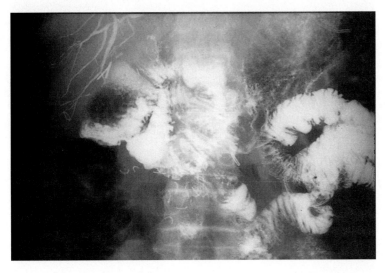

FIGURE 3.42. **Whipple procedure.** Supine view from a post–Whipple procedure upper GI series demonstrating the partial gastrectomy, gastrojejunal anastomosis, and barium entering the biliary tree from the choledochojejunostomy.

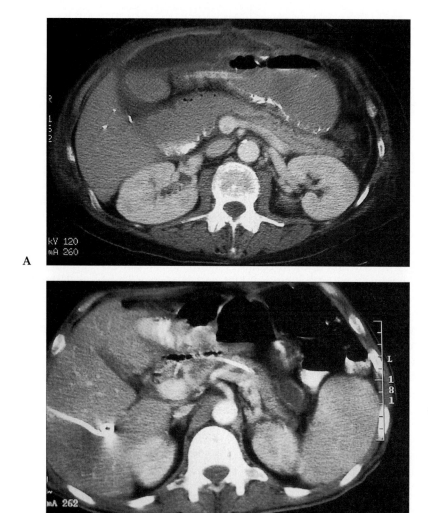

FIGURE 3.43. **Whipple procedure.** (A) CT scan at the level of the pancreas after Whipple procedure showing the gastrojejunal and pancreaticojejunal anastomoses. A nasogastric tube is present. (B) CT scan of a different patient after Whipple procedure showing a stent in the pancreatic duct and an external biliary drain in place.

will show stability or regression over time. Unfilled loops of bowel may simulate adenopathy as well. Increased attenuation of the fat in the surgical bed and surrounding the mesenteric vessels is also an expected postoperative finding, which may persist for up to a year after surgery and should not be confused with tumor infiltration.

The remaining pancreas is often atrophic, and mild dilatation of the pancreatic duct is common. A soft tissue defect at the pancreaticojejunostomy site may be seen secondary to invagination of the pancreas into the bowel loop (the so-called dunking procedure) and may simulate tumor recurrence or intussusception (Fig. 3.44). Bluemke et al. reported thickening of the gastric antrum and proximal duodenum in 64% of patients undergoing the pylorus-preserving Whipple procedure with adjuvant chemotherapy and radiation therapy [42]. These findings were thought to be secondary to the radiation therapy and should not be attributed to metastatic disease.

The most common complication and the leading cause of perioperative mortality following the Whipple procedure is related to leakage or breakdown of the pancreaticojejunostomy. Unfortunately, this anastomosis is the most difficult to visualize with contrast. Trerotola et al. have suggested a preferred method of fluoroscopic visualization of this region by injection of the biliary stent or T tube in a shallow Trendelenburg or left posterior oblique position [45].

Liver infarction is not unusual in patients who have undergone resection of the portal vein and/or superior mesenteric vein, with an incidence of 70% reported in one series [39]. In the later postoperative period, recurrent disease, either in the pancreatic bed or in the liver, is best identified on CT imaging. Recurrent tumor in the region of the surgical bed and liver metastases commonly develop, and the survival rate for pancreatic cancer remains dismal (Fig. 3.45).

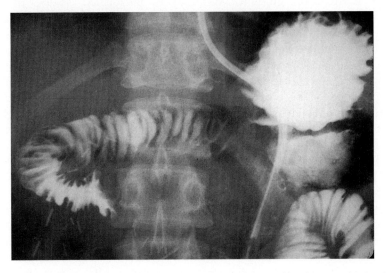

FIGURE 3.44. **Whipple procedure with dunking.** Supine film from an upper GI series showing a defect at the pancreaticojejunostomy site from invagination of the pancreas into the bowel.

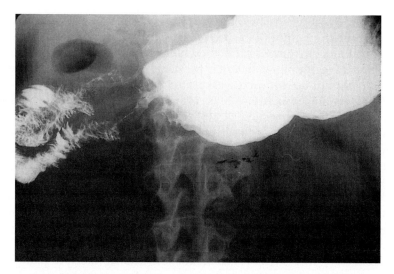

FIGURE 3.45. **Whipple procedure with recurrent tumor.** Supine film from an upper GI series performed 4 months after surgery shows partial gastric outlet obstruction and irregular narrowing of the gastrojejunal anastomosis from recurrent tumor.

Gastrostomy

One of the oldest gastric operations, gastrostomy was first performed in 1876. It is also one of the most commonly performed procedures, usually done for feeding purposes and less commonly for gastric decompression. A Foley, Pezzer, Malecot, or straight Robinson catheter may be employed. The most often used method now is percutaneous endoscopic gastrostomy (PEG), although a percutaneous procedure with fluoroscopic guidance also may be performed [46–49]. In the endoscopic technique, first described in 1979, a gastroscope is placed in the stomach and the stomach is fully inflated. The endoscopic light transilluminates the abdominal wall. An incision is made in the abdomen where the light is best seen. A needle is introduced into the stomach and a suture is passed through it, into the stomach. The suture is grasped with the snare of the endoscope and pulled out of the mouth. The end of the suture is tied to a modified 16F mushroom catheter. Traction is applied to the abdominal end of the suture and the tube is pulled down into the stomach and out of the abdominal wall [50].

The percutaneous fluoroscopic technique was first reported in 1981 [51], and the use of gastropexy devices (T fasteners) was described in 1986 [52]. Simply summarized, with this procedure the stomach is insufflated with air, usually via a nasogastric tube, and punctured under fluoroscopic guidance. A tract with serial dilatations is created over a guide wire, and the tube is then inserted. Although advocated by some, the use of T fasteners is controversial. The T fasteners provide a gastropexy that allows the tract to mature rapidly; moreover, peritonitis and intraperitoneal tube placement is avoided, and in case of tube dislodgment the tube can be easily replaced. The use of larger catheters, which are less likely to occlude, is facilitated by T fasteners. Details of this procedure are available elsewhere [47]. The fluoroscopic procedure is superior to the endoscopic one in terms of feasibility and can be performed in patients who have stenoses and/or tumors of the upper GI tract (preventing the passage of an endoscope) and in obese patients (in whom transillumination of the abdominal wall is not possible). Intravenous sedation is also commonly avoided. Pull-type gastrostomy tubes (placed via an oral route) may also be inserted with radiological guidance [53].

In a small percentage of cases, a surgical approach may be necessary. In patients whose transverse colon and/or liver overlies the stomach or in those whose stomach is high in position under the ribs, the percutaneous methods are not possible. In patients with partial gastrectomies, the percutaneous techniques are more difficult and in some cases may not be successful. When gastrostomy is performed surgically, a gastropexy is done and the stomach is attached to the anterior abdominal wall with a few sutures. In patients who are likely to require long-term gastrostomy feeding, a permanent (Weasel) gastrostomy may be performed surgically. With the Weasel procedure, a seromuscular tunnel is created between the stomach and anterior abdominal wall, and no gastropexy is done.

A variety of complications may develop after gastrostomy tube placement (Table 3.3) [54–56]. The complication rate is between 1% and

TABLE 3.3. Complications of gastrostomy.

Tube dislodgment or migration
  In peritoneal cavity
  In esophagus
  Prolapsed into the duodenum or more distal
    bowel
  In stomach wall
  In anterior abdominal wall
  In colon
  "Lost" (migration out of the stomach)
Gastric outlet obstruction
Small-bowel obstruction
Bowel perforation
Gastric ulcer
Gastric volvulus
Leakage into peritoneal cavity
Peristomal leakage
Gastric pneumatosis
Hemorrhage
Tube blockage
Gastrocutaneous fistula
Gastrocolic fistula [percutaneous endoscopic
  gastrostomy (PEG) technique]
Broken tubes
Tube extrusion
Gastric perforation (PEG technique)

5%. An institutional evaluation and meta-analysis of the literature showed a higher success rate with radiological gastrostomy and less morbidity than with both PEG or surgery [57]. Complications are particularly common in the pediatric population [58–61]. Generally, tube position and complications are evaluated by injection of water-soluble material into the tube, although CT imaging can be helpful. The most common complication of gastrostomy is poor positioning of the tube, either from inadvertent misplacement or from migration. The tube may be identified in the peritoneal cavity, esophagus, colon, stomach wall, or anterior abdominal wall, or it may be prolapsed into the duodenum or more distal bowel (Figs. 3.46–3.52). The additional problem of bowel

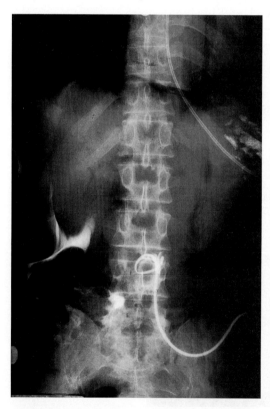

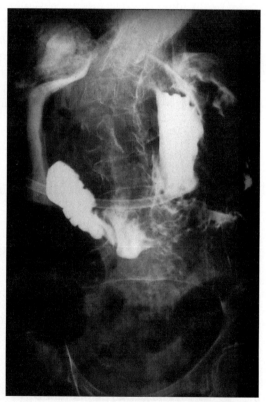

FIGURE 3.46. Gastrostomy tube in the peritoneal cavity. Supine view of the abdomen after injection of contrast into the gastrostomy tube shows malposition of the tube with the tip in the peritoneal cavity with extraluminal contrast.

FIGURE 3.47. Poor positioning of gastrostomy tube. Supine view of the abdomen after water-soluble contrast injection into the gastrostomy tube shows contrast within the stomach, with leakage of contrast into the peritoneal cavity. Portal venous gas is also identified secondary to ischemic bowel due to sepsis and hypotension.

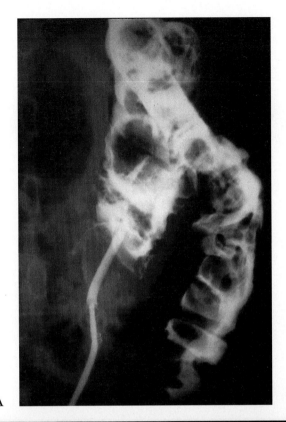

A

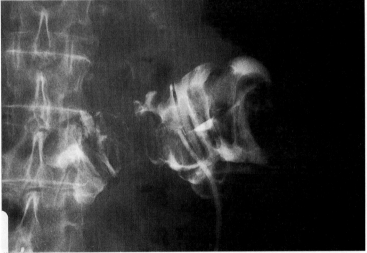

B

FIGURE 3.48. **Gastrostomy tube in transverse colon.** (A, B) Two different patients demonstrating contrast injections of the gastrostomy tube, with the tip in the transverse colon. This complication is more common with PEG placement than with the traditional methods of gastrostomy placement.

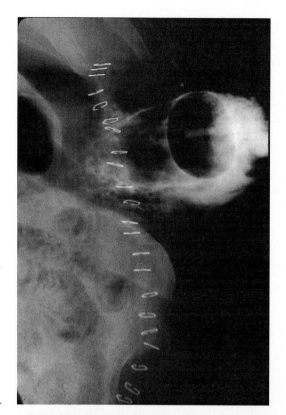

A

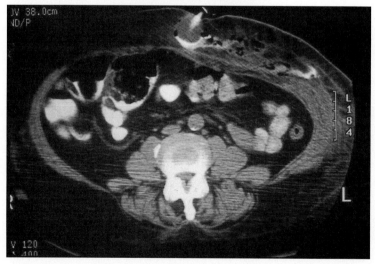

B

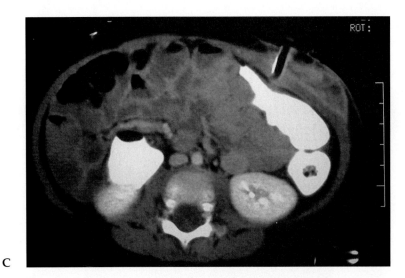

C

FIGURE 3.49. **Gastrostomy tube in the anterior abdominal wall.** (A) Contrast injection of the gastrostomy tube shows it to be outside the stomach in the anterior abdominal wall. (B) CT scan on another patient demonstrating the tip of the gastrostomy tube in the anterior abdominal wall. Contrast medium was injected into the tube in addition to oral contrast administration. (C) CT scan in a different patient with an abscess secondary to positioning of the gastrostomy tube in the anterior abdominal wall.

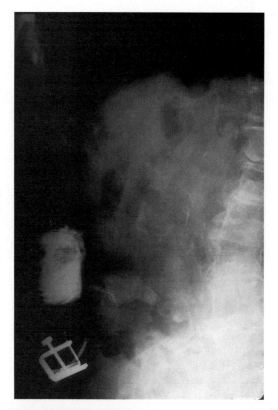

A

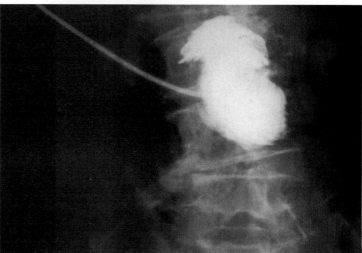

B

FIGURE 3.50. Gastrostomy tube in the peritoneal cavity with abscess.
(A, B) Films from two different patients with injections into the gastrostomy
tube showing a cavity around the tube due to abscesses.

FIGURE 3.51. **Gastrostomy tube in tract communicating with the stomach.** Film from injection of contrast medium into the gastrostomy tube shows the tube to be outside the stomach, filling the stomach via a tract.

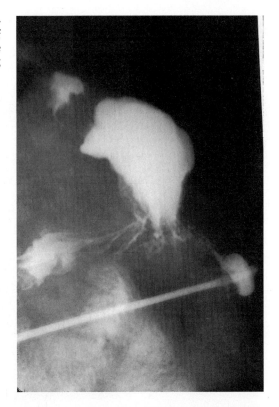

FIGURE 3.52. **Prolapsed gastrostomy tube.** Supine view of the abdomen after injection of contrast medium through the tube shows migration of the gastrostomy tube into the ileum.

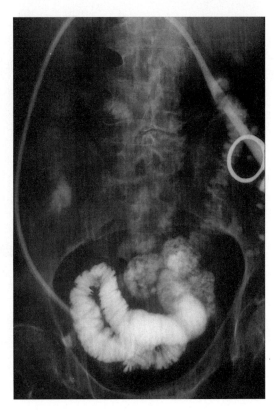

obstruction may develop with prolapse of the tube with an inflated balloon. Gastric outlet obstruction may be a consequence of tube impaction at the pylorus (Fig. 3.53).

Tubes may migrate out of the stomach and beyond and become "lost." Lost tubes, which for the most part are not radiopaque, are often

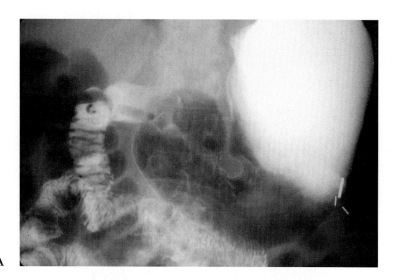

A

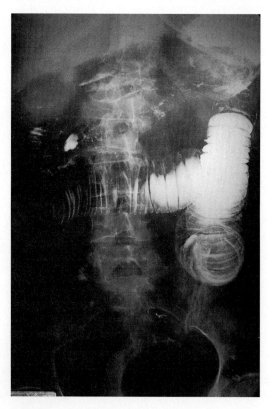

B

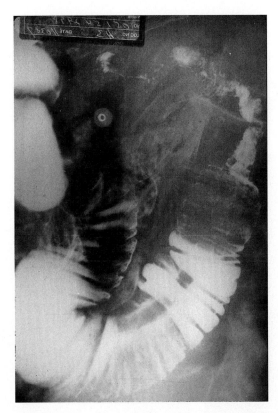

C

FIGURE 3.53. **Gastrostomy tube migration with bowel obstruction.** (A) The gastrostomy tube has migrated into the duodenal bulb and produced partial gastric outlet obstruction. (B, C) Two different patients with migration of the gastrostomy tube into the small bowel with subsequent small-bowel obstruction.

difficult to identify on plain films. A small radiopaque coil in the prox-imal end of the insufflation arm of a Foley catheter is characteristic and may be identified if carefully searched for (Figs. 3.54 and 3.55). "Lost tubes" may be passed through the rectum but intervention may be required for removal. Gastric ulcer may develop secondary to pressure

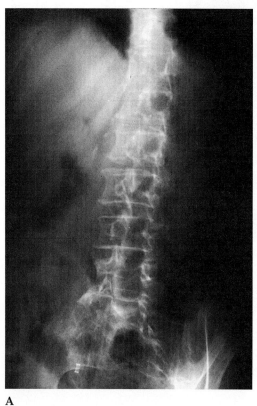
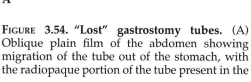

A

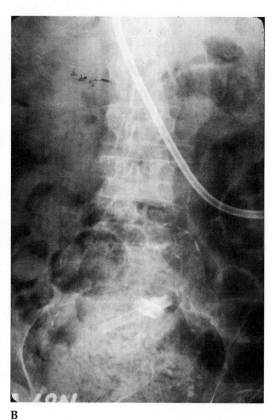

B

FIGURE 3.54. "Lost" gastrostomy tubes. (A) Oblique plain film of the abdomen showing migration of the tube out of the stomach, with the radiopaque portion of the tube present in the right lower quadrant. (B) Another patient with a lost gastrostomy tube; the radiopaque portion is clearly visible in the pelvis. The tube was in the sigmoid colon.

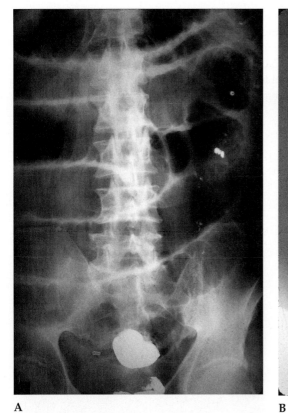

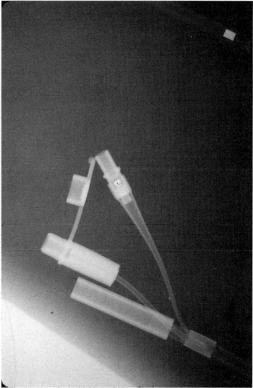

A

B

FIGURE 3.55. "Lost" gastrostomy tube causing small-bowel obstruction. (A) Plain film of the abdomen showing small-bowel obstruction. The radiopaque portion of the tube is present in the right lower quadrant, and difficult to identify. Contrast medium is present in the rectum from a previous examination. (B) Radiograph of the gastrostomy tube showing the radiopaque portion.

necrosis from the balloon (Fig. 3.56). Other rarer complications include gastric pneumatosis, which has been reported in association with gastric outlet obstruction and/or intramural position of the tube (Fig. 3.57), gastrocutaneous fistula after tube removal, gastrocolic fistula (Fig. 3.58), intraperitoneal leakage, and hemorrhage after percutaneous placement. Gastropexy may cause the stomach to assume a character-

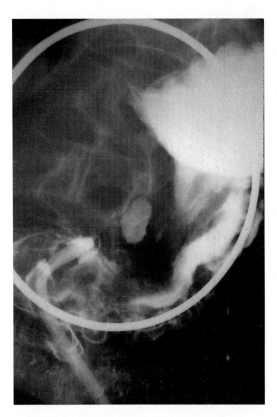

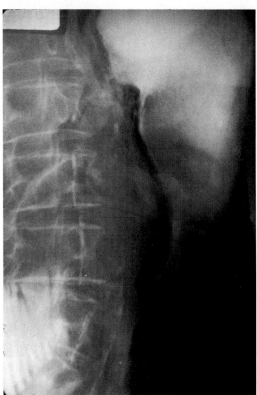

FIGURE 3.56. Gastric ulcer secondary to pressure necrosis from the gastrostomy balloon. View of the stomach after injection of contrast medium through the gastrostomy showing an ulcer along the lesser curvature aspect of the body of the stomach.

FIGURE 3.57. Gastric emphysema secondary to gastric outlet obstruction from gastrostomy tube. Oblique view from a water-soluble contrast study through the gastrostomy tube showing gastric outlet obstruction and gastric emphysema secondary to impaction of the tube at the pyloric channel.

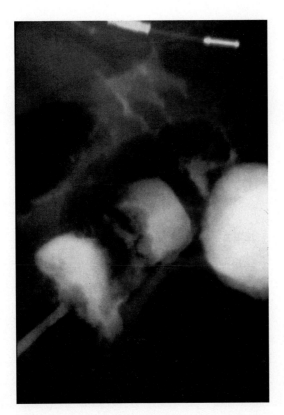

FIGURE 3.58. **Gastrostomy tube in the colon with a gastrocolic fistula.** Film from gastrostomy tube injection shows the tube positioned in the colon with a fistula from the colon to the stomach.

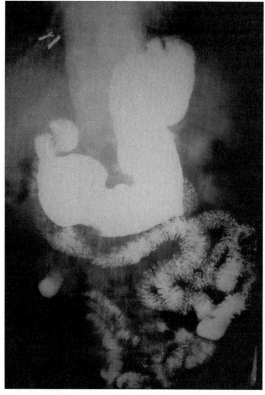

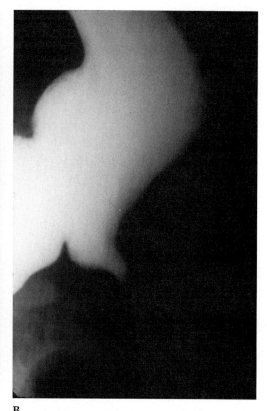

A   B

FIGURE 3.59. **Tenting of the stomach after removal of the gastrostomy tube.** (A) Barium-filled stomach shows the characteristic "tented appearance" along the greater curvature as a result of tacking of the stomach to the anterior abdominal wall. (B) Another patient, showing contrast medium extending into the gastrostomy tube tract.

istic "tented appearance" after tube removal, with tacking of the stomach to the anterior abdominal wall with the surgical approach (Fig. 3.59).

After surgically placed gastrostomy tube removal, a focal, concave deformity along the greater curvature of the stomach may be seen on UGI series [62]. This deformity has been attributed to invaginated gastric mucosa, intentionally produced at the time of surgical gastrostomy placement; it has not been reported with the other tube insertion techniques. It is important not to misinterpret this finding as a neoplasm.

Cystogastrostomy

The traditional surgical method of therapy for pancreatic pseudocysts requiring drainage has been the transgastric cystogastrostomy, although percutaneous drainage of pseudocysts with CT or sonographic guidance is now being performed more frequently. The surgical procedure requires that the pseudocyst have a thick, well-formed wall and be firmly attached to the posterior gastric wall. A communication of 2 to 8cm is made between the posterior gastric wall and the adjacent pseudocyst by stabbing alone, by reinforcement of the margins with sutures, or by excision of a segment of gastric and cyst wall with oversewing of the edges to create a stoma. Occasionally, a temporary drainage tube is left through the opening.

The radiographic findings will vary depending on the surgical technique employed, the size of the communication and the size of the pseudocyst [63]. Barium may enter the cyst on upper GI series during the second or third week after surgery and may be seen up to 6 weeks after surgery when the pseudocysts are large and when reinforced or oversewn anastomoses have been performed (Figs. 3.60–3.62). Some cases will show deformity of the gastric contour and distortion of the

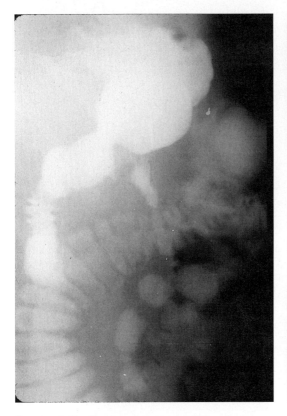

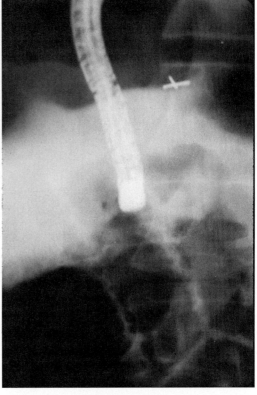

FIGURE 3.60. Cystogastrostomy. Film from an upper GI series 2 weeks after surgery demonstrates the entrance into the pseudocyst of contrast medium from the stomach.

FIGURE 3.61. Cystogastrostomy. Film from an endoscopic retrograde cholangiopancreatogram showing contrast medium entering the pseudocyst from the endoscope passed from the stomach through the surgically created communication to the pseudocyst.

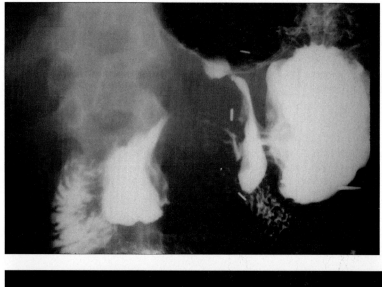

A

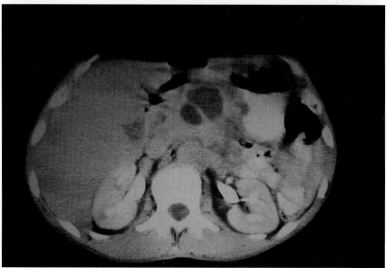

B

FIGURE **3.62. Cystogastrostomy.** (A) Right anterior oblique view from an upper GI series shows extraluminal contrast medium extending from the stomach into the pancreatic pseudocyst. (B) CT scan on the same patient.

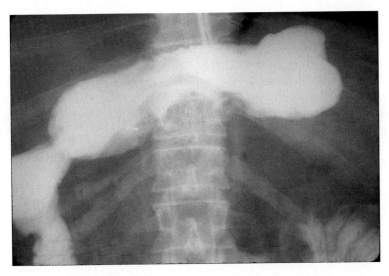

FIGURE 3.63. **Cystogastrostomy.** Supine view from a single-contrast upper GI series shows deformity of the lesser curvature of the body of the stomach following cystgastrostomy.

rugal folds at the site of surgery (Fig. 3.63). In the healing stage, an area of rigidity, which may be flat, smooth, or irregular, may be observed. A localized sacculation or a gastric pseudodiverticulum has also been described.

Radiology of the Stomach After Surgery for Obesity

Morbid obesity is a common problem associated with serious medical complications. Various operative procedures have evolved due to poor success in achieving permanent weight loss in these patients with dietary and behavioral therapy. The number and variety of procedures that have been used reflect the creativity and ingenuity of their developers and attest to the variety of problems and complications associated with each of type of operation.

The rationale behind the surgical approach to obesity (bariatric) surgery is to reduce calories available for fat deposition, either through inducing malabsorption by creating a small-bowel shunt (i.e., jejunoileal bypass) or by calorie deprivation by means of gastric restrictive surgery (i.e., gastric bypass, gastroplasty, bands).

The first surgical therapy for morbid obesity was in the early 1950s when Henriksson treated three patients with resection of a large portion of small bowel, as reported by Linner [64]. Although success was achieved with regard to weight loss, this procedure was not accepted because of its irreversibility. Shortly thereafter, the jejunoileal bypass (JIB) was developed. Various modifications of this operation were made over the next 20 years, with its popularity peaking in the mid-1970s. The general principle is to significantly decrease the amount of functional small bowel by surgically bypassing a large segment of it. Various surgical configurations have been devised to achieve this goal. The radiographic findings will vary depending on which type of operation has been performed. By 1980, however, the JIB had been generally abandoned owing to the development of serious late complications in a fairly high percentage of patients. These included diarrhea, electrolyte disturbances, nephrolithiasis, cholelithiasis, liver abnormalities, and cirrhosis.

Gastric Bypass and Gastroplasty

Gastric restrictive surgery was introduced in the 1960s by Mason and Ito [65]. This type of surgery evolved because of the observation that patients who had undergone gastric resections for other reasons lost weight. With the advent of automatic stapling devices in the 1970s, these procedures became technically easier to perform and they therefore gained in popularity. The rationale for surgery is that with a small gastric pouch that emptied slowly, satiety would occur quickly and oral intake would therefore decrease. The aim of surgery is to limit gastric capacity and restrict gastric outflow while avoiding the long-term serious complications of the JIB. This operation is more difficult to perform than the JIB, however, and the complication rate in the early postoperative period is higher. Comparative studies have shown that gastric bypass procedures achieve weight loss equal to or greater than the JIB [64].

With the gastric bypass (GBP) a small-volume (15–30 ml) gastric pouch is created with an outlet or channel to the small bowel of approximately one centimeter. Approximately 90% of the stomach is excluded. The anastomosis may be either a loop gastrojejunostomy or a Roux-en-Y configuration (Figs. 3.64 and 3.65). The Roux-en-Y procedure is technically easier and decreases the incidence of the late complications of bile reflux gastritis and esophagitis [66]. The gastric pouch is created by using a stapling device. Generally two rows of staples are placed adjacent and parallel to each other, extending completely across the stomach so that the distal stomach is functionally excluded from the pouch. Gastric transaction between the staple lines may be performed if desired. It is important to ensure that the pouch is appropriately sized and accommodates volumes of only about 15 to 30 ml. Some surgeons place a temporary decompressive gastrostomy in the distal stomach, which is removed before hospital discharge.

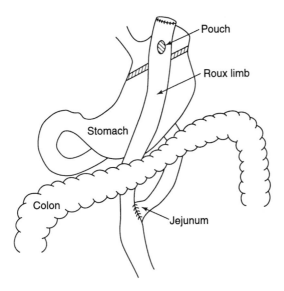

FIGURE 3.64. Gastric bypass for obesity.

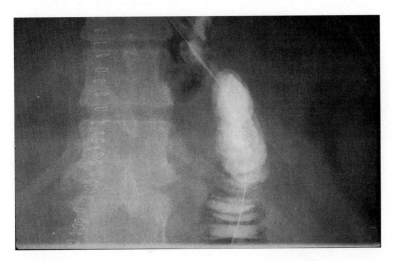

FIGURE 3.65. Gastric bypass for obesity. Water-soluble contrast examination after GBP demonstrating a very small gastric pouch and anastomosis to a Roux-en-Y loop of jejunum.

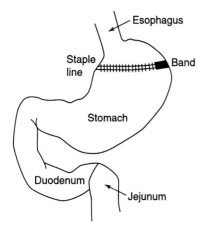

FIGURE 3.66. Horizontal gastroplasty.

Gastroplasty or gastric partition procedures, which create small gastric pouches but without anastomoses, are technically easier to perform than the GBP. Over the years various configurations have been devised. The staples may be placed horizontally or, more commonly currently, vertically. With the horizontal orientation, the channel may be located centrally or along the greater curvature and should measure approximately 1 cm (Figs. 3.66 and 3.67). Reinforcement of the channel is necessary to prevent widening. The vertical banded gastroplasty (VBG) has essentially replaced horizontal stapling because there was a

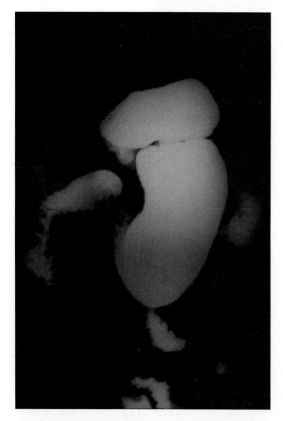

FIGURE 3.67. Horizontal gastroplasty. Single-contrast film from an upper GI series shows the horizontally oriented staples and channel to the remainder of the stomach.

FIGURE 3.68. Vertical banded gastroplasty.

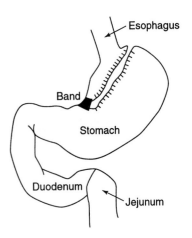

high incidence of failure with the horizontal orientation. In the VBG, staple lines are placed parallel to the lesser curvature so that a pouch 2 to 4 cm wide and 8 to 10 cm long is created. The 1 cm channel must be reinforced with a Silastic or Marlex ring, which may or may not be radioopaque (Figs. 3.68 and 3.69). Most studies comparing the GBP and gastroplasty have found that GBP is more effective and durable than gastroplasty; GBP is technically more difficult, however, and has a higher perioperative morbidity rate.

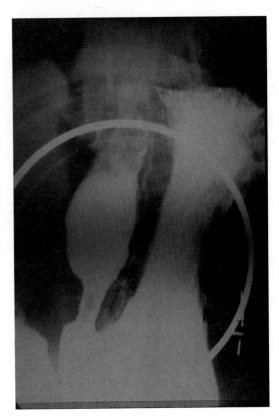

FIGURE 3.69. Vertical banded gastroplasty. Spot film with compression from an upper GI series shows a small gastric pouch with a channel to the remainder of the stomach.

Biliopancreatic Bypass

The biliopancreatic bypass is a malabsorption-producing procedure that includes a subtotal gastrectomy with a long-limb Roux-en-Y distal jejunoileostomy. The gastric remnant is approximately 200 to 400 ml, with a gastroenterostomy to a 250 cm Roux-en-Y limb. The biliopancreatic limb is anastomosed 50 cm from the ileocecal valve, forming a common channel for food and biliopancreatic secretions. A cholecystectomy is also performed. This operation has fewer untoward side effects than the JIB.

Gastric Banding

Gastric banding was developed by Wilkinson about 30 years ago as a simpler alternative to bypass or gastroplasty procedures [67]. In the original operation a prosthetic band is wrapped around the upper stomach, forming a channel between a small proximal pouch and the distal stomach (Fig. 3.70). There are no staple lines or anastomoses. Modifications of the banding technique and the material used have been made over the years. Complications include obstruction and/or narrowing of the channel or too large a channel and pouch dilatation resulting in weight gain.

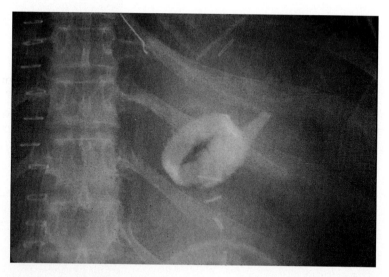

FIGURE 3.70. **Gastric band.** Coned-down view of the left upper quadrant shows a surgically placed band around the stomach creating a small gastric pouch.

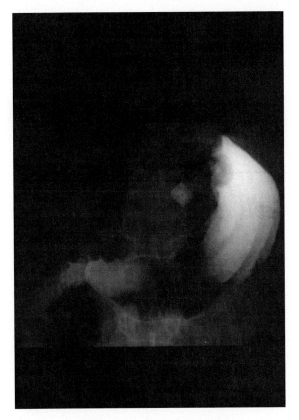

FIGURE 3.71. Laparoscopic band.

An adjustable laparoscopic band technique has been developed in which a gastric pouch is created by laparoscopically placing a silicone band with an inflatable cuff around the proximal stomach (Fig. 3.71). A calibration tube is placed transesophageally during surgery to calibrate the size of the pouch and stoma. The cuff is connected to a port, which is implanted in the rectus muscle, and the cuff size can be increased or decreased via the port. The size of the stoma, which can be adjusted by percutaneous injection or withdrawal of saline solution into the port under fluoroscopic control, is determined by the patient's ability to eat and by the weight loss curve. Reported complications include slippage of the band, erosion of the band into the stomach, and migration of the access port [68–70].

Gastric Bubble and Balloon

The Garren gastric balloon was developed in the early 1980s as a non-invasive alternative to surgical approaches to address obesity [71]. With this procedure a deflated bubble is placed in the stomach via a modified large oral gastric tube and then inflated with room air via an insufflation catheter. The tube and insufflation catheter are removed, leaving

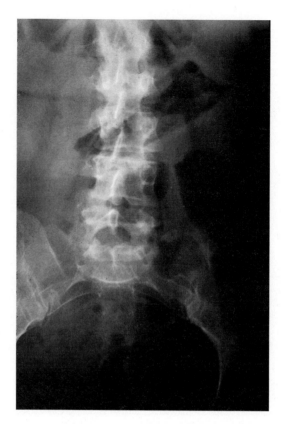

FIGURE 3.72. Garren gastric bubble with migration to the small bowel. Plain film of the abdomen showing the deflated bubble as air-filled tubular structures in the small bowel.

the inflated bubble floating in the stomach. The principle of this procedure is similar to that of the surgical gastric restrictive procedures, and patients experience decreased appetite and early satiety. The main complication is deflation of the balloon with migration beyond the stomach, and rarely subsequent small-bowel obstruction (Fig. 3.72).

Radiographic Evaluation in Obesity

Special challenges face the radiologist studying the morbidly obese patient. Patients may be too large to fit between the table and the fluoroscopic tower, may not fit in the CT gantry, and may be above the weight limits for the fluoroscopic table and CT scanner. Technical factors may prevent adequate exposure technique for plain films and fluoroscopy. Portable technique is generally useless owing to the limited power of the portable generator. The CT image may be degraded by artifacts secondary to beam hardening.

TABLE 3.4. Initial examination position based on staple line geometry (Smith).

Staple geometry	Probable surgery	Optimal initial position
Vertical	Gastroplasty: lesser curvature channel (vertical banded gastroplasty)	Right posterior oblique
Horizontal	Gastroplasty: greater curvature channel	Left posterior oblique
Mixed	Gastric bypass	Left posterior oblique

Obese patients will have difficulty turning rapidly, especially owing to discomfort in the immediate postoperative period, and they may refuse to drink adequate amounts of contrast agent. Smith et al. recommend optimal patient positioning based on the staple geometry identified on the plain scout film of the abdomen (Table 3.4) [72]. Others prefer to start in the upright position if this is technically possible [73]. Smith and her colleagues have also stressed the following points: initial use of small quantities of water-soluble contrast, prompt filming of the first swallow without prolonged fluoroscopy, continued contrast administration only after the anatomy has been determined, and examination of the proximal and distal pouches if present [72,74].

CT imaging has been advocated as an effective method of evaluating the excluded stomach, which is difficult or impossible to visualize with oral contrast examinations [75]. If necessary, contrast medium may be injected percutaneously under CT guidance into the distal stomach [76,77].

Complications of Obesity Surgery

Various complications may develop after bariatric surgery (Table 3.5).

TABLE 3.5. Postoperative complications of gastric restrictive surgery.

Early
  Leak
  Gastric perforation
  Staple line dehiscence
  Channel obstruction
  Distal gastric or afferent limb obstruction
Late
  Staple line dehiscence
  Channel widening
  Channel stenosis
  Distal gastric and afferent limb obstruction
  Pouch dilatation
  Gastric or jejunal ulcer
Small bowel obstruction
  Internal hernia
  Adhesions

Leakage

Leakage may occur from any stapled or sutured anastomosis, partition site, or area of channel reinforcement. The overall risk of leakage is higher in the morbidly obese than in the nonobese population [78]. Leaks are serious complications usually requiring urgent surgery. The incidence of leakage increases with gastric transections as opposed to stapling. Leaks usually occur at the anterior aspect of the staple or suture line and may be difficult to demonstrate with the patient in the supine position [74]. Abscesses may develop as a consequence of leakage. It may be impossible to perform CT because of weight limitations of the equipment, and ultrasonography has limitations in severe obesity. Nuclear scintigraphy may be used to identify abscesses in obese patients; in the early postoperative period, however, normal postsurgical sites will demonstrate increased uptake. To obtain an accurate assessment it is necessary to have a one-week interval from the time of surgery for leukocytes labeled with indium-111 (^{111}In) and a two-week interval for ^{67}[Ga] citrate, unless the site of abscess is remote from the surgical bed.

Pouch Perforation

Perforation of the gastric pouch may occur remote from staple lines or anastomoses. The etiology is unclear but has been attributed to hyperacidity, ischemia, and the use of large nasogastric tubes. The prophylactic use of medications that block or neutralize acid production is advocated to prevent this potential complication.

Staple Line Dehiscence

Early staple line dehiscence is generally attributed to technical failure (i.e., misfiring of the stapling device). Delayed dehiscence is due to staples pulling away from the wall of the stomach, which may be secondary to food impaction in the pouch (Figs. 3.73 and 3.74). For this reason, a diet of liquids only is recommended for 8 weeks following surgery. With partial suture line disruption, an additional channel or channels may form, and subsequent weight gain may ensue. With regard to gastroplasty, staple line dehiscence is more common with horizontal partitioning than with the vertical orientation.

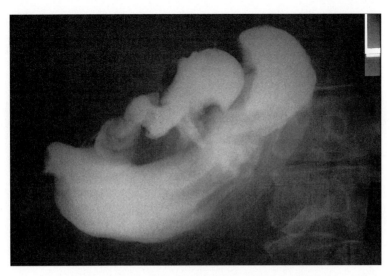

FIGURE 3.73. Gastric bypass with staple dehiscence. Film from an upper GI series showing contrast medium in the pouch and the stomach due to staple line dehiscence. Contrast should be seen only in the pouch and Roux-en-Y loop of jejunum.

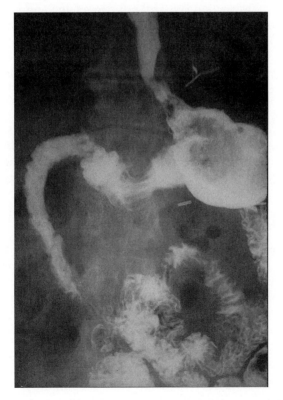

FIGURE 3.74. Gastric bypass with staple line dehiscence, pouch dilatation, and food impaction. Film from an upper GI series shows contrast in a dilated gastric pouch with impacted food and subsequent staple line dehiscence.

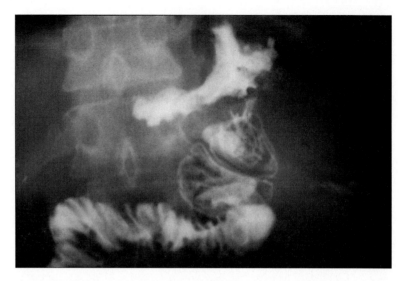

FIGURE 3.75. **Stricture at the anastomotic site after gastric bypass.** Contrast examination shows stricture at the anastomotic site and subsequent staple line dehiscence.

Channel Obstruction and Stenosis

Early channel obstruction is usually due to edema and is usually temporary. Late stenosis, or obstruction may be secondary to food impaction, fibrosis, or channel angulation (Fig. 3.75). Channel stenosis may in turn lead to vomiting and gastroesophageal reflux and/or secondary pouch dilatation and weight gain. Stenosis may be treated by endoscopic dilatation.

Channel Widening

After gastroplasty, channel widening may occur over time, possibly leading to weight gain. The incidence of channel widening has diminished with the standard channel reinforcements now in use and with the creation of smaller channels.

Pouch Dilatation

Pouch size may increase over time, and the change may be identified radiographically. Pouch dilatation may be a cause of weight gain. Numerical measurements of pouch size based on contrast studies have been generally abandoned because of unreliable data. Problems with data are related to difficulties associated with variable magnification and variable distensibility depending on patient cooperation.

Gastric Ulcers

Gastritis and gastric ulcers may rarely develop in the proximal gastric pouch. Gastric ulceration after GBP is a rare complication. Ulcers have also been reported to occur in the distal stomach and may lead to perforation (Fig. 3.76). The classic sign of free intraperitoneal air may not

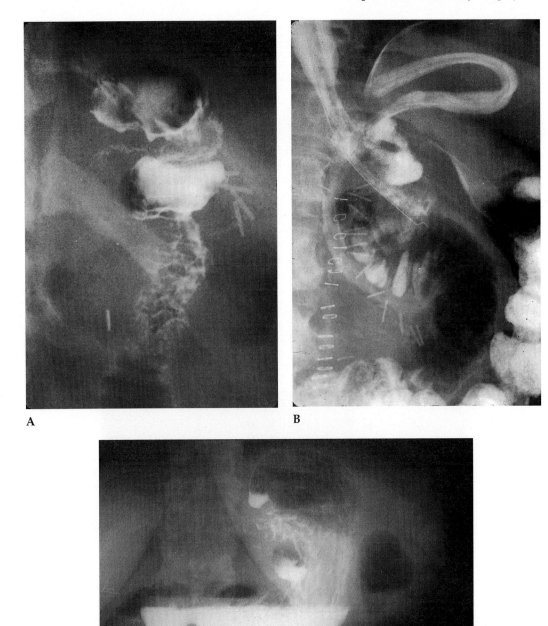

A

B

C

FIGURE 3.76. **Gastric bypass with gastric ulcers.** (A) Water-soluble contrast study shows a large ulcer at the anastomotic site after GBP. (B) Another patient with a perforated ulcer arising from the gastric remnant. (C) Staple line dehiscence and an ulcer on the lesser curvature of the stomach after GBP.

be identified in patients with perforated ulcers in the distal stomach, making the diagnosis more difficult.

Distal Gastric or Afferent Limb Obstruction

Obstruction of the distal stomach may occur after GBP or gastroplasty, and obstruction of the afferent limb may occur after GBP. In the early postoperative period, if a gastrostomy is in place, evaluation of the distal stomach is easily performed by injecting contrast medium into the gastrostomy tube. In the late postoperative period or if a gastrostomy is not present, CT imaging is the examination of choice, since following GBP, the distal stomach and afferent limb will not be visualized with a routine oral contrast examination, especially if a Roux-en-Y anastomosis is employed. Dilatation of the excluded stomach may be due to gastric atony, edema, or preferential filling of the afferent limb. CT imaging readily demonstrates a dilated stomach and/or A limb, although weight limitations of the scanner and/or size limitations of the gantry may render the use of this equipment unfeasible. A dilated excluded stomach could be confused with an abscess, and alternatively an abscess might be mistaken for a distended stomach. Rarely, perforation of the excluded distal stomach may occur secondary to severe dilatation or ulcer (Fig. 3.77).

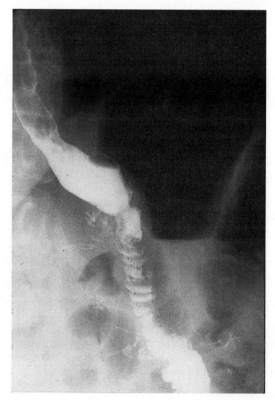

A

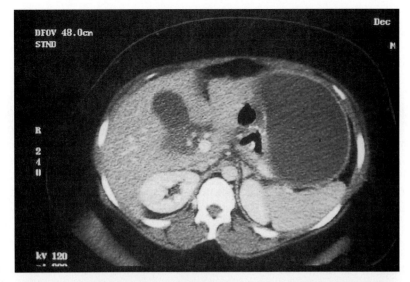

B

C

FIGURE 3.77. **Dilatation of the distal stomach after gastric bypass.** (A) Contrast study shows a dilated air- and fluid-filled bypassed portion of stomach. (B, C) CT scans on a different patient showing a markedly distended bypassed portion of stomach.

Indications for examination of the distal stomach include persistent nausea, vomiting, epigastric pain, and upper GI bleeding. Several percutaneous techniques for examination of the distal stomach have been described [75–77]. The distal stomach can be localized by using CT imaging, fluoroscopy in combination with [^{99}Tc] pertechnetate scanning, or sonography. In the technique described by McNeely et al., the patient is given [^{99m}Tc] pertechnetate and the stomach is visualized on the gamma camera and outlined on the skin with a cotton swab labeled with the isotope and an ink marker [77]. Some surgeons place clips on the greater and lesser curvatures of the antrum at the time of surgery. Assisted by previous barium studies, hemoclip markers, previous gastrostomy scarring, and the radionuclide localization, a 22-gauge needle is advanced under fluoroscopic guidance and water-soluble contrast medium is introduced to identify the stomach. When the needle is in good position, additional contrast medium is administered and spot films obtained. CT imaging and sonography have also been used to localize the distal stomach, and fluoroscopy proceeds once the needle is in place. Gastritis, inflammatory changes of the distal stomach, and ulcers may be identified with these techniques. Endoscopy can also be performed after GBP with a pediatric endoscope, although this procedure is technically difficult.

References

1. Schulman A. Anastomotic, gastrojejunal ulcer: Accuracy of radiological diagnosis in surgically proven cases. Br J Radiol 1971;44(522):422–433.
2. Gabrielsson N. Gastric ulceration revealed only by gastrophotography. Acta Radiol Diagn (Stockh) 1972;12(1):59–68.
3. Gold RP, Seaman WB. The primary double-contrast examination of the postoperative stomach. Radiology 1977;124(2):297–305.
4. Ominsky SH, Moss AA. The postoperative stomach: A comparative study of double-contrast barium examinations and endoscopy. Gastrointest Radiol 1979;4(1):17–21.
5. Gohel VK, Laufer I. Double-contrast examination of the postoperative stomach. Radiology 1978;129(3):601–607.
6. Ott DJ, Munitz HA, Gelfand DW, Lane TG, Wu WC. The sensitivity of radiography of the postoperative stomach. Radiology 1982;144(4):741–743.
7. Jordan Jr PH. Elective operations for duodenal ulcer. N Engl J Med 1972;287(26):1329–1337.
8. Burhenne HJ. Roentgen anatomy and terminology of gastric surgery. Am J Roentgenol Radium Ther Nucl Med 1964;91(4):731–743.
9. Fisher MS. The Hofmeister defect: A normal change in the postoperative stomach. AJR Am J Roentgenol 1965;84(6):1082–1086.
10. Smith C, Gardiner R. Postoperative stomach and recurrent abdominal pain. In: Thompson W, ed. Common Problems in Gastrointestinal Radiology. Chicago: Year Book Medical; 1989:202–211.
11. Bloch C, Wolf BS. The gastroduodenal channel after pyloroplasty and vagotomy: A cineradiographic study. Radiology 1965;84:43–51.
12. Burrell M, Curtis AM. Sequelae of stomach surgery. CRC Crit Rev Diagn Imaging 1977;10(1):17–97.

13. Toye DK, Hutton JF, Williams JA. Radiological anatomy after pyloroplasty. Gut 1970;11(4):358–362.
14. Burhenne HJ. Postoperative defects of the stomach. Semin Roentgenol 1971;6(2):182–192.
15. Jay BS, Burrell M. Iatrogenic problems following gastric surgery. Gastrointest Radiol 1977;2(3):239–257.
16. Burhenne HJ. The retained gastric antrum. Preoperative roentgenologic diagnosis of an iatrogenic syndrome. Am J Roentgenol Radium Ther Nucl Med 1967;101(2):459–467.
17. Beneventano TC, Glotzer P, Messinger NH. The radiology corner. Retained gastric antrum. Am J Gastroenterol 1973;59(4):361–365.
18. Safaie-Shirazi S, Chaudhuri TK, Condon RE. Visualization of isolated retained antrum by using technetium-99m. Surgery 1973;73(2):278–283.
19. Kobayashi S, Prolla JC, Kirsner JB. Late gastric carcinoma developing after surgery for benign conditions. Endoscopic and histologic studies of the anastomosis and diagnostic problems. Am J Dig Dis 1970;15(10):905–912.
20. Feldman F, Seaman WB. Primary gastric stump cancer. Am J Roentgenol Radium Ther Nucl Med 1972;115(2):257–267.
21. Gueller R, Shapiro HA, Nelson JA, Bush R. Suture granulomas simulating tumors: A preventable postgastrectomy complication. Am J Dig Dis 1976;21(3):223–228.
22. Segal AW, Bank S, Marks IN, Rubinstein Z. Bezoars occurring in the gastric remnant after gastrectomy. S Afr Med J 1970;44(41):1176–1180.
23. Szemes GC, Amberg JR. Gastric bezoars after partial gastrectomy. Radiology 1968;90(4):765–768.
24. Strom BG, Beaudry R, Morin F. Yeast overgrowth in operated stomachs. J Can Assoc Radiol 1978;29(3):161–164.
25. Perttala Y, Peltokallio P, Leiviska T, Sipponen J. Yeast bezoar formation following gastric surgery. Am J Roentgenol Radium Ther Nucl Med 1975;125(2):365–373.
26. Licht M, Gold BM, Katz DS. Obstructing small-bowel bezoar: Diagnosis using CT. AJR Am J Roentgenol 1999;173(2):500–501.
27. Bradford JB, Boggs JE. Jejunogastric intussusception—An unusual complication of gastric surgery. Arch Surg 1958;77:201.
28. Seaman WB. Prolapsed gastric mucosa through a gastrojejunostomy. Am J Roentgenol Radium Ther Nucl Med 1970;110(2):304–314.
29. Chaimoff C, Dintsman M, Tiqva P. The long-term fate of patients with dumping syndrome. Arch Surg 1972;105(4):554–556.
30. Gale ME, Gerzof SG, Kiser LC, Snider JM, Stavis DM, Larsen CR, et al. CT appearance of afferent loop obstruction. AJR Am J Roentgenol 1982;138(6):1085–1088.
31. Thomas JL, Cowan RJ, Maynard CD, Wu W. Radionuclide demonstration of small-bowel anatomy in the afferent-loop syndrome: Case report. J Nucl Med 1977;18(9):896–897.
32. Lewicki AM, Kleinhaus U, Brooks JR, Membreno AA. The small bowel following pyloroplasty and vagotomy. Radiology 1973;109(3):539–544.
33. Bar-Natan M, Larson GM, Stephens G, Massey T. Delayed gastric emptying after gastric surgery. Am J Surg 1996;172(1):24–28.
34. Fich A, Neri M, Camilleri M, Kelly KA, Phillips SF. Stasis syndromes following gastric surgery: Clinical and motility features of 60 symptomatic patients. J Clin Gastroenterol 1990;12(5):505–512.
35. Levine MS, Fisher AR, Rubesin SE, Laufer I, Herlinger H, Rosato EF. Complications after total gastrectomy and esophagojejunostomy: Radiologic evaluation. AJR Am J Roentgenol 1991;157(6):1189–1194.

36. Ansel HJ, Wasserman NF. Postsplenectomy gastric deformity. AJR Am J Roentgenol 1982;139(1):99–101.
37. Strasberg SM, Drebin JA, Soper NJ. Evolution and current status of the Whipple procedure: An update for gastroenterologists. Gastroenterology 1997;113(3):983–994.
38. McGrath PC, Sloan DA, Kenady DE. Surgical management of pancreatic carcinoma. Semin Oncol 1996;23(2):200–212.
39. Furukawa H, Kosuge T, Shimada K, Yamamoto J, Ushio K. Helical CT of the abdomen after pancreaticoduodenectomy: Usefulness for detecting postoperative complications. Hepatogastroenterology 1997;44(15):849–855.
40. Lepanto L, Gianfelice D, Dery R, Dagenais M, Lapointe R, Roy A. Postoperative changes, complications, and recurrent disease after Whipple's operation: CT features. AJR Am J Roentgenol 1994;163(4):841–846.
41. Coombs RJ, Zeiss J, Howard JM, Thomford NR, Merrick HW. CT of the abdomen after the Whipple procedure: Value in depicting postoperative anatomy, surgical complications, and tumor recurrence. AJR Am J Roentgenol 1990;154(5):1011–1014.
42. Bluemke DA, Fishman EK, Kuhlman J. CT evaluation following Whipple procedure: Potential pitfalls in interpretation. J Comput Assist Tomogr 1992;16(5):704–708.
43. Bluemke DA, Abrams RA, Yeo CJ, Cameron JL, Fishman EK. Recurrent pancreatic adenocarcinoma: Spiral CT evaluation following the Whipple procedure. Radiographics 1997;17(2):303–313.
44. Tamm EP, Jones B, Yeo CJ, Maher MM, Cameron JL. Pancreaticogastrostomy and the Whipple procedure: Radiographic appearance and complications. Radiology 1995;196(1):251–255.
45. Trerotola SO, Jones B, Crist DW, Cameron JL. Pylorus-preserving Whipple pancreaticoduodenectomy: Postoperative evaluation. Radiology 1989;171(3):735–738.
46. Saini S, Mueller PR, Gaa J, Briggs SE, Hahn PF, Forman BH, et al. Percutaneous gastrostomy with gastropexy: Experience in 125 patients. AJR Am J Roentgenol 1990;154(5):1003–1006.
47. De Baere T, Chapot R, Kuoch V, Chevallier P, Delille JP, Domenge C, et al. Percutaneous gastrostomy with fluoroscopic guidance: Single-center experience in 500 consecutive cancer patients. Radiology 1999;210(3):651–654.
48. Dewald CL, Hiette PO, Sewall LE, Fredenberg PG, Palestrant AM. Percutaneous gastrostomy and gastrojejunostomy with gastropexy: Experience in 701 procedures. Radiology 1999;211(3):651–656.
49. Halkier BK, Ho CS, Yee AC. Percutaneous feeding gastrostomy with the Seldinger technique: Review of 252 patients. Radiology 1989;171(2):359–362.
50. Ponsky JL, Gauderer MW. Percutaneous endoscopic gastrostomy: A nonoperative technique for feeding gastrostomy. Gastrointest Endosc 1981;27(1):9–11.
51. Preshaw RM. A percutaneous method for inserting a feeding gastrostomy tube. Surg Gynecol Obstet 1981;152(5):658–660.
52. Brown AS, Mueller PR, Ferrucci Jr JT. Controlled percutaneous gastrostomy: Nylon T-fastener for fixation of the anterior gastric wall. Radiology 1986;158(2):543–545.
53. Szymski GX, Albazzaz AN, Funaki B, Rosenblum JD, Hackworth CA, Zernich BW, et al. Radiologically guided placement of pull-type gastrostomy tubes. Radiology 1997;205(3):669–673.
54. Vade A, Jafri SZ, Agha FP, Vidyasagar MS, Coran AG. Radiologic evaluation of gastrostomy complications. AJR Am J Roentgenol 1983;141(2):325–330.

55. Wolf EL, Frager D, Beneventano TC. Radiologic demonstration of important gastrostomy tube complications. Gastrointest Radiol 1986;11(1):20–26.

56. Connar RG, Sealy WC. Gastrostomy and its complications. Ann Surg 1956;143(2):245–250.

57. Wollman B, D'Agostino HB, Walus-Wigle JR, Easter DW, Beale A. Radiologic, endoscopic, and surgical gastrostomy: An institutional evaluation and meta-analysis of the literature. Radiology 1995;197(3):699–704.

58. Holder TM, Leape LL, Ashcraft KW. Gastrostomy: Its use and dangers in pediatric patients. N Engl J Med 1972;286(25):1345–1347.

59. Gallagher MW, Tyson KR, Ashcraft KW. Gastrostomy in pediatric patients: An analysis of complications and techniques. Surgery 1973;74(4):536–539.

60. Campbell JR, Sasaki TM. Gastrostomy in infants and children: An analysis of complications and techniques. Am Surg 1974;40(9):505–508.

61. Haws EB, Sieber WK, Kiesewetter WB. Complications of tube gastrostomy in infants and children. 15-year review of 240 cases. Ann Surg 1966;164(2):284–290.

62. Hammerman AM, Shady K, Fry R, Cohen E. Postgastrostomy tube deformity on upper GI series. Gastrointest Radiol 1991;16(1):13–14.

63. Balthazar EJ. Radiographic examination of the stomach following surgery for pancreatic pseudocyst. A source of diagnostic error. Gastrointest Radiol 1979;4(1):23–28.

64. Linner JH. Overview of surgical techniques for the treatment of morbid obesity. Gastroenterol Clin North Am 1987;16(2):253–272.

65. Mason EE, Ito C. Gastric bypass in obesity. Surg Clin North Am 1967;47(6):1345–1351.

66. Griffen Jr WO, Young VL, Stevenson CC. A prospective comparison of gastric and jejunoileal bypass procedures for morbid obesity. Ann Surg 1977;186(4):500–509.

67. Wilkinson LH, Peloso OA. Gastric (reservoir) reduction for morbid obesity. Arch Surg 1981;116(5):602–605.

68. Hainaux B, Coppens E, Sattari A, Vertruyen M, Hubloux G, Cadiere GB. Laparoscopic adjustable silicone gastric banding: Radiological appearances of a new surgical treatment for morbid obesity. Abdom Imaging 1999;24(6):533–537.

69. Wiesner W, Schob O, Hauser RS, Hauser M. Adjustable laparoscopic gastric banding in patients with morbid obesity: Radiographic management, results, and postoperative complications. Radiology 2000;216(2):389–394.

70. Szucs RA, Turner MA, Kellum JM, DeMaria EJ, Sugerman HJ. Adjustable laparoscopic gastric band for the treatment of morbid obesity: Radiologic evaluation. AJR Am J Roentgenol 1998;170(4):993–996.

71. Edell SL, Wills JS, Garren LR, Garren ML. Radiographic evaluation of the Garren gastric bubble. AJR Am J Roentgenol 1985;145(1):49–50.

72. Smith C, Gardiner R, Kubicka RA, Dieschbourg JJ. Gastric restrictive surgery for obesity: Early radiologic evaluation. Radiology 1984;153(2):321–327.

73. Baer JW. Radiology of obesity surgery. Gastroenterol Clin North Am 1987;16(2):349–375.

74. Smith C, Gardiner R, Kubicka RA, Dieschbourg JJ. Radiology of gastric restrictive surgery. Radiographics 1985;5(2):193–216.

75. Zingas AP, Amin KA, Loredo RD, Kling GA. Computed tomographic evaluation of the excluded stomach in gastric bypass. J Comput Tomogr 1984;8(3):231–236.

76. Barmeir EP, Solomon H, Charuzi I, Hirsch M. Radiologic assessment of the distal stomach and duodenum after gastric bypass: Percutaneous CT-guided transcatheter technique. Gastrointest Radiol 1984;9(3):203–205.

77. McNeely GF, Kinard RE, Macgregor AM, Kniffen JC. Percutaneous contrast examination of the stomach after gastric bypass. AJR Am J Roentgenol 1987;149(5):928–930.

78. Moody FG, McGreevy JM. Complications of gastric surgery. In: Greenheld LJ, ed. Complications in Surgery and Trauma. Philadelphia: JB Lippincott, 1990.

4

The Biliary Tree

Gallstones and associated biliary tract disorders are commonly encountered problems. Approximately 10 to 15% of the adult population has gallstones, and each year about 1% of this group will develop complications, often requiring surgery.

Cholecystectomy

Cholecystectomy is the most commonly performed general surgical procedure in the United States. Approximately 600,000 cholecystectomies are performed each year, and the number has been increasing with the advent of laparoscopic cholecystectomy. Indications for cholecystectomy include acute and chronic calculous and acalculous cholecystitis, symptomatic gallstones, gallstone pancreatitis, gallbladder polyps, porcelain gallbladder, gallstones in patients with sickle cell disease, and large gallstones (>3 cm) [1].

Cholecystectomy was first performed in 1882 and has traditionally been done by the conventional open technique. Laparoscopic cholecystectomy (LC) was developed in 1987 and has become the surgical procedure of choice, now being employed in over 80% of cases. The advantages of LC over open cholecystectomy include a significant reduction in hospitalization time and recovery period, less pain, and minimal scarring. Overall postoperative complications rates for LC are comparable to those for open cholecystectomy, although there is a slightly higher incidence of biliary injury with LC. Contraindications to LC include peritonitis, sepsis, bowel distention, and advanced pregnancy. Some surgeons would prefer open cholecystectomy in cases of acute cholecystitis, cholangitis, common duct stones, acute pancreatitis, previous upper abdominal surgery, morbid obesity, and portal hypertension [1].

Laparoscopic cholecystectomy is performed under general anesthesia by specialized surgical instruments placed through four trocars placed through the abdominal wall (Fig. 4.1). The surgery is done with visualization of the surgical field on a video monitor.

Complications of laparoscopy in general differ somewhat from those encountered with standard laparotomy and usually occur secondary to trauma from the trocar insertions. These include abdominal wall and omental bleeding, abdominal and retroperitoneal injury, gastrointestinal and bladder perforation, solid visceral injury, and hernias at the trocar incision sites. Rarely, implantation of tumor cells into the abdominal wall at the port sites can occur in patients with unsuspected gallbladder carcinoma [2].

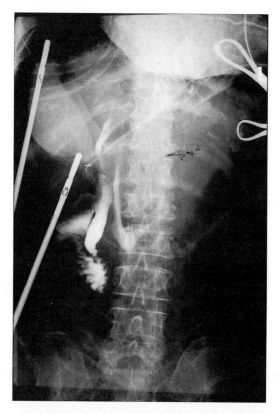

FIGURE 4.1. **Intraoperative cholangiogram during laparoscopic cholecystectomy.** Supine view of the abdomen at the time of laparoscopic cholecystectomy with contrast medium injected into the biliary tree shows the trocars used for this procedure. A large amount of intraperitoneal air is introduced during surgery.

Normal Postcholecystectomy Appearance

The normal postcholecystectomy findings have been investigated using sonography and computed tomography (CT) [3–6]. Small amounts of fluid in the gallbladder fossa are commonly identified in the gallbladder bed on CT images and sonograms and may be seen up to at least 5 days after surgery (Fig. 4.2). The fluid should be only minimal in amount and poorly circumscribed, without distinct or bulging contours [7]. Fluid in the gallbladder fossa is generally considered to be due partly to small accumulations of bile that resolve spontaneously. Such fluid may result from interruption of accessory cystohepatic ducts, which are persistent embryological remnants between the liver and the biliary system, usually involving the gallbladder, found in approximately 30% of the population. One type of

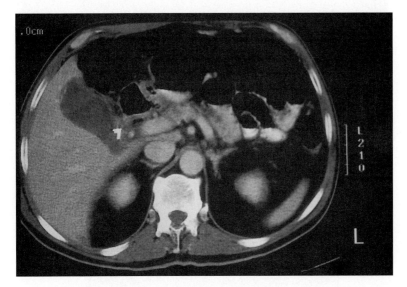

FIGURE 4.2. **Normal postcholecystectomy CT appearance.** CT scan through the upper abdomen shows fluid in the gallbladder fossa after cholecystectomy. Fluid may be observed normally for up to at least 5 days after surgery.

cystohepatic duct; the duct of Luschka, is a persistent congenital con-
nection between the biliary ducts in the right lobe of the liver and the
gallbladder (Figs. 4.3 and 4.4) [8]. In one study, extrabiliary accumulation of radiotracer was identified in 44% of patients who had
hepatobiliary scintigraphic (DISIDA) scanning 2 to 4 hours after open
cholecystectomy, but only one patient developed a clinically significant
bile leak [9]. This suggests, as other have speculated, that some cystic
duct leaks heal spontaneously and some small leaks go undetected [7].
After cholecystectomy, no distinct or well-marginated fluid collections
should be found in the gallbladder fossa, and the presence of such
(the "pseudogallbladder sign"), or increasing fluid collections, should

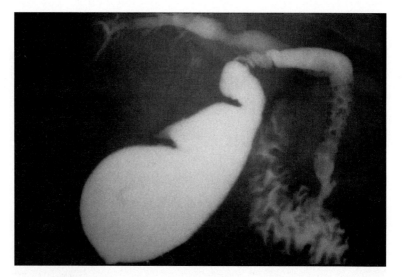

FIGURE 4.3. Duct of Luschka. Cholecystostomy study demonstrates a short
tubular structure extending from the superior aspect of the gallbladder extending toward the liver.

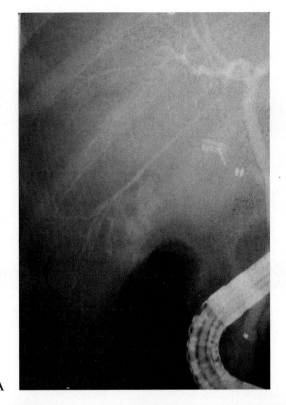

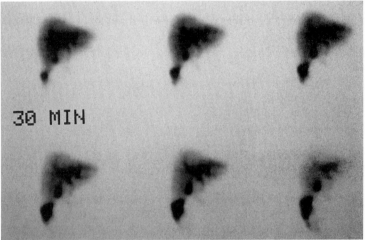

FIGURE 4.4. **Leak from duct of Luschka.** (A) Film from an ERCP demonstrates extraluminal contrast medium extending from peripheral ducts at the edge of the liver. (B) DISIDA scan in the same patient showing radioactive tracer in the same location.

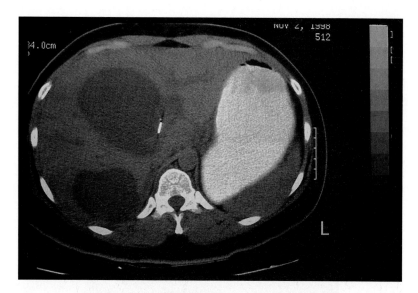

FIGURE 4.5. Biliary intravenous leak with "pseudogallbladder sign." CT scan
of the upper abdomen without contrast medium, shows a large fluid collection
with bulging contours in the gallbladder fossa. Fluid is also present in the right
subhepatic space.

suggest a biliary leak or biloma (Fig. 4.5). Subhepatic fluid collections
have been identified by sonography in 20% of asymptomatic patients
after open cholecystectomy [10]. The fluid may consist of bile, blood,
serous fluid, or lymph, owing to oozing from surgical trauma from
patients with gallbladders partially or completely intrahepatic or
adherent to the liver due to chronic cholecystitis. The persistence of this
material depends on the efficiency of peritoneal absorption and the
external drainage provided.

The use of Penrose drains is controversial, but subhepatic fluid collections have been demonstrated in only 5% of patients after open
cholecystectomy with drains as opposed to 20% without them [11].
Small amounts of pelvic or intra-abdominal fluid may also be observed
normally following LC. Small amounts of free intraperitoneal air
are commonly identified after LC, since carbon dioxide is introduced
into the peritoneal cavity during surgery. The gas is usually rapidly
absorbed. Subcutaneous emphysema, due to dissection of carbon
dioxide around the trocar sites, is also commonly identified (Fig. 4.6).

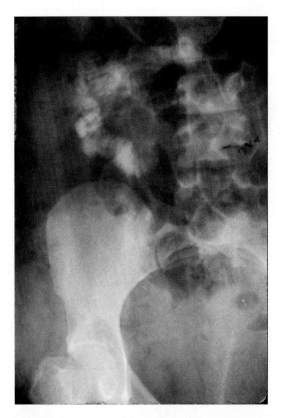

FIGURE 4.6. Subcutaneous emphysema after laparoscopic cholecystectomy. Supine view of the abdomen after laparoscopic cholecystectomy shows subcutaneous emphysema in the lateral abdominal wall.

Complications of Cholecystectomy

The reported overall complication rate after cholecystectomy ranges from 4.5 to 21% [12–15]. There is an increase in the rate of complications with increasing age. Complications of cholecystectomy are listed in Table 4.1. Imaging studies play a crucial role in delineating and defining the complications of cholecystectomy [3,6,7,16–22]. In recent series of LCs, bile duct injuries, the most serious complication reportedly occurred with an incidence of approximately 0.5% [23,24]. The incidence of bile duct injury is slightly higher with LC than with conventional cholecystectomy, with a complication rate of 0.1 to 0.2% [25]. The actual incidence of biliary complications after LC may be underestimated, however, since up to 40% of postoperative biliary strictures

TABLE 4.1 Complications of cholecystectomy.

Bile duct injury
  Leak
  Stricture
Biliary obstruction
Biloma
Bile peritonitis
Biliary cutaneous fistula
Choledocholithiasis
Retained calculi in cystic duct remnant
Dropped stones
Abscess
Intrahepatic ductal rupture and ectasia
Hemorrhage
Drainage tube problems
Pancreatitis
Neuroma
Choledochoduodenal fistula

may not develop until 6 months to 25 years after surgery. In addition, if patient selection is considered, the incidence of biliary injury with LC may actually be higher than it is with open cholecystectomy since the more complicated cases usually are performed by the open method. Since the greatest number of complications generally is observed during the learning curve for the procedure, the surgeon who lacks experience may have a higher complication rate [23,26]. It is suggested that bile duct injury may be less likely if intraoperative cholangiography is performed during LC [27]. Intraoperative cholangiography is more difficult to perform laparoscopically than open and has a higher failure rate [28]. Some surgeons perform intraoperative cholangiography routinely, while others do it selectively or rarely.

Bile Duct Injuries

The most common site of injury during cholecystectomy is the common hepatic duct followed by, in decreasing order, the common bile duct, the ductal confluence, the right hepatic duct, and the left hepatic duct [29]. The bile ducts can be injured as a result of ligation, laceration, or resection, potentially causing biliary leak, obstruction, or stricture. The most common cause of biliary leak following LC is leakage from the cystic duct remnant (Fig. 4.7). During cholecystectomy the cystic duct is ligated with clips or sutures. The clips or knot may become dislodged, may be loose or improperly placed, or may cause necrosis of the cystic duct remnant and a subsequent leak, perhaps leading to the

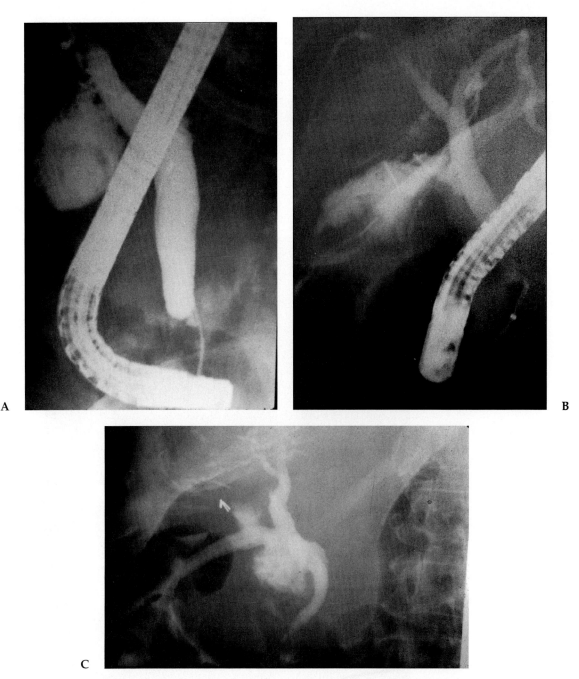

FIGURE 4.7. **Leaks from cystic duct remnant after laparoscopic cholecystectomy.** (A) Film from an ERCP demonstrating contrast medium in the gallbladder bed secondary to leak from the cystic duct remnant. (B) Another patient with contrast medium accumulating in the gallbladder bed and the subhepatic space. (C) Another patient with contrast medium accumulating in the gallbladder bed, subhepatic space, and peritoneal cavity.

development of a biloma and/or bile peritonitis. If distal bile duct obstruction is present from overlooked common bile duct (CBD) stones or stricture, the leak will be aggravated (Figs. 4.8 and 4.9). Hepatobiliary scintigraphy is useful in the evaluation of a suspected biliary leak and has the advantage of being noninvasive [30]. The site of leakage and the presence of retained stones or distal strictures can be more definitively identified by endoscopic retrograde cholangiopancreatography (ERCP). In uncomplicated cases of leakage from the cystic duct remnant, treatment with an endoscopically placed biliary stent is usually successful.

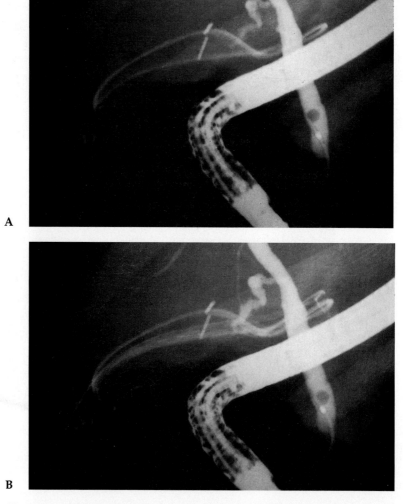

A

B

FIGURE 4.8. **Leak from cystic duct remnant with CBD stone.** (A) Postoperative ERCP film from a recent cholecystectomy showing extraluminal contrast medium extending from the cystic duct remnant. A stone is present with CBD. (B) Same patient showing contrast medium accumulating in the drain.

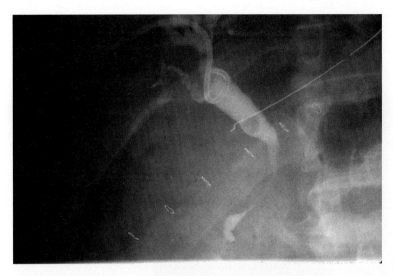

FIGURE 4.9. **Leak from cystic duct remnant with choledocholithiasis and CBD stricture.** Cholangiogram performed via an external biliary drainage catheter shows leakage of contrast medium from the cystic duct remnant, a stone in the CBD, and a stricture of the distal CBD due to pancreatitis.

Biliary leakage may also be secondary to inadvertent transection of the common duct or an accessory bile duct. Transection of the common duct can occur if a segment of the common hepatic duct is mistaken for the cystic duct and is excised along with the gallbladder (Fig. 4.10). Under this circumstance, the proximal duct lies free and the distal portion is clipped. ERCP will demonstrate only the distal portion of the distal system (Fig. 4.11) Percutaneous transhepatic cholangiography

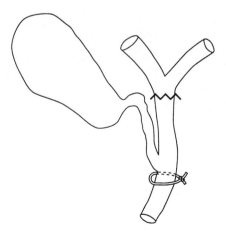

FIGURE 4.10. **Common duct injury.** The common duct was mistaken for the cystic duct and excised along with the gallbladder.

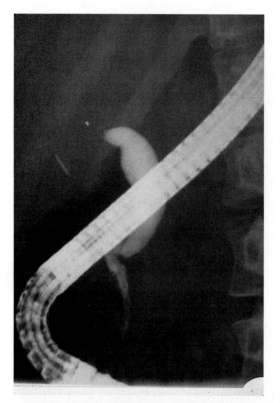

A

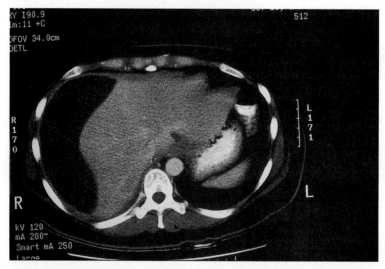

B

FIGURE 4.11. **Common duct injury.** (A) Film from an ERCP shows the common duct to be clipped. (B, C) CT scan on the same patient demonstrates fluid due to bile leak from the proximal duct in the gallbladder fossa and subhepatic and right subphrenic spaces. (D) Sonogram in the same patient showing the fluid collection in the gallbladder bed. (E) Filling of the collection with communication to the biliary tree in the same patient upon injection of contrast medium via and drainage catheter.

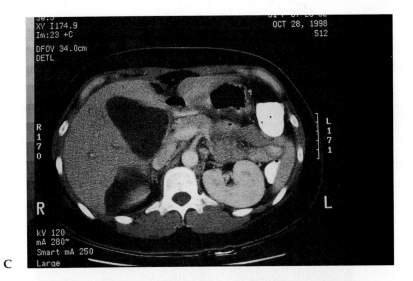

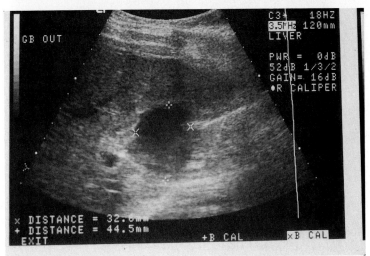

FIGURE 4.11. (*Continued*)

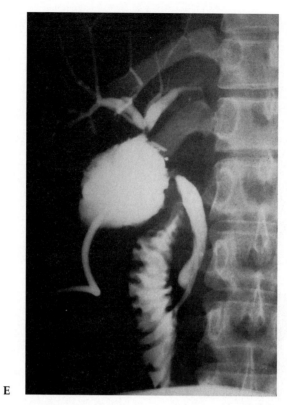

E

FIGURE 4.11. (*Continued*)

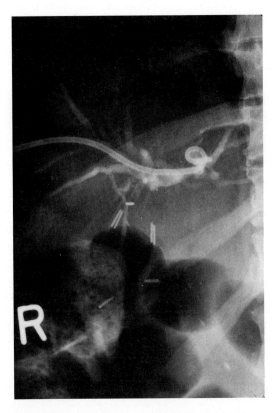

FIGURE 4.12. **Biliary injury.** Film from a cholangiogram via an external biliary drainage catheter reveals obstruction at the level of the bifurcation of the left and right intrahepatic ducts due to bile duct injury during cholecystectomy.

(PTC) is generally necessary to identify the proximal ducts and to provide important information for planning therapy (Fig. 4.12). Inadequate identification of the junction of the cystic duct and common duct may lead to tenting, ligation, or partial excision of a segment of common duct when the gallbladder is removed [31]. Simple lacerations can be successfully repaired after conversion to open technique. These injuries to the common duct occur more frequently with LC than with conventional cholecystectomy because visualization of the portal triad is more limited with LC. Deziel and others state that bile duct injuries during LC are best avoided by maintaining a low threshold for conversion to open cholecystectomy in cases where the anatomy cannot be precisely delineated [24]. Unrecognized Mirizzi syndrome can also lead to inadvertent ligation of the common bile duct.

Moossa et al. [25] identified four ways in which the bile duct may be injured at the time of cholecystectomy:

Ligating or transecting the wrong duct

Occluding the lumen of the common duct during "flush ligation" of the cystic duct

Excessive dissection to "expose" the common duct, with compromise of the blood supply and subsequent ischemic stricture

Trauma to the common duct during common duct exploration by forceful manipulation or "dilatation"

Common duct perforation may occur secondary to technical problems during T-tube placement. Blind clamping of bleeding vessels may lead to common duct injury as well.

Anatomic variants are commonly found in the biliary tree, some of which predispose patients to bile duct injury. An accessory right hepatic duct, coursing along the gallbladder fossa draining into the extrahepatic biliary tree or cystic duct, is present in approximately 2 to 3% of the population. Anomalous ducts may be ligated, transected, or torn during extraction of the gallbladder, and subsequent bile leakage may ensue. Such anomalies may not be appreciated at the time of surgery, particularly if inflammatory changes are present. Since there is less exposure of the common duct with LC than with open cholecystectomy, there is an increased risk of this type of injury. For this reason, as well as others, some advocate preoperative ERCP, magnetic resonance cholangiopancreatography (MRCP), or intraoperative cholangiography to identify any unusual anatomical features.

Clinically, bile leaks usually present with shoulder pain, abdominal pain, bloating, leukocytosis, and fever with mildly elevated bilirubin and transaminase levels, or bilious drainage from a drain, if present. Bile collections usually accumulate in the gallbladder fossa and in the subhepatic and right subphrenic spaces, but bile can accumulate in other locations as well, such as the cul-de-sac.

"Biloma" is the term used to describe an encapsulated bile collection. Biloma may be treated with percutaneous drainage. Bile peritonitis, which may result when bile leakage is rapid and not contained by peritoneal adhesions, can be a cause of postoperative mortality [20]. Bile increases the permeability of the peritoneum and causes exudation of fluid, which if not recognized and treated may lead to fluid and electrolyte imbalance, hypotension, and oliguria. Bile peritonitis may be identified on CT imaging by ascites associated with engorged mesenteric vessels and diffuse inflammatory changes [32]. CT imaging and sonography are sensitive for identification of fluid collections; however they cannot usually differentiate between a postoperative seroma, lymphocele, hematoma, abscess, or bile leak, and CT and sonography are unable to determine the precise site of leakage in most cases (Fig. 4.13). Hepatobiliary scintigraphy is specific for bile leak, demonstrating the so-called choleperitoneum unless the leak has sealed at the time of the study, but owing to poor anatomic resolution it is not precise in determining the site of leakage (Fig. 4.14). ERCP is generally necessary for this purpose.

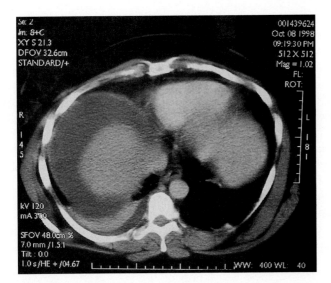

FIGURE 4.13. **Biliary leak.** CT scan of the upper abdomen shows fluid around the liver from biliary leak. The exact etiology cannot be determined on CT imaging.

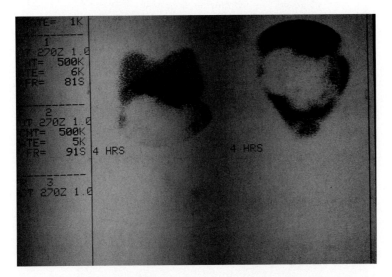

FIGURE 4.14. **Biliary leak on DISIDA scan: "choleperitoneum."** Radiotracer is seen to accumulate in the peritoneal cavity in this patient with a biliary leak.

Biliary obstruction may develop if the common duct is ligated but not transected (Fig. 4.15). These patients will present with progressive obstructive jaundice. Postoperative jaundice may be secondary to ligated ducts, retained stones, or biliary leak with peritoneal absorption of bile. Differentiation of these conditions can be made by ERCP, or ERCP in combination with CT or radionuclide scintigraphy. The consequences of ligation of an aberrant duct will depend on the volume of liver parenchyma drained by the duct. An aberrant right hepatic duct is the most common biliary anomaly [33]. If the segment is small and there is normal liver function, jaundice is unlikely but cholangitis may occur, and isolated dilatation of the posterior segment of the right lobe (usually segment VI) may be identified. In chronic obstruction, segmental biliary cirrhosis may develop along with segmental atrophy. Recognition of a ligated aberrant right hepatic duct can be difficult on cholangiography on account of underfilling.

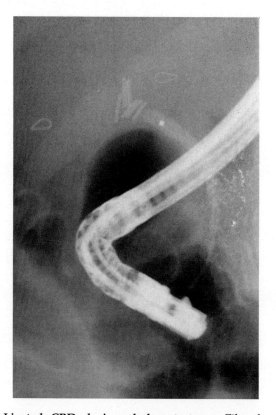

FIGURE 4.15. Ligated CBD during cholecystectomy. Film from an ERCP demonstrates abrupt termination of the common duct at the level of the clips due to inadvertent ligation of the duct during cholecystectomy.

Biliary Stricture

Biliary strictures occur in approximately 0.5 to 1% of open cholecystectomies (Fig. 4.16) [17]. Injury during cholecystectomy is the most common cause of a benign biliary stricture of the extrahepatic system. Since strictures are often not clinically apparent until months or years after surgery, their incidence with LC is not yet determined. Strictures tend to develop when the cystic duct is clamped or ligated near the junction with the common duct, and a portion of the wall of the common duct is included in the clips or subjected to trauma, with subsequent scarring. Patients with short cystic ducts are prone to this

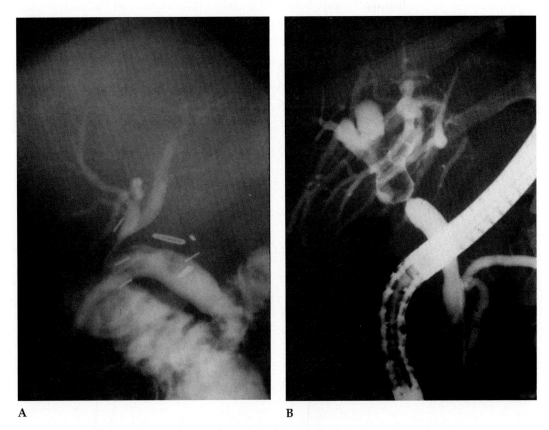

A   B

FIGURE 4.16. **Biliary stricture after cholecystectomy.** (A) Film from a cholangiogram demonstrates a focal stricture in the proximal hepatic duct from injury at the time of cholecystectomy. (B) An ERCP from another patient showing a stricture in a similar location with proximal calculi.

complication. With the progression of fibrosis and scarring, luminal narrowing develops and an elevated alkaline phosphatase level ensues, followed by jaundice. Thermal injury from cautery or laser may also cause stricture formation. The usual presentation is 3 to 10 years after surgery. Surgical repair is often unsuccessful. The success rate is related to the level of stricture, the number of previous repairs, and the type of surgical reconstruction. The prognosis is worse for high strictures. Biliary strictures may be treated with balloon dilatation in some cases. The earlier the treatment is performed, the better is the prognosis. Stenting after balloon dilatation is controversial [34]. The long-term patency of biliary strictures treated with balloon dilatation is 65 to 75% which is comparable to the results of surgical repair [28,35].

Bile duct injuries are categorized according to the Bismuth classification (Fig. 4.17). Originally used to describe only the level of a stric-

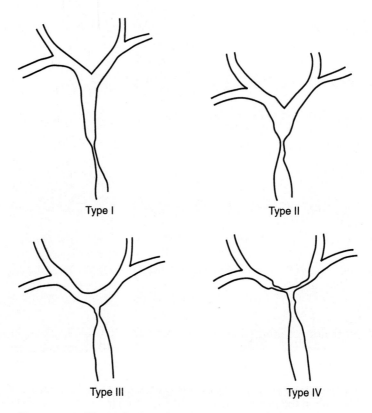

FIGURE 4.17. Bismuth classification of bile duct stricture/injury.

ture, this classification is now commonly used to describe any biliary injury, including stricture, transection, tear, and ligation. Bismuth type I strictures involve the distal common bile duct in which the length of the duct proximal to the stricture is greater than 2 cm. In type II, the proximal duct is less than 2 cm. In type III there is a high hilar stricture, and in type IV the stricture extends to involve the bifurcation into the main left and right ducts. In patients with high ductal injuries PTC may be necessary to identify the proximal extent of the injury or stricture. The prognosis is poorer for high strictures (Bismuth III and IV). High injuries are usually inflicted during cholecystectomy (open or LC), while the low injuries usually occur during common duct exploration. Bismuth type II, III, and IV strictures require a hepatojejunostomy if surgical repair is necessary.

Choledocholithiasis

The incidence of choledocholithiasis in patients with gallstones is approximately 10 to 15%. In patients undergoing LC, common duct stones should generally be removed preoperatively by endoscopic means, since removal at the time of laparoscopic surgery is often difficult or not possible. Those at highest risk for the presence choledocholithiasis are those with biliary dilatation (CBD >8 mm on sonography) elevated bilirubin, or cholangitis. With modern ultrasound equipment and techniques, common duct stones can be identified in 70 to 90% of patients, depending on stone location. Common duct stones may be primary or secondary. Primary common duct stones are formed in the duct itself, whereas secondary stones are formed in the gallbladder and migrate into the common duct. Although an answer may not be found, it is important to try to determine whether stones are primary or secondary because the therapeutic implications may be different. In general, primary stones are softer, less well formed, and darker than retained stones [36]. Stasis is usually necessary for secondary stones to form, so it is necessary to perform a sphincteroplasty or choledochoduodenostomy on these patients in addition to stone removal.

Choledocholithiasis is considered to be a complication of cholecystectomy if not recognized at the time of surgery (Fig. 4.18). Approximately 2 to 5% of postcholecystectomy patients will develop symptoms due to choledocholithiasis, most of which are retained calculi. Symptoms may be immediate or delayed up to months or years after surgery. Choledocholithiasis is a common cause of jaundice after

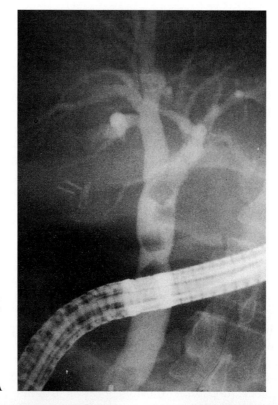

A

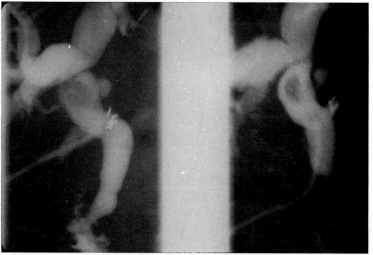

B

FIGURE **4.18. Retained common duct stones.** (A) Film from on ERCP demon-strates biliary dilatation with multiple stones in the common duct after chole-cystectomy. (B) T-tube cholangiogram on another patient after cholecystectomy shows a retained stone in the common hepatic duct and biliary dilatation.

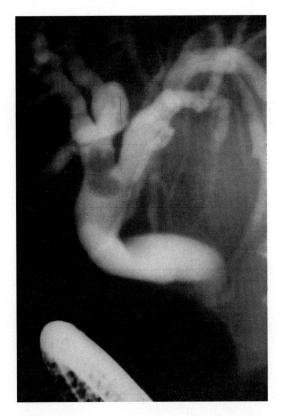

FIGURE 4.19. Surgical clip as nidus for a common duct stone. Film from an ERCP demonstrates a figure eight-shaped defect due to a calculus in the proximal common hepatic duct. After stone removal, the nidus of the stone was found to be a surgical clip.

cholecystectomy. Occasionally, a clip or suture may serve as a nidus for stone formation (Fig. 4.19). Care must be taken not to mistake a pseudocalculus for a true calculus. The "pseudocalculus sign" may be observed as a transient phenomenon during cholangiography, caused by contraction of the internal choledochal sphincter. Radiographically, a meniscus-shaped defect is seen at the distal CBD (Fig. 4.20A), but it usually disappears rapidly (Fig. 4.20B). In some cases, the defect may persist, becoming difficult to distinguish from a true calculus. The administration of glucagon may relax the sphincter under this circumstance [37,38].

Complications Associated with the Cystic Duct Remnant

A successful cholecystectomy includes resection of the gallbladder and a portion of the cystic duct. Theoretically, the entire cystic duct should be removed. This is generally not possible, however, and often not advisable owing to anatomic and technical considerations.

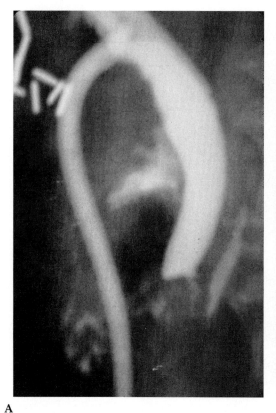

A

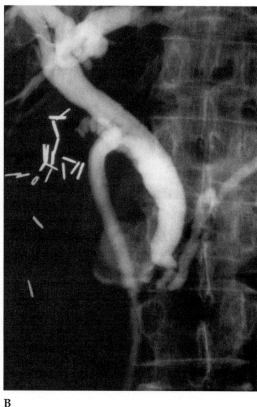

B

FIGURE 4.20. Pseudocalculus sign. (A) Film from an ERCP shows a meniscus-shaped defect in the distal CBD simulating a stone. (B) Additional film from the ERCP in the same patient taken moments later shows the defect to have disappeared. The pseudo-calculus sign is due to contraction of the choledochal sphincter.

The cystic duct's length, course, and angulation are variable and will determine the optimum site for ligation. Anatomically, the cystic duct has two portions; the convoluted juxtacholecystic segment, which contains the valves of Heister, and the smooth juxtacholedochal segment. Since particulate matter is more likely to be found in the proximal convoluted segment than in the distal smooth segment, it is desirable to remove the entire convoluted segment, but not necessarily the entire smooth segment.

The cystic duct may join the common duct at an acute angle, may course parallel to the common duct for a variable distance, or may course over or under the common duct to enter on its left-hand side (Figs. 4.21 and 4.22). In the latter circumstances, the walls of the cystic and common bile ducts are firmly bound together, and their junction lies deep within the hepatoduodenal ligament. Dissection in this region is associated with a high rate of bile duct injury. Complete excision of

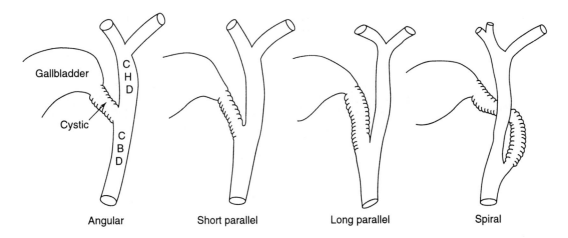

Angular   Short parallel   Long parallel   Spiral

FIGURE 4.21. Variations in the insertion of the cystic duct.

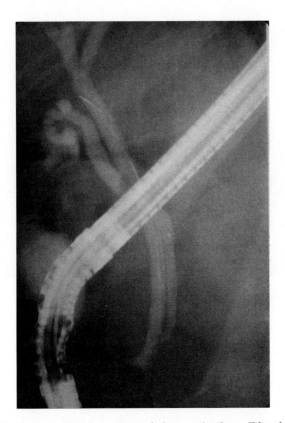

FIGURE 4.22. **Low medial insertion of the cystic duct.** Film from an ERCP demonstrates the spiral or low medial insertion variant of cystic duct insertion. The walls of the cystic duct and common duct are usually firmly bound together.

the cystic duct is not advised, even when the junction is clearly seen at surgery, because the traction necessary for excision of the cystic duct may lead to common duct stricture. Optimally, the cystic duct remnant should be long enough to allow for adequate ligature without tenting the choledochus. With the angular configuration, it is generally advised to leave a cystic duct stump of 5 mm, although some surgeons feel that up to 1 cm is safe [20]. With long remnants, stasis occurs and stones tend to re-form (Fig. 4.23). In patients with configurations other than the angular one, which occur in about 25% of the population, the cystic duct should be ligated at a site distal to the cholecystic ampulla (neck of the gallbladder), and the absence of stones in the stump should be verified.

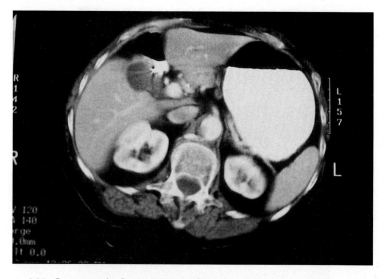

FIGURE 4.23. **Long cystic duct remnant.** CT scan of the upper abdomen after cholecystectomy reveals a long dilated cystic duct remnant.

The retention of calculi is the most common complication associated with the cystic duct remnant. Stones may be overlooked at the time of surgery or may form at a later date (Fig. 4.24). With long cystic duct remnants, stasis occurs, stones tend to re-form, and inflammatory changes may develop. Since most stumps will be located dorsal or posteromedial to the common duct and difficult to visualize in the anteroposterior projection, it is important to obtain films in the lateral or right posterior oblique projections during cholangiography to demonstrate stones in the cystic duct remnant [20]. Mirizzi's syndrome can occur secondary to a large stone impacted in the cystic duct, remnant causing compression and obstruction of the common duct.

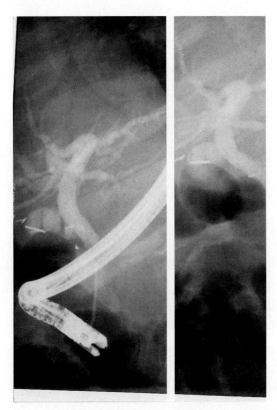

FIGURE 4.24. **Stone in cystic duct remnant.** Film from an ERCP demonstrates a long cystic duct remnant that contains stones.

An excessively long cystic duct remnant with a bulbous dilatation of its proximal portion has been termed a "re-formed gallbladder"(Fig. 4.25). This can be a source of stone disease and subsequent choledo-cholithiasis. Retention of part of the gallbladder after cholecystectomy

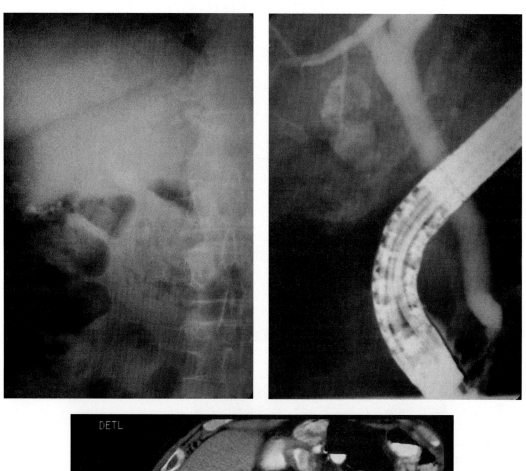

A

B

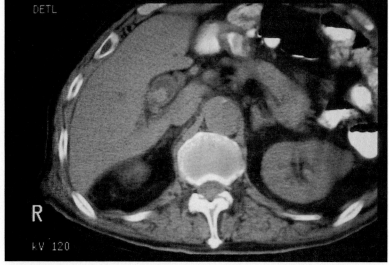

C

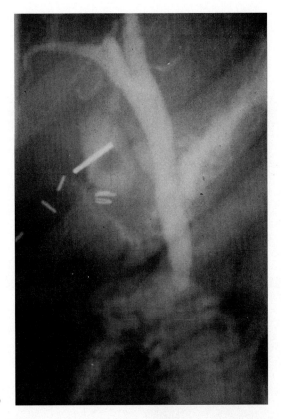

D

FIGURE **4.25. "Re-formed gallbladder."** (A) Plain film of the abdomen shows a stone in the right upper quadrant after cholecystectomy. (B) Film from the ERCP demonstrates a "re-formed gallbladder" containing calculi. (C) CT image in the same patient shows the dilated remnant and a calculus. (D) ERCP from another patient reveals a long cystic duct remnant with bulbous dilatation containing a stone.

has been called gallbladder remnant disease or cystic stump syndrome (Fig. 4.26).

Rarely, a fistula may develop between the cystic duct remnant and the adjacent duodenum, transverse colon, or stomach [19]. The pathogenesis may be similar to that of gallstone perforation or gallstone ileus, or the cause may be operative trauma.

Also referred to as amputation neuromas, cystic duct neuromas may form after cholecystectomy. They are due to a reactive disorganized proliferation of damaged nerve fibers at the margin of the cystic duct stump. Radiographically, they may present as a nodular mass protruding into the lumen of the stump or they may obliterate the lumen entirely (Fig. 4.27).

Postcholecystectomy Syndrome

After cholecystectomy, about 10 to 30% of patients will develop recurrent or persistent symptoms, such as right upper quadrant pain, biliary colic, fatty food intolerance, or jaundice. The onset of the so-called postcholecystectomy syndrome can occur from 3 months to years after

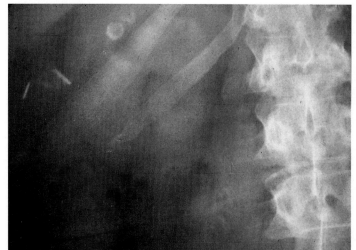

A

FIGURE 4.26. **Retention of part of the gallbladder after cholecystectomy.** (A) Plain film of the abdomen shows a calculus in the right upper quadrant. (B) CT image of the upper abdomen in the same patient shows the calculus in the region of the gallbladder fossa. (C) Film from an ERCP in the same patient demonstrates contrast filling a large portion of retained gallbladder.

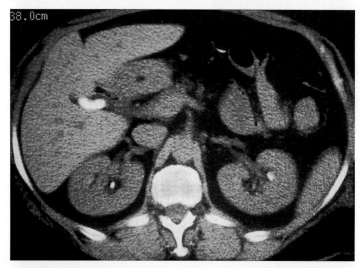

B

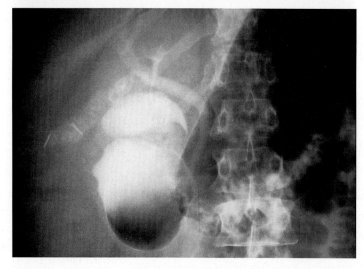

C

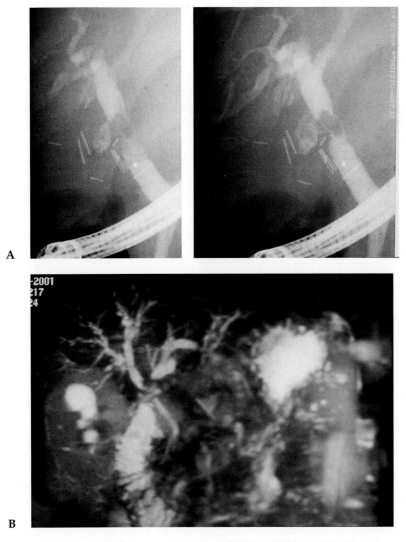

FIGURE 4.27. **Cystic duct neuroma after cholecystectomy.** (A) Films from an ERCP shows a nodular defect at the level of the cystic duct insertion projecting into the common duct. At surgery this proved to be a neuroma. (B) MRCP image of the same patient showing similar findings.

surgery. In some cases, the symptoms will be identical to the presenting complaints prior to cholecystectomy. This syndrome has been shown to be due to a variety of causes, although the precise cause of symptoms sometimes remains unclear. A higher incidence of post-cholecystectomy symptoms has been reported in women and in younger patients. Also, the length of time of the preoperative symptoms correlates with the likelihood of postoperative symptoms. One study showed 27% of patients operated on after the initial attack of gallbladder disease had recurrent symptoms, whereas 50% of those with preoperative symptoms of over 5 years' duration had postoperative symptoms [29].

In one study of the postcholecystectomy syndrome, over half the patients had abnormalities related to the biliary tree, including choledocholithiasis, ampullary stenosis, and pancreas divisum [39]. The syndrome is often attributed to problems related to the cystic duct remnant. In a study of 500 postcholecystectomy patients, those with cystic duct stumps greater than 1 cm experienced a higher incidence of postoperative pain [40]. In another study, 70% of patients with severe postoperative complaints had long cystic duct remnants [41]. Although it has been reported that cystic duct neuromas often cause symptoms and can lead to postcholecystectomy pain, this is probably not the case. It is controversial whether a long cystic duct remnant alone can lead to recurrent symptoms. It is probable that only cystic duct remnants that contain calculi cause symptoms. Some patients without definitive pathology respond favorably to sphincterotomy. Nonbiliary disease such as peptic ulcer disease, irritable bowel syndrome, and reflux esophagitis can cause abdominal pain following cholecystectomy. A thorough history and physical examination must be performed to identify these conditions.

Some use the term "postcholecystectomy syndrome" to describe the condition in patients in whom the etiology of symptoms is uncertain. There is some physiological or pathological evidence that papillary stenosis, biliary dyskinesia, or phantom pain may be responsible for symptoms in some patients [29].

Postoperative Biliary Dilatation

At one time it was thought that the common duct dilated after cholecystectomy to serve as a reservoir for bile; however, several sonographic studies have documented that this does not occur [42–44]. The development of biliary dilatation, or an increase in ductal diameter after cholecystectomy, should be considered to be abnormal and perhaps indicative of the presence of biliary obstruction from choledocholithiasis, stricture, ampullary stenosis, or tumor. In patients with preoperative biliary dilatation due to stone disease or tumor, decompression of the ductal system should lead to a decrease in ductal diameter, although if the obstruction and dilatation have been present for a long time, the duct generally will not revert to normal caliber [45].

Focal intrahepatic biliary dilatation may occur after cholecystectomy if an aberrant duct has been ligated inadvertently; such dilatation also may be due to overlooked intrahepatic calculi. This diagnosis may be missed on ERCP if it is not appreciated that a portion of the intrahepatic ductal system is not opacified, but it can be identified clearly on CT images. In the case of ductal ligation, there will be focal atrophy of the affected segment.

Intraperitoneal Gallstones ("Dropped" or "Spilled" Stones)

With the advent of LC, spillage of gallstones into the peritoneal cavity due to perforation of the gallbladder or spillage during removal of the gallbladder itself has become a recognized complication of cholecystectomy, one rarely seen with open cholecystectomy. Initial opinion was that stones left in the peritoneal cavity were harmless. However it is now accepted that there are potential complications from dropped stones, including abscess, sinus tracts, septicemia, and adhesions. Improvements in instrumentation, improved video systems, and modifications in technique have been developed which have helped to prevent stone spillage. When spillage is noted to occur, attempts to retrieve dropped stones should be made [46]. In selected cases, open retrieval should be considered if a large number of stones or large stones have been spilled. Stones or stone fragments can lodge in any site in the peritoneal cavity and may even migrate into the pleural space and pulmonary parenchyma, resulting in empyema or lithoptysis [47,48]. Stones may also be trapped in trocar sites. The incidence of dropped stones has been reported to range from 6 to 16% [46,49]. It is believed that less than 1% of these patients will develop an abscess or other complication requiring reoperation, although the true incidence is unknown because of delayed presentation. The average time from surgery to presentation due to a complication from a dropped stone is 27.3 weeks [50].

The development of abscesses from dropped stones is probably related to the significant bacterial content gallstones [51]. It has been shown that bacteria also have an adhesive property that facilitates pigment stone formation [52]. This correlates with the finding that most abscesses due to dropped stones are found in association with calcified stones. Another explanation may be that infected bile causes these abscesses.

The diagnosis is often made by CT imaging. A calcified nidus is often identified within the abscess (Figs. 4.28–4.30). If the stone is not calcified, the etiology of the abscess may be initially unclear.

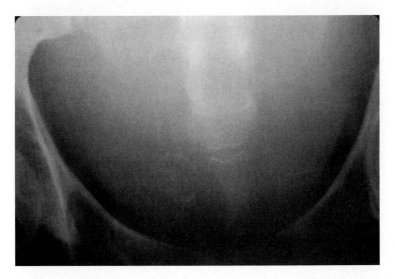

FIGURE 4.28. "Dropped stone" after cholecystectomy. Coned-down view of the pelvis reveals a calcific density due to a dropped stone postcholecystectomy. (Courtesy of R. Wachsberg, M. D., Newark, NJ)

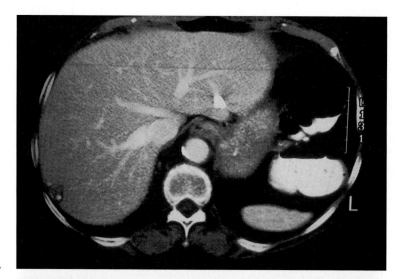

A

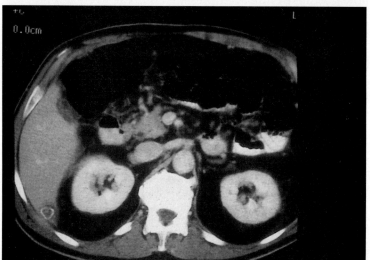

B

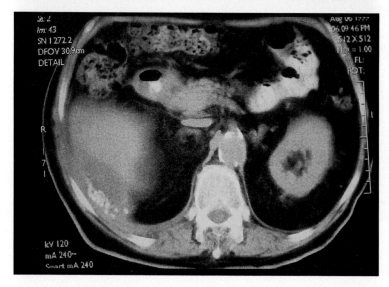

C

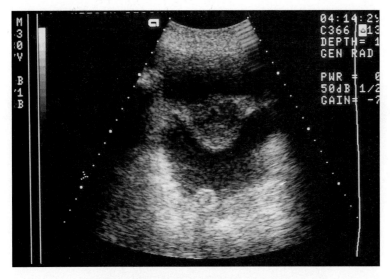

D

FIGURE 4.29. "Dropped stones" after cholecystectomy. (A) CT scan of the upper abdomen demonstrates calcific densities due to calculi in the perihepatic space with associated small amount of fluid. (B) Another patient with similar findings. (C) CT scan of the upper abdomen in another patient with multiple calculi and fluid in the right subhepatic space. (D) Sonogram in a fourth patient demonstrating fluid and a calculus in the pelvis.

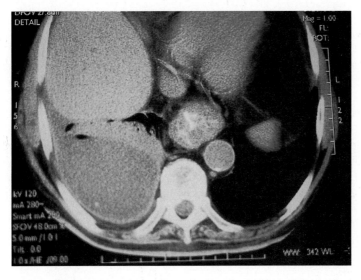

FIGURE 4.30. "Dropped stones after cholecystectomy. "Dropped stones" migrating into the pleural space with empyema.

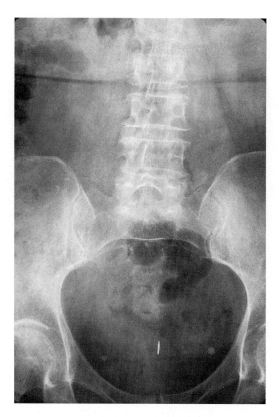

FIGURE 4.31. "Dropped clip" after cholecystectomy. Plain film of the abdomen shows a closed surgical clip in the pelvis that had "dropped" from the right upper quadrant.

Abscesses may be drained percutaneously, and associated percutaneous dropped stone removal has also been reported [53]. Stones less than 1 cm in diameter usually can be removed by a 30F sheath, whereas stones greater than 1 cm must be fragmented before removal.

"Dropped" clips after LC are also fairly common, with 19 patients in a series of 52 demonstrating one or more ectopic clips on intraoperative or postoperative radiographs [54] (Fig. 4.31). Most of these clips were closed, although some were open. The most common location was the right lower quadrant. The significance, if any, of "dropped" clips is yet to be determined.

Intrahepatic Ductal Rupture and Ectasia

Intrahepatic ductal rupture is a complication that occurs secondary to intraoperative extraction of biliary calculi with Fogarty balloon catheters [55]. With this technique, the catheter is often advanced blindly into the intrahepatic ducts through a choledochotomy. The balloon is inflated and then withdrawn to remove calculi. Intrahepatic ducts may rupture if the balloon is distended beyond the luminal capacity of the duct. The use of fluoroscopy would help to prevent this

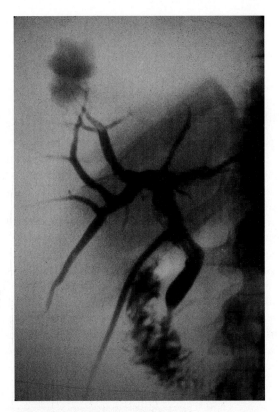

FIGURE 4.32. **Intrahepatic ductal rupture.** Film from a T-tube cholangiogram demonstrate an amorphous collection of contrast medium in the liver parenchyma due to intrahepatic ductal rupture from extraction of calculi with a Fogarty balloon catheter.

problem, but the necessary equipment may not be available in the oper-ating room. Radiographically, large or small irregular collections of contrast medium can be identified in the liver parenchyma associated with focally dilated intrahepatic ducts (Fig. 4.32). Hepatic abscess may be a sequela of this problem in patients with cholangitis and infected bile. Focal or segmental ductal ectasia, rather than rupture, may result if the balloon is deflated before frank rupture has occurred [19]. The radiographic findings in this circumstance may simulate Caroli's disease.

Hemorrhage

Bleeding after cholecystectomy may be secondary to avulsion or tear of the cystic artery, slippage of the cystic artery sutures, injury to the hepatic artery, laceration of the liver, bleeding from the gallbladder bed after surgery for acute cholecystitis, and rarely, injury to the inferior vena cava or iatrogenic fistulas between the hepatic artery and portal vein [17,20]. One angiographic study showed evidence of vascular injury in 57% of patients with biliary strictures [29]. The presence of portal hypertension increases the risk of vascular injury.

The right hepatic artery is particularly susceptible to injury because of its course, running almost parallel to the cystic duct along the edge of the hepaticoduodenal ligament. Variations in the anatomy of the right hepatic artery also predispose patients to injury. Accidental ligation of the hepatic artery may lead to hepatic infarction [20].

Drainage Tube Problems

T tubes are commonly placed in the common duct after common duct exploration. Since most common duct stones are now removed endoscopically, the number of patients requiring ductal explorations and T tubes is diminishing. Complications related to T tubes include faulty placement, dislodgment, obstruction, extrusion, breakage, and disintegration. A long proximal arm of a T tube can lead to obstruction, cause biliary obstruction from a portion of the liver, or prevent retained stone passage. Blood clots, calculi, gravel, encrusted material, or kinking can lead to obstruction of the T tube. Obstruction by encrusted material is related to the length of time the T tube has been in place. T tubes may also cause biliary perforation if a limb penetrates the walls. The limbs of the T tube are usually cut obliquely, and the sharp end can erode the bile duct wall, especially if cholangitis has rendered it friable [19].

Plain films of the abdomen may suggest an abnormal position of the tube, and contrast medium can be injected for confirmation (Fig. 4.33).

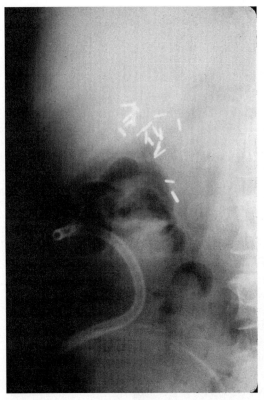 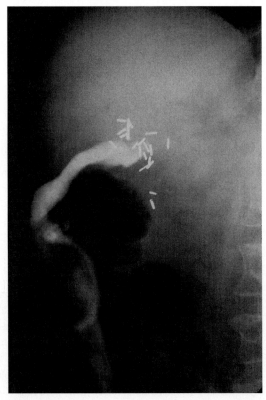

A   B

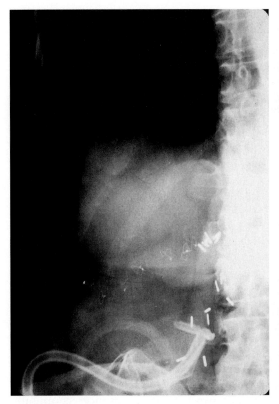

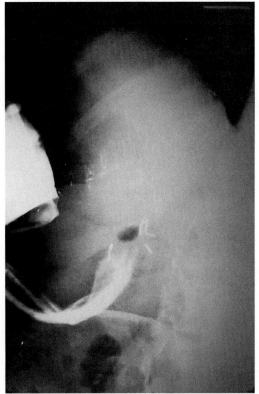

C

D

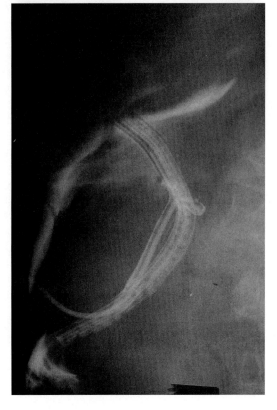

FIGURE 4.33. **Malposition of T tubes.** (A) Plain film of the right upper quadrant shows a T tube in a low and horizontal orientation suggesting malposition. (B) Injection of contrast medium into the T tube in the same patient reveals the tube to be outside the biliary tree. Contrast medium fills a tract in the subhepatic space leading toward the biliary tree. (C, D) Another patient demonstrating similar findings. (E) Another patient shows contrast medium in the subhepatic space after T-tube injection. Contrast is also accumulating in the drain left in at the time of surgery.

E

With T tube dislodgment, bile may spill into the peritoneal cavity. If the tube has been present long enough for a tract to form along the course of the tube, a biliary–cutaneous fistula may develop.

Tubes may become partially or completely occluded by blood clots or gravel, or with long-standing indwelling catheters, encrusted material. Rarely, broken pieces of the T tube or catheter used for intraoperative cholangiography are retained in the ductal system. Rubber T tubes may disintegrate if left in place for prolonged periods. Depending on their size and position, retained fragments may lead to symptoms. All retained fragments should be removed when identified, regardless of symptoms.

Technical problems at the time of T-tube placement can lead to mucosal dissection of the common duct. Tubes may also be malpositioned or in an extraluminal position; a limb may penetrate through one wall of a bile duct, which may in turn lead to bile leak or hemobilia; and a long proximal limb can obstruct biliary drainage from a part of the liver.

Pancreatitis

Hyperamylasemia, seen in 4 to 8% of patients after cholecystectomy, is generally not clinically significant in and of itself. Postcholecystectomy pancreatitis is an uncommon complication, reported in between 0.7 and 2.4% of patients in the older literature [56]. It occurs more commonly after cholecystectomy with common duct exploration than after cholecystectomy alone. The etiology is likely to be related to trauma from instrumentation and manipulation. Reflux of bile into the pancreatic duct during intraoperative cholangiography has been implicated as a cause of pancreatitis; this etiology is generally felt to be unlikely, however.

Choledochoduodenostomy

Choledochoduodenostomy, first performed in 1891, has been used as an effective technique to provide biliary drainage in selected circumstances. It circumvents the problems of retained common duct stones and the sequelae of benign obstructive disease in the distal CBD. Indications for this procedure include choledocholithiasis and concomitant biliary stricture, giant stones, retained stones, large number of stones, ampullary stenosis, and a markedly dilated common duct. This procedure is performed less frequently than in the past because common duct stones are now more likely to be successfully removed endoscopically, and endoscopic sphincterotomy has become available.

In candidates for choledochoduodenostomy, the common duct should be at least 1.2 cm in diameter, preferably 1.4 cm. A cholecystectomy should be performed if the gallbladder is still present, since the choledochoduodenostomy renders the gallbladder atonic, and it would become inflamed if not removed. Generally, a side-to-side anastomosis is made between the common duct and the duodenum at the level where the common duct crosses the duodenum (Fig. 4.34). The stoma must be at least 2.5 to 3 cm to allow effective biliary drainage and passage of any residual calculi. This procedure has been performed laparoscopically [57,58]. On upper GI series the biliary tree should fill freely and empty completely by 12 hours (Figs. 4.35 and 4.36). Air in the biliary tree does not necessarily indicate an adequate anastomosis and can be identified even if a stricture is present.

Complications, which occur in 5% of patients, include cholangitis, the sump syndrome, and loss of stomal patency secondary to stricture at the anastomotic site. A theoretical problem is cholangitis secondary to regurgitation into the biliary tree of intestinal contents with bacteria. Cholangitis in fact is an uncommon problem, and when it does occur, it is usually in association with technical problems and/or a strictured anastomosis [59].

The sump syndrome, defined as a collection of debris and/or lithogenic bile in the distal stagnant portion of the common duct, results in intermittent obstruction of the choledochoduodenal anastomosis that

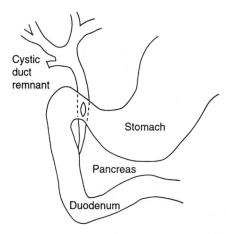

FIGURE 4.34. **Choledochoduodenostomy.** A side-to-side anastomosis is created between the common duct and the duodenum at the level where the common duct crosses the duodenum.

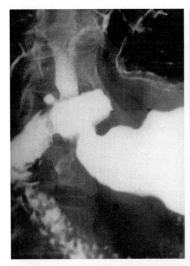
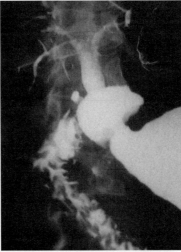

A

FIGURE 4.35. Choledo-
choduodenostomy. (A)
Right anterior oblique view
from an upper GI series
demonstrates contrast
medium entering the biliary
tree via a choledochoduo-
denostomy. There is preferential filling of the proximal
biliary system. (B) Film from
an upper GI series in
another patient reveals
filling of the biliary tree via
the choledochoduodenos-
tomy. Stricture in that region
prevents opacification of the
distal CBD.

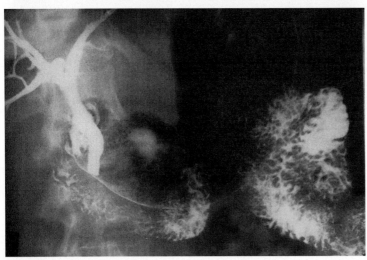

B

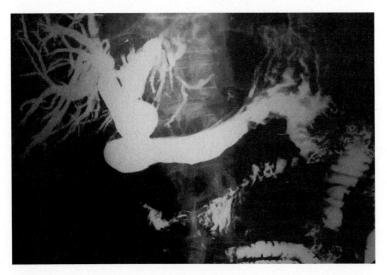

FIGURE 4.36. Choledo-
choduodenostomy with
poor emptying of the
biliary tree. Film taken 4
hours after completion of an
upper GI series demon-
strates a large amount of
barium in a dilated biliary
tree. The biliary tree failed
to empty normally.

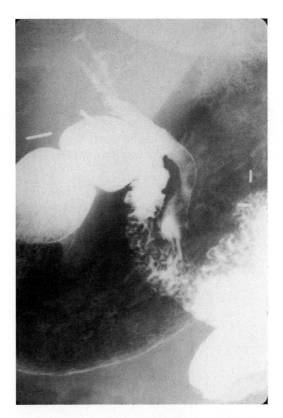

FIGURE 4.37. **Sump syndrome after choledochoduodenostomy.** Oblique film from a double-contrast upper GI series shows filling of the biliary tree via a choledochoduodenostomy with filling defects in the common bile duct due to debris. Debris and/or lithogenic bile in the distal stagnant portion of the CBD may result in intermittent obstruction of the choledochoduodenal anastomosis, resulting in pain, cholestasis, and/or pancreatitis.

produces pain, cholestasis, and/or pancreatitis (Fig. 4.37). In some cases, the stoma remains adequate, but the debris itself produces symptoms. Treatment is often successful with antibiotics alone. Endoscopic sphincterectomy and bile duct clearance with a balloon catheter or basket may be necessary [60].

Stricture at the anastomotic site may occur after choledochoduodenostomy. The stoma usually decreases in diameter following surgery, but it may become strictured or occluded. Endoscopic percutaneous balloon dilatation may be used as an effective therapy, although reoperation may be required.

Hepaticojejunostomy

Hepaticojejunostomy is performed when the common duct is strictured, usually because of tumor or biliary injury. Typically, an anastomosis is created between the common hepatic duct and a Roux-en-Y loop of jejunum (Figs. 4.38 and 4.39). A Roux-en-Y anastomosis, although more complicated to perform than a loop anastomosis, has the advantage of preventing reflux of intestinal contents into the biliary tree. It should therefore be done for benign disease where the long-term

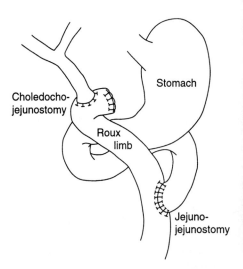

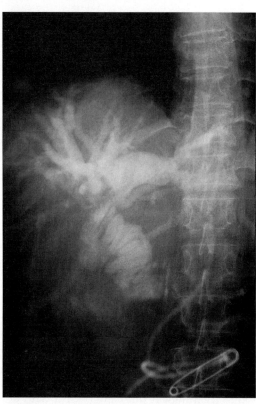

FIGURE 4.38. Hepaticojejunostomy. An anastomosis is created between a Roux-en-Y loop of jejunum and the common hepatic duct.

FIGURE 4.39. Hepaticojejunostomy. Supine view from a cholangiogram performed via an external biliary drainage catheter shows filling of the intrahepatic biliary tree and anastomosed Roux-en-Y loop of jejunum.

prognosis for survival is good. The usual technique is a direct anastomosis of the jejunum to the common duct above the strictured segment.
An alternative method is the Rodney Smith procedure, a sutureless
technique in which the jejunal mucosa is made to approximate the
biliary ductal epithelium by passage of a transhepatic catheter or
catheters, which also serve as temporary stents (Fig. 4.40). Complications include leak and anastomotic stricture. The results depend on the
level of the initial biliary narrowing, with higher lesions having a
poorer prognosis [25].

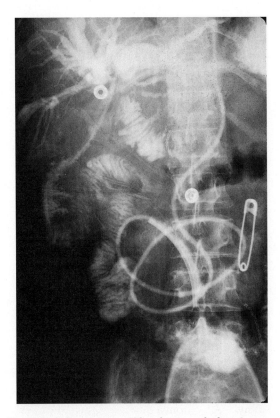

FIGURE 4.40. **Hepaticojejunostomy.** Film from a cholangiogram in a patient
following the Rodney Smith procedure shows stents in the left and right
hepatic ducts entering the jejunal anastomosis.

Cholecystojejunostomy

Cholecystojejunostomy is generally not recommended as a biliary decompression procedure for benign disease because the cystic duct frequently causes a relative obstruction. The gallbladder is often used for biliary bypass in malignant disease if the insertion of the cystic duct is sufficiently proximal to the obstructing tumor. The use of stents for biliary drainage has obviated the need for this procedure in many circumstances. After cholecystojejunostomy, barium should fill the biliary tree during upper GI examination. The gallbladder can be readily identified as distinct from small bowel by its characteristic mucosal pattern (Fig. 4.41).

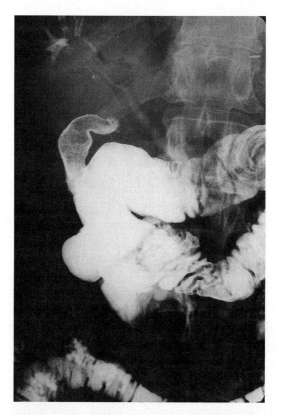

FIGURE 4.41. **Cholecystojejunostomy.** Supine view from a small-bowel series demonstrates both contrast medium in the gallbladder and biliary tree filling via a cholecystojejunal anastomosis.

Cholecystostomy

Cholecystostomy is now performed primarily percutaneously. Generally, cholecystostomy is indicated in elderly or debilitated, poor-surgical-risk patients with acute cholecystitis, where emergent cholecystectomy with general anesthesia may be considered to be risky (since cholecystostomy can be performed with local anesthesia). A cholecystostomy is also sometimes performed when a cholecystectomy has been planned but is deemed hazardous for reasons of poor exposure and technical difficulties. When the procedure is performed surgically, a large bore catheter, such as a Foley or a Malecot, is inserted through a purse-string suture and secured to the skin to prevent bile leakage into the peritoneal cavity. Gallstones may be removed at the time of tube placement as well. The cholecystostomy tube is generally left in place for approximately 6 weeks. Contrast studies via the tube may be performed to determine whether stones are present and to evaluate for patency of the cystic duct (Figs. 4.42 and 4.43).

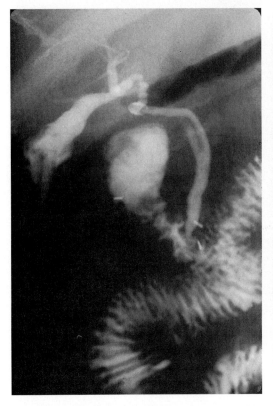

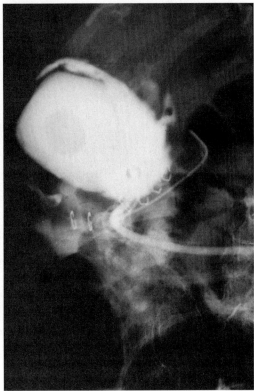

FIGURE 4.42. Cholecystostomy. Film from an injection of contrast medium into a cholecystostomy tube placed for acute cholecystitis in an elderly high risk patient shows filling of the gallbladder and common duct with free flow into the GI tract.

FIGURE 4.43. Cholecystectomy with leak, as well as stone and cystic duct obstruction. Cholecystostomy tube injection shows a distended gallbladder containing a large stone, extraluminal contrast due to leak, and nonfilling of the common duct.

Biliary Stents

Biliary stents and endoprostheses may be used for the treatment of both benign and malignant disease. Stents are commonly placed endoscopically, but they may be placed by the interventional radiologist by percutaneous methods or at the time or surgery. Stents are generally placed to provide biliary drainage in patients with both benign and malignant obstruction, tone disease, or cholangitis, to treat cystic duct leaks after cholecystectomy, and to protect surgically created anastomoses. For the long-term treatment of biliary obstruction, removable endoprostheses may be made of plastic, whereas metal stents are permanent. The most common indication for stent placement in malignant disease is pancreatic cancer, although central cholangiocarcinoma and metastatic disease may be amenable to treatment with multiple stents (Fig. 4.44).

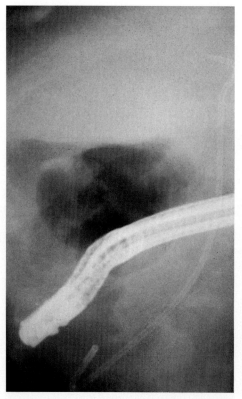

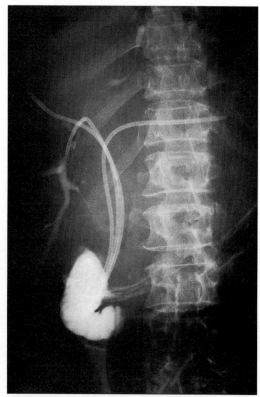

A   B

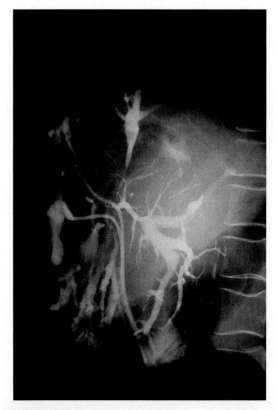

C

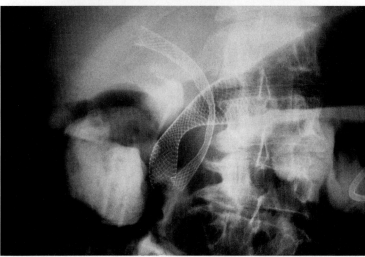

D

FIGURE 4.44. **Biliary stents.** (A) Temporary stent inserted into the common duct endoscopically. (B, C) Multiple biliary stents in a patient with metastatic disease from colon cancer. (D) Metallic stents in the common duct and duodenum in a patient with pancreatic carcinoma.

References

1. Gadacz TR, Talamini MA. Traditional versus laparoscopic cholecystectomy. Am J Surg 1991;161(3):336–338.
2. Garcia FR, Diaz TM, Lapena Villarroya JA, Armesto Fernandez MJ, Gonzalez Rodriguez AA, Arguelles PM. Port site metastases after laparoscopic cholecystectomy for an unexpected gallbladder carcinoma. Abdom Imaging 1999;24(4):404–406.
3. Moran J, Del Grosso E, Wills JS, Hagy JA, Baker R. Laparoscopic cholecystectomy: Imaging of complications and normal postoperative CT appearance. Abdom Imaging 1994;19(2):143–146.
4. Kang EH, Middleton WD, Balfe DM, Soper NJ. Laparoscopic cholecystectomy: Evaluation with sonography. Radiology 1991;181(2):439–442.
5. McAllister JD, D'Altorio RA, Snyder A. CT findings after uncomplicated percutaneous laparoscopic cholecystectomy. J Comput Assist Tomogr 1991; 15(5):770–772.
6. McAllister JD, D'Altorio RA, Rao V. CT findings after uncomplicated and complicated laparoscopic cholecystectomy. Semin Ultrasound Comput Tomogr Magn Reson 1993;14(5):356–367.
7. Quinn SF, Sangster W, Standage B, Schuman E, Gross G. Biliary complications related to laparoscopic cholecystectomies: Radiologic diagnosis and management. Surg Laparosc Endosc 1992;2(4):279–286.
8. Javors BR, Simmons MZ, Wachsberg RH. Cholangiographic demonstration of the cholecystohepatic duct of Luschka. Abdom Imaging 1998;23(6): 620–621.
9. Gilsdorf JR, Phillips M, McLeod MK, Harness JK, Hoversten GH, Woodbury D, et al. Radionuclide evaluation of bile leakage and the use of subhepatic drains after cholecystectomy. Am J Surg 1986;151(2):259– 262.
10. Neff CC, Simeone JF, Ferrucci Jr JT, Mueller PR, Wittenberg J. The occurrence of fluid collections following routine abdominal surgical procedures: Sonographic survey in asymptomatic postoperative patients. Radiology 1983;146(2):463–466.
11. Maull KI, Shirazi KK, Whitley RE, Halloran LG, Gayle WE, Haynes Jr BW. The effect of prophylactic drainage on subhepatic fluid collections after elective cholecystectomy: A prospective randomized ultrasonographic study. Am Surg 1981;47(2):85–88.
12. Kovalcik PJ, Burrell MJ, Old Jr WL. Cholecystectomy concomitant with other intra-abdominal operations. Assessment of risk. Arch Surg 1983; 118(9):1059–1062.
13. Gilliland TM, Traverso LW. Modern standards for comparison of cholecystectomy with alternative treatments for symptomatic cholelithiasis with emphasis on long-term relief of symptoms. Surg Gynecol Obstet 1990; 170(1):39–44.
14. Glenn F, McSherry CK, Dineen P. Morbidity of surgical treatment for nonmalignant biliary tract disease. Surg Gynecol Obstet 1968;126(1):15–26.
15. Scher KS, Scott-Conner CE. Complications of biliary surgery. Am Surg 1987;53(1):16–21.
16. Ward EM, LeRoy AJ, Bender CE, Donohue JH, Hughes RW. Imaging of complications of laparoscopic cholecystectomy. Abdom Imaging 1993;18(2): 150–155.
17. Burhenne HJ, Cooperberg P. Complications of biliary tract surgery. In: Meyers MA, Ghahremani GG, eds. Iatrogenic Gastrointestinal Complications. New York: Springer-Verlag; 1981:197–210.

18. Walker AT, Shapiro AW, Brooks DC, Braver JM, Tumeh SS. Bile duct disruption and biloma after laparoscopic cholecystectomy: Imaging evaluation. AJR Am J Roentgenol 1992;158(4):785–789.

19. Ghahremani GG, Crampton AR, Bernstein JR, Caprini JA. Iatrogenic biliary tract complications: Radiologic features and clinical significance. Radiographics 1991;11(3):441–456.

20. Ghahremani GG. Postcholecystectomy complications. Crit Rev Diagn Imaging 1984;23(2):119–149.

21. Trerotola SO, Savader SJ, Lund GB, Venbrux AC, Sostre S, Lillemoe KD, et al. Biliary tract complications following laparoscopic cholecystectomy: Imaging and intervention. Radiology 1992;184(1):195–200.

22. Ray Jr CE, Hibbeln JF, Wilbur AC. Complications after laparoscopic cholecystectomy: Imaging findings. AJR Am J Roentgenol 1993;160(5):1029–1032.

23. A prospective analysis of 1518 laparoscopic cholecystectomies. The Southern Surgeons Club. N Engl J Med 1991;324(16):1073–1078.

24. Deziel DJ, Millikan KW, Economou SG, Doolas A, Ko ST, Airan MC. Complications of laparoscopic cholecystectomy: A national survey of 4,292 hospitals and an analysis of 77,604 cases. Am J Surg 1993;165(1):9–14.

25. Moossa AR, Mayer AD, Stabile B. Iatrogenic injury to the bile duct. Who, how, where? Arch Surg 1990;125(8):1028–1030.

26. Davidoff AM, Pappas TN, Murray EA, Hilleren DJ, Johnson RD, Baker ME, et al. Mechanisms of major biliary injury during laparoscopic cholecystectomy. Ann Surg 1992;215(3):196–202.

27. Phillips EH, Berci G, Carroll B, Daykhovsky L, Sackier J, Paz-Partlow M. The importance of intraoperative cholangiography during laparoscopic cholecystectomy. Am Surg 1990;56(12):792–795.

28. Wright TB, Bertino RB, Bishop AF, Brady TM, Castaneda F, Berkman WA, et al. Complications of laparoscopic cholecystectomy and their interventional radiologic management. Radiographics 1993;13(1):119–128.

29. Preoperative and postoperative biliary problems. In: Meyers WC, Jones RS, eds. Textbook of Liver and Biliary Surgery. Philadelphia: Lippincott-Raven; 1990:373–390.

30. Weissmann HS, Gliedman ML, Wilk PJ, Sugarman LA, Badia J, Guglielmo K, et al. Evaluation of the postoperative patient with ^{99m}Tc-IDA cholescintigraphy. Semin Nucl Med 1982;12(1):27–52.

31. Love L, Kucharski P, Pickleman J. Radiology of cholecystectomy complications. Gastrointest Radiol 1979;4(1):33–40.

32. Ghahremani GG. Postsurgical and traumatic lesions of the biliary tract. In: Gore RM, Levine MS, Laufer I, eds. Textbook of Gastrointestinal Radiology. Philadelphia: WB Saunders, 1994:1762–1778.

33. Christensen RA, van Sonnenberg E, Nemcek Jr AA, D'Agostino HB. Inadvertent ligation of the aberrant right hepatic duct at cholecystectomy: Radiologic diagnosis and therapy. Radiology 1992;183(2):549–553.

34. Boland GW, Mueller PR, Lee MJ. Laparoscopic cholecystectomy with bile duct injury: Percutaneous management of biliary stricture and associated complications. AJR Am J Roentgenol 1996;166(3):603–607.

35. Mueller PR, van Sonnenberg E, Ferrucci Jr JT, Weyman PJ, Butch RJ, Malt RA, et al. Biliary stricture dilatation: Multicenter review of clinical management in 73 patients. Radiology 1986;160(1):17–22.

36. Madden JL. Primary common bile duct stones. World J Surg 1978;2(4):465–471.

37. Beneventano TC, Schein CJ. The pseudocalculus sign in cholangiography. Arch Surg 1969;98(6):731–733.

38. Martin MB, Kon ND, Ott DJ, Sterchi JM. Pseudocalculus sign. A pitfall of static cholangiography. Am Surg 1986;52(4):197–200.
39. Cooperman M, Ferrara JJ, Carey LC, Thomas FB, Martin Jr EW, Fromkes JJ. Endoscopic retrograde cholangiopancreatography. Its use in the evaluation of nonjaundiced patients with the postcholecystectomy syndrome. Arch Surg 1981;116(5):606–609.
40. Bodvall B, Overgaard B. Cystic duct remnant after cholecystectomy: Incidence studied by cholegraphy in 500 cases, and significance in 103 reoperations. Ann Surg 1966;163(3):382–390.
41. Larmi TK, Mokka R, Kemppainen P, Seppala A. A critical analysis of the cystic duct remnant. Surg Gynecol Obstet 1975;141(1):48–52.
42. Graham MF, Cooperberg PL, Cohen MM, Burhenne HJ. Ultrasonographic screening of the common hepatic duct in symptomatic patients after cholecystectomy. Radiology 1981;138(1):137–139.
43. Graham MF, Cooperberg PL, Cohen MM, Burhenne HJ. The size of the normal common hepatic duct following cholecystectomy: An ultrasonographic study. Radiology 1980;135(1):137–139.
44. Mueller PR, Ferrucci Jr JT, Simeone JF, Wittenberg J, van Sonnenberg E, Polansky A, et al. Postcholecystectomy bile duct dilatation: Myth or reality? AJR Am J Roentgenol 1981;136(2):355–358.
45. Vogel H, Segebrecht P, Schreiber HW. [Postoperative retonisation of dilatated bile ducts (author's transl)]. ROFO Fortschr Geb Roentgenstr Nuklearmed 1980;132(5):522–526.
46. Schafer M, Suter C, Klaiber C, Wehrli H, Frei E, Krahenbuhl L. Spilled gallstones after laparoscopic cholecystectomy. A relevant problem? A retrospective analysis of 10,174 laparoscopic cholecystectomies. Surg Endosc 1998;12(4):305–309.
47. DeVincenzo R, Haramati LB, Wolf EL, Klapper PJ. Gallstone empyema complicating laparoscopic cholecystectomy. J Thorac Imaging 2001; 16(3):174–176.
48. Downie GH, Robbins MK, Souza JJ, Paradowski LJ. Cholelithoptysis. A complication following laparoscopic cholecystectomy. Chest 1993;103(2): 616–617.
49. Memon MA, Deeik RK, Maffi TR, Fitzgibbons Jr RJ. The outcome of unretrieved gallstones in the peritoneal cavity during laparoscopic cholecystectomy. A prospective analysis. Surg Endosc 1999;13(9):848–857.
50. Chin PT, Boland S, Percy JP. "Gallstone hip" and other sequelae of retained gallstones. HPB Surg 1997;10(3):165–168.
51. Stewart L, Smith AL, Pellegrini CA, Motson RW, Way LW. Pigment gallstones form as a composite of bacterial microcolonies and pigment solids. Ann Surg 1987;206(3):242–250.
52. Horton M, Florence MG. Unusual abscess patterns following dropped gallstones during laparoscopic cholecystectomy. Am J Surg 1998; 175(5):375–379.
53. Trerotola SO, Lillemoe KD, Malloy PC, Osterman Jr FA. Percutaneous removal of "dropped" gallstones after laparoscopic cholecystectomy. Radiology 1993;188(2):419–421.
54. Rawson JV, Klein RM, Hodgson J. "Dropped" surgical clips following laparoscopic cholecystectomy. Surg Endosc 1996;10(1):77–78.
55. Goldman SM, Diamond A, Salik JO. Intrahepatic rupture secondary to duct exploration demonstrated by cholangiography. Radiology 1976; 118(1):13–17.
56. White MT, Morgan A, Hopton D. Postoperative pancreatitis. A study of seventy cases. Am J Surg 1970;120(2):132–137.

57. Gurbuz AT, Watson D, Fenoglio ME. Laparoscopic choledochoduodenos-
    tomy. Am Surg 1999;65(3):212–214.
58. Tinoco R, El Kadre L, Tinoco A. Laparoscopic choledochoduodenostomy.
    J Laparoendosc Adv Surg Tech A 1999;9(2):123–126.
59. Schein CJ, Shapiro N, Gliedman ML. Choledochoduodenostomy as an
    adjunct to choledocholithotomy. Surg Gynecol Obstet 1978;146(1):25–32.
60. Mavrogiannis C, Liatsos C, Romanos A, Goulas S, Dourakis S, Nakos A,
    et al. Sump syndrome: Endoscopic treatment and late recurrence. Am J
    Gastroenterol 1999;94(4):972–975.

5

The Small Bowel

Adhesions

In discussing small-bowel obstruction, one must take into account that adhesions are either the first [1,2] or second [3] most common cause. One study states that up to 70% of small-bowel obstructions in the United States are secondary to adhesions [4], while other studies showed that the rate may vary between 49 [5,6] and 80% [7]. A prospective study showed that at surgery, 93% of patients with prior abdominal surgery had evidence of adhesions even if they were not obstructed [8]. In patients with previous abdominal surgery there is a 33% rate of readmission within a 10-year period for a possibly adhesion-related problem [9]. Among patients with one episode of small-bowel obstruction secondary to adhesions, 15 to 30% will develop a recurrence of that problem [10–12]. More significantly, the National Center for Health Statistics estimated that 344,000 operations were performed for the lysis of adhesions in 1992 [13]. Other adhesion-related problems cause between 3 and 5% of all laparotomies [8,9,14]. Patients who had had an appendectomy had an 11% rate of adhesive small-bowel obstruction during a 5-year follow-up period [15]. This compares with a 5% rate of the same period for patients with prior cholecystectomies. Total colectomy with ileal anal reservoir creation resulted in a rate of adhesive small-bowel obstruction slightly greater than 25% [16].

Intraperitoneal adhesions are formed by the transudation of serosanguinous fluid that is rich in protein [2]. This fluid coagulates during the first several postoperative hours [2]. Aiding in the production of adhesions is a reduction in fibrinolytic activity within the peritoneal cavity [17]. These two factors combine to allow the formation of fibrinous bands between adjacent intraperitoneal organs [18]. Collagen deposition and fibroblast proliferation is noted in these adhesions within 5 days [19].

The struggle to prevent adhesions is an ongoing one. As the preceding statistics demonstrate, even a small decrease in the rate of adhesions and subsequent small-bowel obstruction would have a major impact on health care and the course of providing it. Three different tactics have been or are being used to possibly prevent lesions. These are fibrinolytic therapy, anti-inflammatory medication, and physical separation of tissues [2].

Formerly, hyperosmolar solutions of dextran were used to help prevent lesions. Complications including occasional anaphylaxis as well as doubts of its efficacy have led to the abandonment of this technique [20,21]. Another older technique that led to serious and unexpected complications was the instillation into the peritoneum of mineral oil or other lipoid substances [22]. In 1908 Bake instilled sterile olive oil [23], and eventually mineral oil, Vaseline, animal fat, and paraffin were also tried [22]. By 1934, it had been noted that lipids not only failed to prevent adhesions but also caused an increase in them [24]. The oil resulted in the formation of dense adhesions, and the droplets were encapsulated by fibrous tissue containing foreign body giant cells, as well [22]. Calcification occurred within the fibrous stroma and in the periphery of these nodules. This could occur as early as 4 months after instillation [24] or as late as 30 years postoperatively [22].

On conventional radiography, calcified plaques may be seen outlining the serosal surfaces of the intraperitoneal organs. When actual lipid droplets are surrounded by fibrous tissues that calcify, ringlike calcifications, either incomplete or continuous, are noted (Figs. 5.1 and 5.2A). These may reach up to 3.5 cm in diameter. On computerized tomography (CT), the low density lipid center is easily demonstrated (Fig. 5.2B,C) and helps to differentiate this entity from pseudomyxoma peritonei, in which ringlike intraperitoneal calcifications may also be noted [22].

Current research centers on absorbable and nonabsorbable barriers [25–28]. Gore-Tex (polytetrafluoroethylene) is sutured in place and acts as a nonabsorbable barrier preventing adhesions from bridging from one organ to adjacent viscera [25,26]. Another approach, combining fibrinolytic therapy with a barrier mechanism, is the infusion of methylcellulose mixed with hyaluronidase, has proven effective in decreasing the rate of adhesions seen at second-look procedures or at the time of stomal closures [27,28]. Sodium carboxymethylcellulose instillation has shown no deleterious effects on wound or anastomosis healing in an animal model [2].

The role of the conventional or plain film of the abdomen in small-bowel obstruction is still a controversial one. Sensitivities of 50 to 60% in cases of complete small-bowel obstruction and even lower in partial obstruction have been reported [29,30]. Other studies report sensitivities and accuracy similar to that seen with computerized tomography [31,32].

Baker and Cho have written extensively on the plain film findings of small-bowel obstruction [3]. These signs may include abnormal dilatation of the small bowel (>2.5 cm), disproportionate dilatation compared with the colon, and the "stretch" sign in which air is caught between the valvulae conniventes, creating thin lucencies perpendicular to the long axis of the small-bowel loop. Radiographs utilizing a horizontal beam, either upright or decubitus films, transformed the stretch sign into the "string of pearls" sign in which small bubbles of air are caught between the valvulae at the top of fluid-filled small-bowel loops.

The upright film may also demonstrate differential air fluid levels in the small bowel. This sign of small-bowel obstruction was championed by Frimman-Dahl in his groundbreaking work [33]. However, Frimman-Dahl was commenting on dynamic fluoroscopic evaluation of the small bowel, not a single static image of the abdomen. More recent work on plain film analysis shows that differential air fluid levels do not help differentiate a small-bowel obstruction from an ileus [34,35].

Another, and very significant problem with the interpretation of the plain film of the abdomen is the reporting of the results. Many referring physicians and radiologists use the term "nonspecific bowel gas pattern" [36]. Emergency room physicians often interpret this as meaning a normal-appearing abdomen [37]. Yet radiologists attach various meanings to the term, which is used by 70% of a group of radiologists who were polled in the past decade [36]. Of these, 65% meant that the bowel gas pattern is normal or probably normal, 22% meant that at the bowel gas pattern is abnormal or normal, while only 13% meant that although the bowel gas pattern was abnormal the respondents could not determine whether an ileus or obstruction was present. Because of the

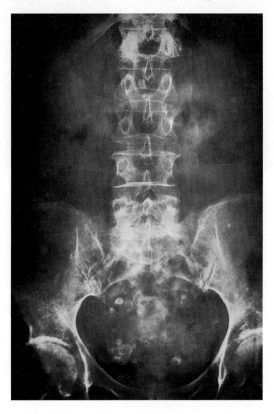

FIGURE 5.1. **Mineral oil globulosis.** Supine film of the abdomen shows small ringlike calcific densities throughout the abdomen. These represent small globules of mineral oil and their encapsulation.

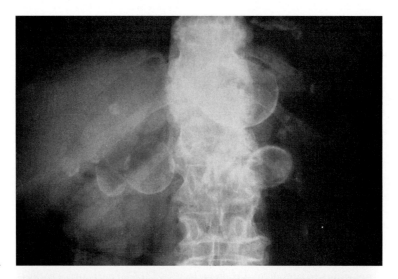

A

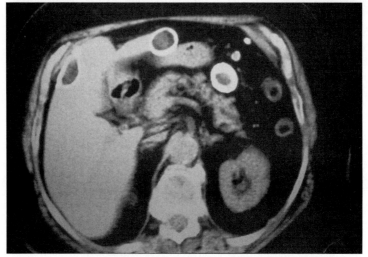

B

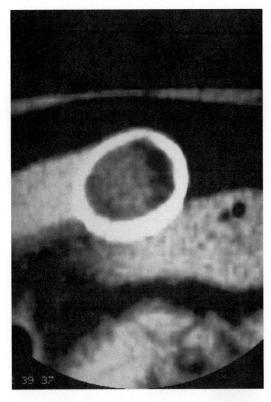

C

FIGURE 5.2. **Mineral oil globulosis.** (A) Supine film of the abdomen of another
patient reveals large masses with cyst wall calcifications in the upper abdomen.
(B) CT scan on the same patient shows the thick calcified wall encompassing
a mixed attenuation center. (C) Magnified view on one of these lesions demonstrates some of the low density lipid material within the pseudocyst. (Courtesy
of S.R. Baker, MD, Newark, NJ)

confusion among radiologists themselves, let alone between radiologists and referring physicians, the term "nonspecific bowel gas pattern"
should be banished from the medical lexicon.

Another problem for all imaging modalities is posed when the
patient is treated with a nasogastric or long intestinal tube for decompression. Follow-up examinations are often requested to evaluate
the results of the treatment. As Baker and Cho have stated, the tube
removes the contrast (air and fluid) that we depend upon for our
diagnosis [3]. The decreased dilatation gives rise to pain relief [38,39].
The improved radiographic picture is the "beneficial consequence of
the treatment of symptoms, not necessarily a manifestation of cure" [3].

The detection of a strangulated small-bowel obstruction via plain
film analysis is even more difficult. A gasless abdomen or a severe
paucity of bowel gas is a common presentation. However, a gasless
abdomen may also be seen with persistent vomiting, with esophageal
or gastric outlet obstruction, or even as a variant of normal [3]. One
review found that in 18 gasless abdomens, only one third had evidence
of strangulation [40]. Another plain film finding is that of distended

small-bowel loops surrounded by a rim of fat (mesenteric or serosal in origin) [41]. These loops may be fixed in position on serial films.

Conventional barium studies still play a limited role in the detection and evaluation of small-bowel obstruction. Enteroclysis has certain advantages over the conventional small-bowel series. These are based on bypassing a fluid-filled stomach, not depending on gastric empty-ing, and stressing the small bowel to its maximal diameter. This latter advantage allows demonstration of minor or relative narrowings that are easily missed on conventional small-bowel series that do not fully distend every loop of small bowel. The intermittent fluoroscopic eval-uation utilized in enteroclysis further adds to its utility [42]. However, the authors disagree with a statement that one of the drawbacks to enteroclysis is the need for conscious sedation. One of the authors (BRJ) has performed more than 500 small-bowel enemas without once using conscious sedation.

On conventional small-bowel studies or enteroclysis, adhesions may be noted by acute angulation (Fig. 5.3) or traction on the bowel wall (Fig. 5.4) [43]. When multiple loops are acutely angulated in the same

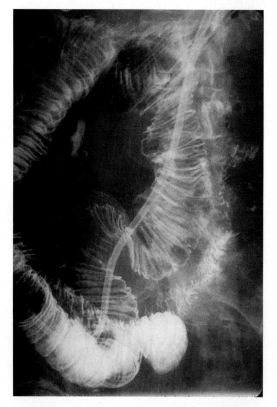

FIGURE 5.3. Small-bowel adhesions. Spot film from a double-contrast enteroclysis demonstrates an abrupt change in direction of the small bowel secondary to adhesions in this patient with a prior Whipple's procedure. Also note that the folds have lost their normal transverse orientation.

FIGURE 5.4. **Traction deformity from small-bowel adhesions.** Spot film from a double-contrast small-bowel enema shows a traction deformity pulling on and acutely angulating a loop of small bowel deep in the pelvis.

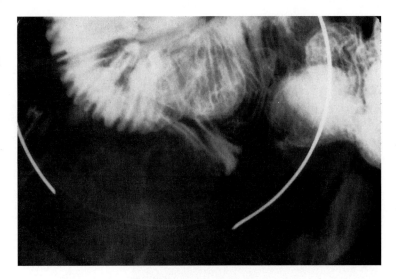

general area, a stellate appearance may result (Fig. 5.5). The valvulae conniventes, which are normally perpendicular to the long axis of the small bowel, may become canted or tethered together (Fig. 5.6), thereby indicating an extrinsic process. Pseudosacculations may form when

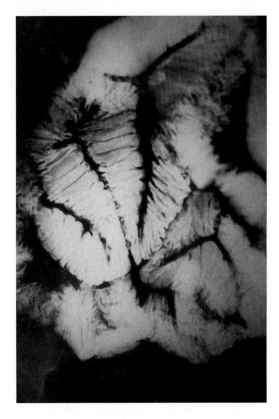

FIGURE 5.5. **Marked small-bowel adhesions.** Coned-down film from an enteroclysis examination reveals the stellate appearance of multiple small-bowel loops as they are acutely angulated to a central point by adhesions.

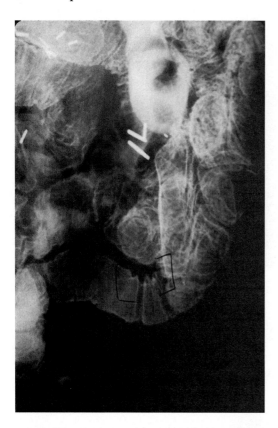

FIGURE 5.6. **Minimal deformity from small-bowel adhesions.** Double-contrast small-bowel enema demonstrates a small area of pleating of the mesenteric border of a loop of ileum in the pelvis (enclosed in brackets). This was thought to represent a "drop" or serosal metastasis from an ovarian primary. At surgery, a small area of scar tissue and adhesion was noted in the area without evidence of recurrent disease.

one wall of the bowel becomes tethered as the opposite side distends. Occasionally, a well-marginated straight or curvilinear crossing defect may be seen, representing a fibrinous band as it crosses the small bowel (Figs. 5.7 and 5.8) [5,42,43]. Rarely, the adhesions may become dense

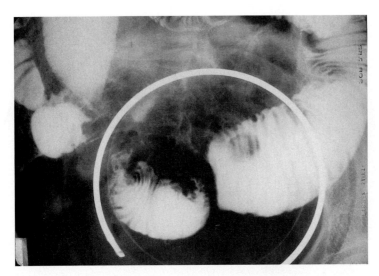

FIGURE 5.7. **Small-bowel adhesion with enterolith formation.** Spot film from a small-bowel enema shows a high grade small-bowel obstruction secondary to a crossing adhesion. Just proximal to the adhesion is the round filling defect of an enterolith secondary to this long-standing obstruction.

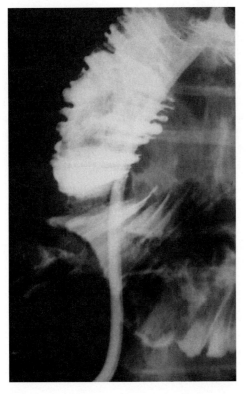

FIGURE 5.8. **Crossing defect from small-bowel adhesion.** Spot film from a single-contrast enteroclysis shows a thick crossing defect from a small-bowel adhesion. The small bowel is dilated downstream from the adhesion because of multiple other adhesions causing a multifocal small bowel obstruction.

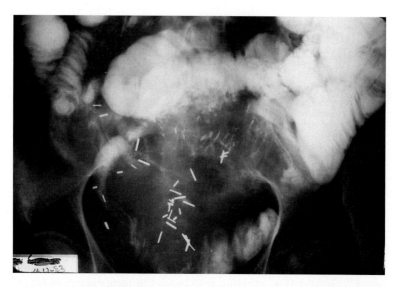

FIGURE 5.9. **Small-bowel adhesions mimicking a mass.** Conventional small-bowel series reveals marked narrowing and deviation of small bowel loops deep in the pelvis. Recurrent neoplasm was suspected, but at surgery, only marked adhesions were found.

and numerous enough to simulate a mass (Fig. 5.9). When adhesions become obstructive, there may be an abrupt change in caliber of the small bowel. The folds in the prestenotic segments may be normal, or they may become stretched and thinned as the bowel distends proximal to the obstruction. Radiographic depiction of adhesions involving the colon is seen less frequently, probably because the wall of that organ is significantly thicker. Similarly, obstruction is rarely encountered. However, the radiographic appearance is the same (Figs. 5.10 and 5.11).

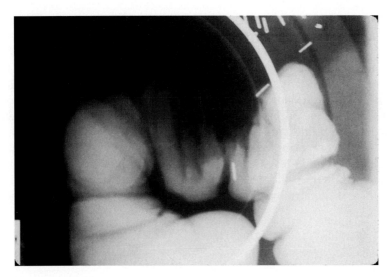

FIGURE **5.10. Colonic adhesions.** Compression spot film of the hepatic flexure reveals mild deformity of the superior aspect of the colon with pleating and slightly decreased distensibility secondary to pericolonic adhesions.

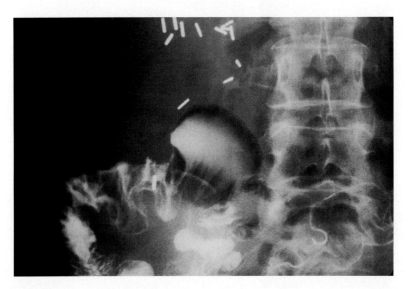

FIGURE **5.11. Colonic adhesions.** Double-contrast enema shows marked distortion of the hepatic flexure with a large pseudodiverticulum. This was secondary to a partial hepatectomy with severe adhesions in the right upper quadrant.

A recent study compared the diagnostic qualities of two different barium suspensions utilized for small-bowel series [44]. Although the authors found significant differences between the two products, they did not study the consequences on diagnostic results. In addition, the barium product that suffered in the comparison was not an up-to-date formulation of a dedicated small-bowel product, while the other one was. At the time of this writing, therefore, no definite reason to prefer one barium product to another can be found.

A study comparing CT and enteroclysis images in diagnosing small-bowel obstruction revealed that the small-bowel enema was far better than CT imaging in detecting obstruction and was only slightly less accurate in determining the cause of the obstruction (Figs. 5.12 and

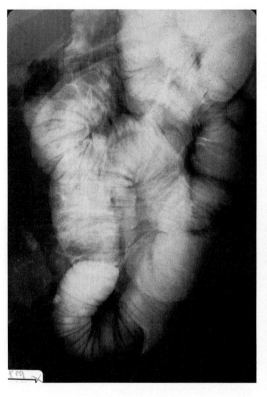

A

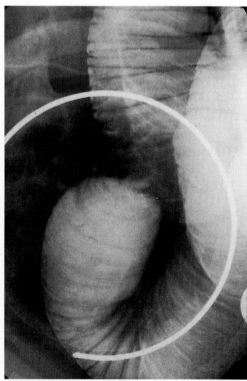

B

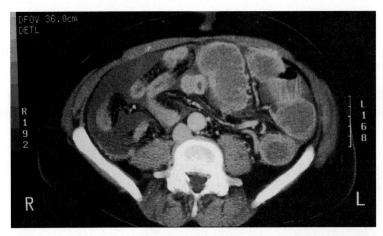

C

FIGURE 5.12. **Adhesive small-bowel obstruction.** (A) Overhead film from a single-contrast enteroclysis shows marked dilatation of the jejunum and some ileum, with no visualization of the distal small bowel or colon consistent with a small-bowel obstruction. (B) Spot film from the same examination demonstrates that the obstruction is due to a crossing defect from an adhesion. (C) CT scan on the same patient demonstrates the dilated small bowel with a mild degree of hazy mesentery at the transition point to relatively collapsed distal small bowel. The bowel at this point shows slight mural thickening and enhancement consistent with a mild degree of ischemia. Other loops of small bowel demonstrate an irregular degree of mural enhancement.

5.13) [45]. The small-bowel enema was also far more accurate than CT imaging in determining the level of the obstruction. Fewer false positive examinations were also noted in patients examined with enteroclysis.

The role of CT imaging in small-bowel obstruction is multifold. First, CT images are needed to make the diagnosis of small-bowel obstruction and to determine its level and etiology. Second, its roles are to

A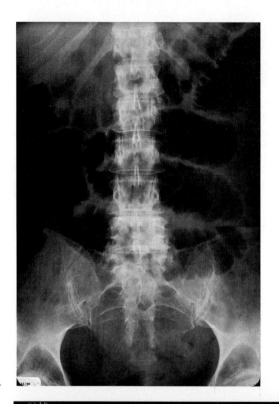

B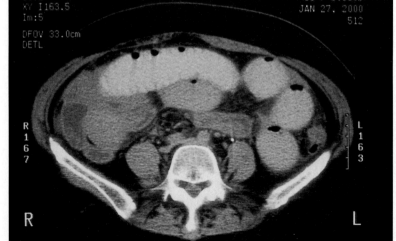

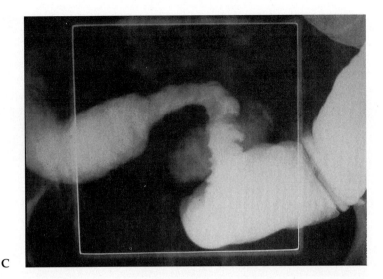

C

FIGURE 5.13. **Small-bowel obstruction with adhesions and ischemic stricture.**
(A) Supine plain film of the abdomen shows multiple dilated small-bowel
loops having the same diameter as the colon, diagnostic of an incomplete small-
bowel obstruction. (B) CT scan shows a relatively collapsed loop of small bowel
just distal to the dilated small bowel (both without significant oral contrast).
(C) Spot film from a single-contrast small-bowel enema demonstrates acute
angulation consistent with adhesions. In addition, the angulated loop is strictured by ischemic changes.

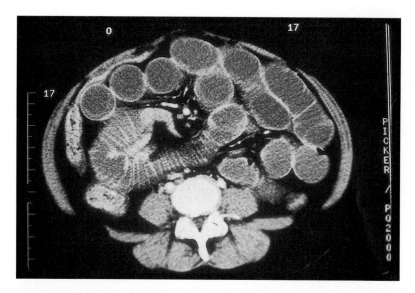

FIGURE 5.14. **Closed-loop obstruction with a "beak" sign.** CT scan at the level of the lower abdomen demonstrates multiple dilated fluid-filled loops of small bowel consistent with a small-bowel obstruction. Just to the right of midline there is an abrupt change in caliber of the small bowel, with two loops being collapsed and high in density. One of these loops comes to an angulated and abrupt end, representing the "beak" of a closed-loop obstruction. (Courtesy of D. Frager, M.D., New York City)

detect the presence of a closed-loop obstruction, and last, but certainly not least, to detect the complications of a closed-loop obstruction, strangulation, and ultimately intestinal ischemia and necrosis.

In the evaluation of the subset of small-bowel obstruction caused by adhesions, CT imaging can reach a sensitivity of 100% and a specificity of 90% [46]. Most often, the lesions themselves are not seen, and the diagnosis of adhesive small-bowel obstruction is one of exclusion. Another study of patients with suspected small-bowel obstruction showed that CT made the correct diagnosis of small-bowel obstruction in 34 of 43 patients with similar accuracy for the level and cause of the obstruction [45].

Balthazar and colleagues described multiple finding suggestive of a closed-loop obstruction [47]. These included incarcerated small bowel with a radial distribution in which the mesenteric vessels were noted to be stretched and converged on the point of torsion. There, two adjacent collapsed round or oval loops could be seen with sharp tapering and constitute the "beak" sign (Fig. 5.14). A "whirl" sign is seen when a central loop of collapsed small bowel surrounds a whirlpoollike arrangement of mesentery [46] (Fig. 5.15). The fixed position of the small-bowel loops in a closed-loop obstruction can be demonstrated by

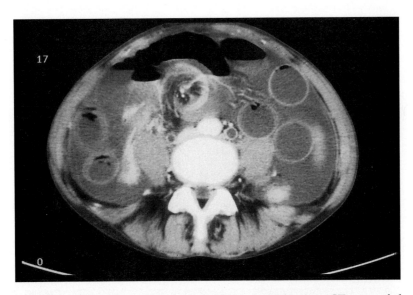

FIGURE 5.15. Closed-loop obstruction with a "whirl" sign. CT scan of the lower abdomen reveals marked ascites and multiple dilated loops of small bowel. A spiral configuration to the mesenteric vessels is seen in the midline representing the "whirl" of a closed-loop obstruction. (Courtesy of D. Frager, M.D., New York City)

scanning the patient in supine and either prone or decubitus positions (Fig. 5.16).

CT criteria for strangulation include slight (but not defined) circumferential bowel wall thickening (Fig. 5.17), increased attenuation of the bowel wall (Fig. 5.17), a "target" or "halo" sign (Fig. 5.18), pneumatosis intestinalis, and a lack of homogeneous enhancement of the bowel wall following intravenous contrast enhancement [47] (Fig. 5.18). Additional findings may include mesenteric edema (haziness of vessels) (Figs. 5.17–5.19) and hemorrhage. Mesenteric ischemia is characterized by arterial blockage, mesenteric or portal venous thrombosis, thickened

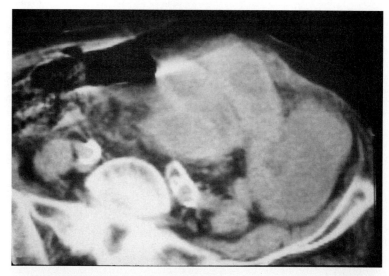

A

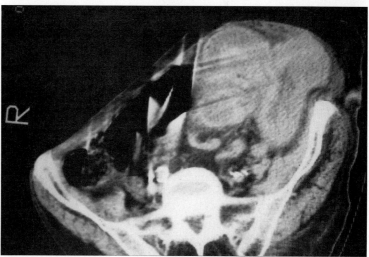

B

FIGURE 5.16. **Closed-loop obstruction.** (A) Supine and (B) left lateral decubitus CT scans of the abdomen reveal multiple dilated fluid-filled loops of small bowel in a constant configuration, diagnostic of a closed-loop obstruction. Note the acute curvature of the mesenteric vessels in the decubitus scan representing their entry into the closed loop. (Courtesy of K. Cho, M.D., Newark, NJ)

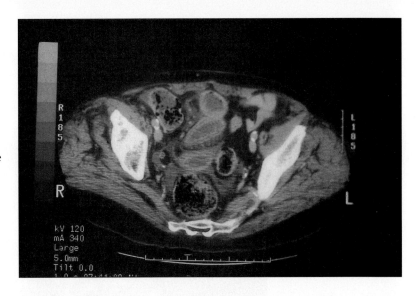

FIGURE 5.17. Closed-loop obstruction. CT scan through the pelvis shows three loops of mildly dilated small-bowel with a thickened small-bowel wall with increased attenuation. The prominent mesenteric vascularity of the middle loop is the result of arterial inflow, but no venous outflow, in a closed-loop obstruction.

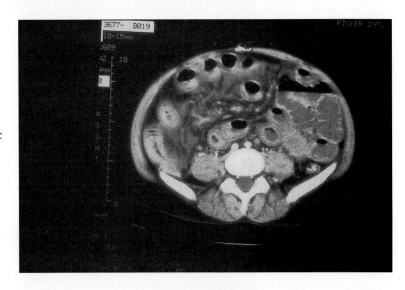

FIGURE 5.18. Small-bowel obstruction with ischemic changes. CT scan reveals evidence of mesenteric ischemia with hazy mesentery and interloop fluid. The loops of small bowel show varying degrees of the "halo" sign as well as differing amounts of contrast enhancement.

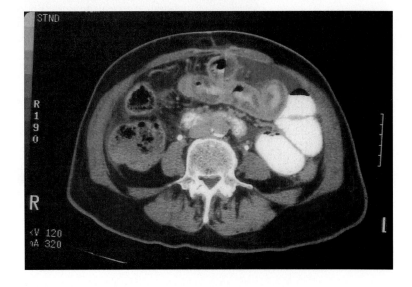

FIGURE 5.19. Small-bowel obstruction with bowel ischemia. CT scan of the midabdomen shows a loop of small bowel with a very thickened, edematous wall and a narrow lumen. Considerable edema is noted in the adjacent omentum.

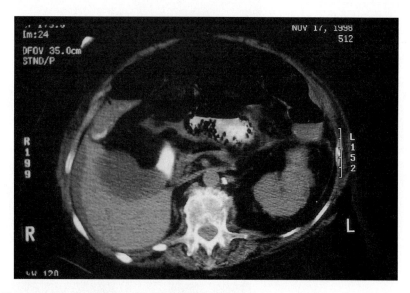

FIGURE 5.20. Small-bowel obstruction with bowel necrosis. CT scan of the abdomen demonstrates a loop of dilated small bowel in the midabdomen with pneumatosis. Directly posterior to this loop is air in the splenic vein (just anterior to the superior mesenteric artery).

small-bowel wall (again not defined), pneumatosis intestinalis (Figs. 5.20–5.22), and portal (Fig. 5.23) and/or mesenteric venous gas [47] (Fig. 5.21).

Ha et al. have reported that multiple phenomena combine to account for the development of strangulation [48]. First is the presence of a

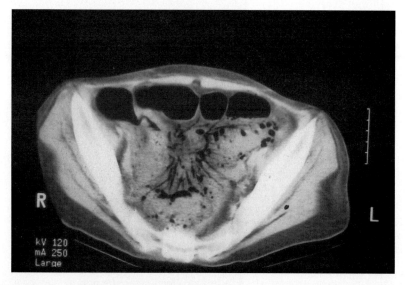

FIGURE 5.21. Small-bowel obstruction with bowel necrosis. CT scan through the pelvis reveals multiple loops of dilated small bowel. Innumerable linear collections of air are seen from gas within mesenteric veins. Severe pneumatosis is also seen.

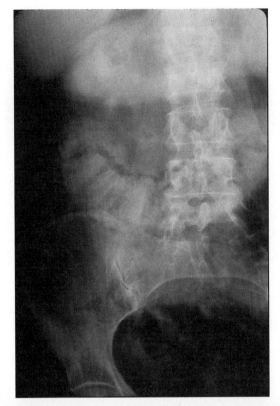

A

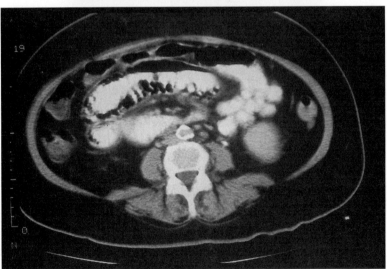

B

FIGURE 5.22. **Adhesive small-bowel obstruction with ischemia.** (A) Supine film of the abdomen demonstrates residual contrast medium in dilated small-bowel loops from a recent CT series. Pneumatosis of one loop of bowel in the left midabdomen is indicative of ischemia. (B) Section from a CT scan on the same patient better demonstrates the air collections in the nondependent portions of the small-bowel wall. The obstruction and ischemia were secondary to adhesions.

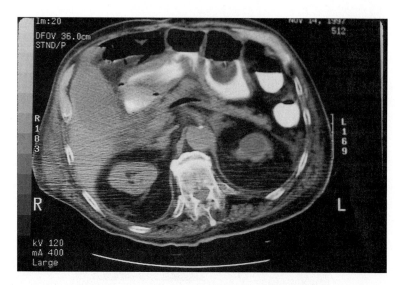

FIGURE 5.23. **Small-bowel obstruction with bowel necrosis.** CT scan of the upper abdomen reveals a loop of small bowel with a thickened, edematous wall. Two foci of intramural air represent air within necrotic bowel or in mesenteric veins. Air is also seen in larger mesenteric veins at the splenoportal confluence.

mechanical small-bowel obstruction with resultant small-bowel dilatation proximal to the involved loop. Then, the loop becomes torted, changing from a simple to a closed-loop obstruction. Finally venous congestion develops within the loop [49]. As the venous return is compromised, arterial inflow is not. This accounts for the presence of distended blood vessels in the mesentery noted on CT examinations (Fig. 5.24). Ultimately, frank hemorrhage into the wall or lumen develops. A transudate or exudate that crosses the serosa accounts for the development of peritoneal fluid [50] (Fig. 5.25).

Various authors have used some of the same and some differing CT findings to differentiate ischemic or necrotic bowel from viable tissue [30,47,48,51]. Ha found the highest specificity for decreased contrast enhancement and the serrated "beak" sign [48]. Unfortunately, both radiographic signs are low in sensitivity. Of the signs with relatively high specificity and sensitivity were any unusual course of the mesenteric vessels, mesenteric vascular engorgement, a large amount of ascites, and a hazy mesentery [48]. Somewhat similarly, Frager et al. found that abnormal small-bowel wall enhancement and the local presence of mesenteric edema or fluid were the best indicators of ischemia [30]. The analysis of Makita et al. revealed that the combined presence of increased mesenteric attenuation (due to hemorrhage or edema), a radial distribution of mesenteric vessels and bowel loops, and ascites were the best discriminators between necrotic and nonnecrotic bowel [51]. When they were present, the CT imaging was both sensitive and specific.

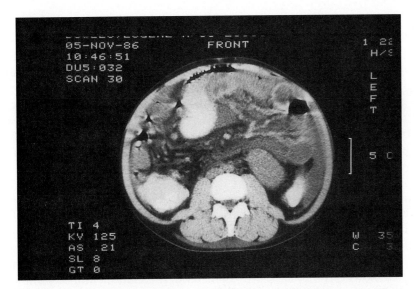

FIGURE 5.24. Closed-loop obstruction with prominent mesenteric vessels. CT scan through the midabdomen shows dilated small bowel from an obstruction. Very prominent mesenteric vessels represent the slow flow from a closed-loop obstruction.

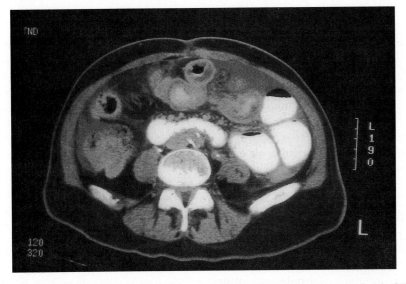

FIGURE 5.25. Ischemic bowel with mesenteric and intraperitoneal fluid. CT scan (of the patient seen later, in Fig. 5.40) reveals free intraperitoneal fluid, interloop or mesenteric fluid, and infiltration of the adjacent omentum in the left midabdomen. Also note the "target" or "halo" appearance of the small-bowel loops due to ischemia.

The importance of correlating imaging findings with appropriate clinical information is exemplified in the evaluation of the postoperative abdomen. Small-bowel obstructions, which occur in the immediate postoperative period, do not usually develop ischemic changes and can be treated conservatively [52,53].

More recent studies have suggested some utility for magnetic resonance (MR) imaging of the small bowel. HASTE imaging, utilizing a Half-Fourier Acquisition Single-shot Turbo spin Echo, allows subsecond imaging per section, resulting in complete examinations in a 20-second breath hold [54]. Normal patients showed a wide range of small-bowel fluid content, from none in 8% of patients to less than 25% of loops filled in 40% of patients to 25 to 50% of loops filled in another 40% of patients. Only 12% of patients had more than half their bowel loops filled with fluid [54]. The jejunum either had more fluid than the ileum (32%) or the same amount of fluid (60%), reflecting the increasing water resorption that occurs as one progresses downstream in the small bowel. The small-bowel diameter in the jejunum ranged from 1.5 to 2.7 cm (mean 2.1 cm), and the ileum somewhat less, ranging from 1.3 to 2.5 cm (mean 1.9 cm). The high signal intensity intestinal contents contrasted well with the medium signal intensity wall, even allowing visualization of the valvulae conniventes [54].

A study of the efficacy of HASTE imaging in patients with suspected small-bowel obstruction revealed that the presence of a small-bowel obstruction could be identified correctly by MR images in 26 of 29 cases (90%) [55]. The actual level was correctly identified in 19 of 26 patients (73%). HASTE imaging was much less successful in identifying the cause of the obstruction, being correct in only half these patients [55]. However, when a subgroup of patients with postoperative complications were selected and analyzed separately, the results varied somewhat. The rate of detection of the obstruction remained high (13 of 15, or 87%), while successful determination of the level of the obstruction dropped off to slightly less than half (7 of 15). The detection of the actual cause of the obstruction decreased to only 27% (4 of 15) [55]. Even more recent investigations are centered upon combining MR imaging with enteroclysis, but the results are far too preliminary to report at this time.

Contrast Agents for Ileus and Obstruction

Following abdominal pelvic surgery, intestinal activity may be considerably decreased or even absent. This may be secondary to a postoperative ileus or an early small-bowel obstruction. Various studies have shown that postoperative electrical activity in the GI tract is recovered most rapidly in the small bowel, then the stomach, and finally in the colon [56–59]. This correlates well with multiple-contrast studies that showed the colon recovering last as well [60–64]. Therefore, there is good physiological basis for the postoperative appearance of an air- and fluid-distended small bowel with little or no colonic contents. The differentiation between ileus, incomplete and complete small-bowel obstruction is an important although difficult one. As many as 58% of patients with small-bowel obstruction in the early postoperative period require reoperation [65]. The administration of hyperosmolar water-soluble contrast medium has been proposed as a way of differentiating ileus from small-bowel obstruction [66–69] as well as a means of separating incomplete from complete small-bowel obstructions [70].

In addition, some authors have studied the possibility of a therapeutic effect of hyperosmolar water-soluble contrast medium in cases of small-bowel obstruction [70–72]. This hypothesis is based on the shift of fluid into the gut due to an osmotic gradient. The increased liquid content stimulates bowel motility, helping transport contents distally [73–75]. The results from this and other studies are disparate and contradictory. In addition, anecdotal reports of success and failure are almost as numerous as the number of surgeons and radiologists queried.

One large prospective but nonrandomized trial concluded that high osmolarity, water-soluble contrast medium did not aid in the resolution of ileus following gynecological surgery [69]. Another randomized trial revealed that high osmolarity, water-soluble contrast medium significantly shortened the hospital stays of patients with adhesive small-bowel obstruction [72]. Less surgical intervention was needed in patients receiving these contrast agents as well.

Another, albeit noncontrolled study showed that high osmolarity, water-soluble contrast media help differentiate incomplete from complete small-bowel obstructions [70]. The authors stated that contrast medium appearing in the colon in less than 8 hours from its administration had sensitivity of 90%, specificity of 100%, and accuracy of 93% in predicting nonsurgical outcome of these patients. However, contradicting these reports is another prospective, randomized trial that found no difference in length of stay, relief of symptoms, or rate of surgical intervention in patients given high osmolarity water-soluble contrast medium versus those treated conservatively [71].

Crohn's Disease

Crohn's disease is not an uncommon disease that frequently recurs following surgical intervention. Clinical recurrence rates have been estimated by the National Cooperative Crohn's Disease Study to be 78% after 20 years [76] or as high as 60% at 5 years and 94% at 15 years [77]. Recurrence necessitating surgery is estimated at 15 to 40% at 10 years and 50 to 70% at 20 years following the initial resection [78–80]. Several studies have demonstrated that although the radiographic appearance of Crohn's may wax and wane over time in a given bowel segment, there is no significant progression longitudinally over time [81–83].

Many studies have tried to analyze the predictive factors for the extremely high and alarming recurrence rates. The involvement of the terminal ileum and the neoterminal ileum following surgery raises the possibility of reflux of colonic contents through the ileocecal valve as an etiological factor [84]. D'Haens et al. found that the duration of recurrent disease in the neoterminal ileum correlated with the extent of disease on presurgical studies [84]. Other studies showed that patients with ileocolic disease preoperatively had a higher rate of recurrence than those without terminal ileal involvement [79,85]. These patients also came to surgery earlier than those with more limited disease. A study from Norway suggested that younger patients (both at the onset of symptoms as well as the time of surgery) were at higher risk for recurrence than their more senior counterparts [86]. Yet another study contradicted this finding and found no relationship between the age of the patient and the rate of recurrence [87]. Distal colonic [86] and perianal disease [79] were also negative predictors for a disease-free postoperative course.

Another area of study has been the length of resected small bowel and the histological appearance of the margins of resection. The presence of granulomas or other evidence of inflammation at the margins of resection should be expected to lead to an increased rate of postoperative recurrence. This has been verified in at least two studies [86,88] but surprisingly refuted in at least one other [89]. Another study showed that resections of more than 25 cm of ileum and more than 50 cm of combined small and large bowel resulted in decreased rates of rehospitalization and reoperation [87]. Greater lengths of colon along with at least 25 cm of small-bowel resection did not result in an improved clinical outcome.

Some studies have suggested that there are two subgroups of patients with Crohn's disease [80,90,91]. In the more aggressive type, perforation may be part of the initial presentation. Those patients are more prone to early relapse postoperatively [90]. In the second group, patients with symptoms appearing less than 6 months prior to surgery had a 50% higher recurrence rate than those with a 10-year history of symptomatology [80]. The presence of postoperative complications following the initial surgery was also a predictor of early recurrence of the disease.

The postoperative appearance of Crohn's disease is similar to that seen preoperatively [92–96] (Fig. 5.26). Enteroclysis revealed evidence of submucosal disease in more than 60% of patients studied postoperatively [82]. This submucosal disease was evidence by a progression of changes from thickened to irregular to complete effacement of folds. Mucosal disease was evidence by superficial ulcerations in two-thirds of patients. Transmural disease was evidence by decreased pliability and reduced peristaltic activity in the intestinal segments. True stricture formation, a cobblestone appearance, and deep ulcerations and/or sinus tracts were also evidence of transmural disease. There was good correlation of the clinical activity of the disease and the radiographic appearance. Patients with transmural disease had a high rate of clinical symptoms when compared with those only having mucosal or submucosal disease. Patients with normal postoperative small-bowel enemas had no clinical evidence of recurrence [82].

Transabdominal sonography has already been shown to be of value in selecting patients with suspected Crohn's disease for barium studies.

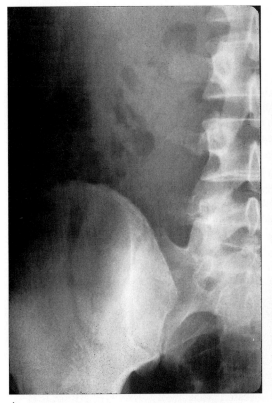

A

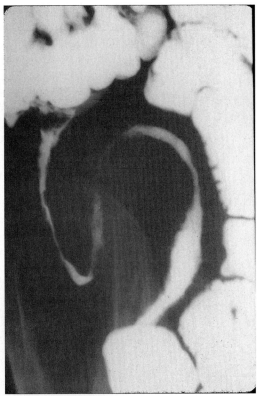

B

FIGURE 5.26. Recurrent Crohn's disease. (A) Plain film of the abdomen shows a very narrow, irregular loop of air-filled small bowel in the right lower quadrant. (B) Corresponding film from a small-bowel series reveals the abnormal loop to be recurrent Crohn's disease in the neoterminal ileum proximal to an ileotransverse colostomy.

Sensitivity, specificity, accuracy, and positive and negative predictive values were all in excess of 90% in at least one study [97]. Results from evaluating postoperative patients have not been quite as accurate, with reported sensitivities from 78 to 82% and specificities ranging from 91 to 100%, respectively [98,99]. Findings included a bowel wall thickness exceeding 5 mm, luminal narrowing with a hyperdense rim, decreased compressibility of the wall, decreased peristalsis, and a gradual transition from normal to abnormal appearing bowel. All layers of the bowel wall were symmetrically thickened in patients with Crohn's disease, and this was a good differentiator of inflammatory bowel disease from neoplastic processes [99]. Mural stratification, similar to that described shortly for CT imaging, allows visualization of the mucosal, submucosal, and muscularis propria layers [100] (Fig. 5.27). When seen, mural stratification means that edema, not fibrosis, is still present and that the

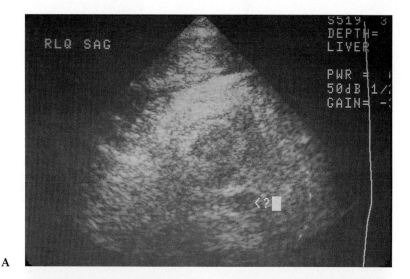

A

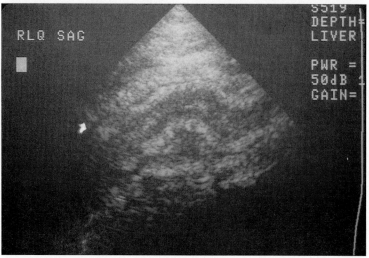

B

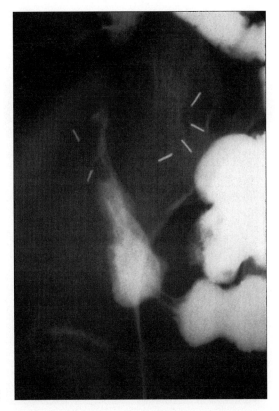

C

FIGURE 5.27. Recurrent Crohn's disease. (A) Transverse and (B) longitudinal sonograms of the right lower quadrant reveal an abnormal loop of small bowel characterized by an echogenic mucosal layer in the center of the bowel, and surrounding alternating layers of sonolucency and echogenicity. These are non-specific changes of Crohn's or other inflammatory disease of the small bowel. (C) Small-bowel series on the same patient shows typical findings of Crohn's disease in the neoterminal ileum. (Courtesy of R. Wachsberg, M.D., Newark, NJ)

narrowing may still be reversible [101,102]. In time, the loops of bowel may become matted together. Based on these and other studies, ultrasound may play an important role in limiting radiation exposure for patients with a chronic disease that can reach from childhood to patients with advanced maturity [97–99].

The postoperative CT appearance of Crohn's disease [103] parallels that seen preoperatively [100]. Increased bowel wall thickness, inflammatory masses, so-called fibrofatty changes in the mesentery and regional adenopathy were most commonly encountered (Fig. 5.28).

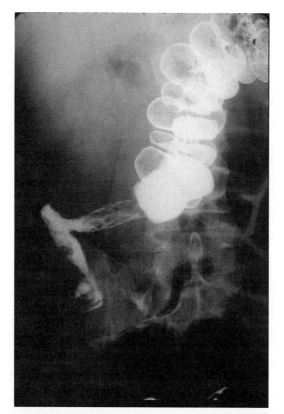

A

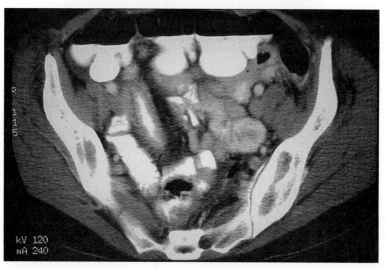

B

FIGURE 5.28. Recurrent Crohn's disease. (A) Frontal film from a double-contrast barium enema shows that the patient has undergone a right hemi-colectomy with an ileotransverse colostomy. The neoterminal ileum shows classic findings of Crohn's disease with narrowing and a cobblestone appearance. (B) CT scan at the level of the neoterminal ileum shows narrowing of the lumen, a thickened wall, and slight infiltration of the surrounding mesentery correlating well with the conventional contrast examination.

Gore et al. noted that the change from mural stratification to homogeneous enhancement heralded the change from edema to fibrosis [100]. Similarly, this loss of the target appearance was seen in postoperative patients who would eventually need strictureplasty [103]. Regional lymph nodes less than 8 m in diameter may be seen in Crohn's disease, but nodes larger than that may indicate associated lymphoma or carcinoma [100]. The appearance of sinus tracts and fistulas, as well as extraintestinal changes, should be similar in postoperative patients to that in newly diagnosed patients.

When small-bowel strictures occur, they may be resected and bowel continuity restored. However, strictureplasty may be performed maintaining bowel lengths with similar postoperative outcomes [91]. Two different types of strictureplasty result in radically different radiologic appearances. The Heineke–Mikulicz technique is used for strictures that are less than 7 cm long [104]. The bowel is opened longitudinally through the stricture and then closed transversely, thereby increasing the effective diameter of the small bowel (as well as causing very minimal foreshortening of the gut) (Fig. 5.29). The Finney strictureplasty is used for longer strictures [104]. In this technique the bowel is configured to form a loop similar in shape to the Greek letter omega (Ω) with the stricture at the apex. The two loops are sutured together apposing the loops both proximal and distal to the small-bowel narrowing. A longitudinal incision is then made, opening the stricture. Next, the posterior walls of the two apposed limbs are sutured together, and ultimately the two anterior walls are brought together. The resulting configuration is that of an upside-down U-shaped loop in which the two limbs come together near the apex into a dilated area, replacing the stricture (Fig. 5.30). The Heineke–Mikulicz and Finney strictureplasties can be performed together in cases of stenoses and skip areas of involvement [104] (Fig. 5.31).

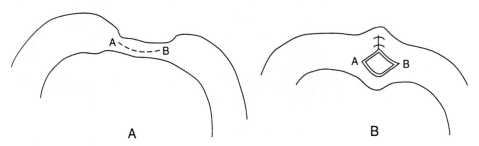

FIGURE 5.29. **Heineke–Mikulicz strictureplasty.** Schematic drawings show the longitudinal incision in the strictured region (A) and their subsequent closure in a transverse manner (B).

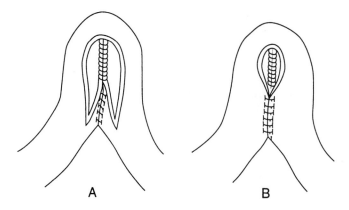

FIGURE 5.30. Finney strictureplasty. (A) Schematic drawing shows the formation of an omega-shaped loop from a strictured segment of small bowel with closure of the common posterior walls. (B) Subsequent closure of the anterior wall.

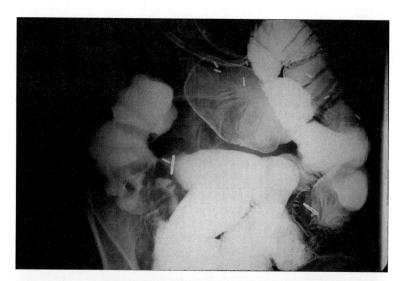

A

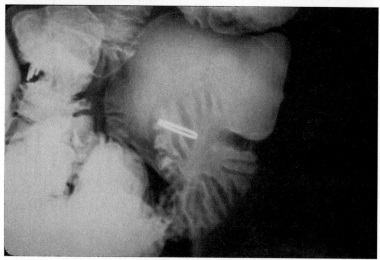

B

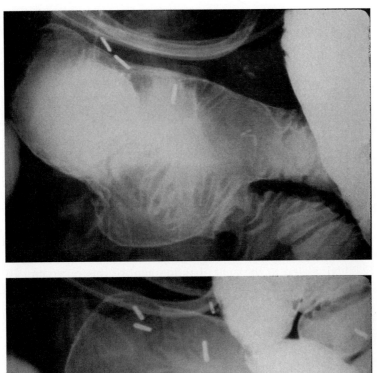

C

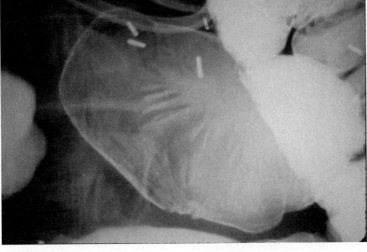

D

FIGURE 5.31. **Crohn's disease with two different strictureplasties.** (A) Single supine film from a double-contrast enteroclysis of a patient with Crohn's disease and multiple operations in the past for obstruction. In the left lower quadrant, a small deformity is seen secondary to a prior Heineke–Mikulicz procedure. In the upper abdomen a larger, almost saccular appearance is noted secondary to a prior Finney strictureplasty. (B) Spot film of the Heineke–Mikulicz strictureplasty showing saccular dilatation with interruption of the normally transverse valvulae conniventes. The seam of the strictureplasty is noted as an area devoid of folds. (C) Another spot film from the same examination demonstrates the sequelae of a Finney strictureplasty. The previously strictured loop is folded back upon itself with the two lumina joined into a common one. The seam of this longitudinal anastomotic line is evident on another spot film (D) from the small-bowel enema.

Another surgical technique utilized in cases of multiple strictures, long strictures, and lesions longer than 30 cm is that of a side-to-side isoperistaltic strictureplasty [104]. In this very complex technique, the bowel is divided in the middle of the diseased area. The two segments are lain together side by side in an isoperistaltic arrangement. Each bowel loop is then opened longitudinally along its antimesenteric border and joined together along this enterotomy [104] (Fig. 5.32).

There is some evidence that Crohn's disease leads to an increased rate of carcinoma in the small bowel [105]. It tends to develop in a younger age group than other small-bowel carcinomas [106]. Patients usually have had Crohn's disease for 15 to 20 years before malignancy develops [106]. Some patients undergo bypass of severely involved bowel without resection of these loops. Since the long-standing inflammatory process remains in situ with this type of procedure, carcinoma may develop within the bypassed but retained segments [107]. This has led to the near abandonment of this procedure [105]. Carcinoma may also develop at sites of chronic fistula formation [105].

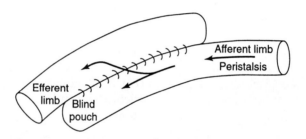

FIGURE 5.32. Side-to-side isoperistaltic enteroenterostomy. Schematic drawing shows how this technique may be used to bypass long strictures or to reestablish continuity of the small intestine following a segmental resection. A blind pouch may result at the distal end of the afferent limb.

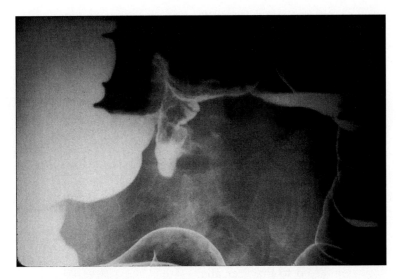

FIGURE 5.33. **Carcinoma in bypassed loop of small bowel.** Coned down view of the transverse colon from a double-contrast barium enema reveals reflux into a loop of small bowel. The loop ends at an annular constricting lesion, a carcinoma that arose in a bypassed limb of small bowel in this patient with Crohn's disease.

Visualizing carcinomas in bypassed loops of small bowel must usually depend on the use of CT or other cross-sectional imaging modalities [105]. Occasionally, reflux into a bypassed segment may afford demonstration of a carcinoma (Fig. 5.33). However, the best clue to its presence is that of change in a stricture or fistula over a period of time, demonstrated on serial examinations [105].

Diversion Procedures

Ileostomies may be performed for multiple reasons including temporarily diverting the stream of intestinal contents in patients with surgery involving the more distal small bowel or colon. Removal of the colon may necessitate creation of a permanent stoma. Everting the distal end of the ileum and bringing it through the anterior abdominal wall creates a permanent stoma. Various abnormalities of the stoma may include adhesions, prolapse (Fig. 5.34), parastomal herniation, and recurrent disease (especially Crohn's disease) at the stomal site.

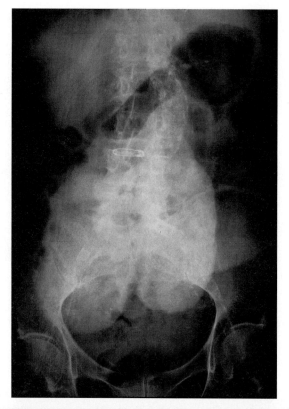

A

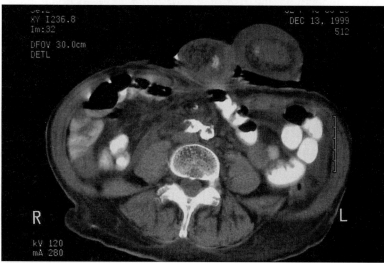

B

FIGURE 5.34. **Prolapsed ileostomy.** (A) Supine film of the abdomen shows a bilobed soft tissue density overlying the lower abdomen and pelvis. Its high density represents the sharp boundary with the surrounding air and not increased density of the mass itself. (B) CT scan of the same patient demonstrates the two prolapsed loops of small bowel lying on the anterior abdominal wall. The extent of the prolapse is very unusual.

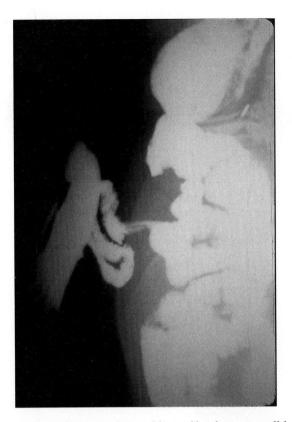

FIGURE **5.35. Parastomal hernia.** Steep oblique film from a small-bowel series demonstrates multiple loops of small bowel coiled within the anterior abdominal wall at the site of an ileostomy.

Parastomal hernias may be detected on routine contrast studies (Fig. 5.35) or CT images. The key to the diagnosis on routine contrast studies is the use of a steep oblique or even lateral position to bring the stoma and prestomal loop into tangential view [108] (Fig. 5.36). In addition, the use of a cone stomal appliance (Fig. 5.37) makes performance of the exam easier and avoids the use of a balloon catheter that could cause damage to the prestomal loop or the stoma itself [108]. On CT imaging, the finding of loops of small bowel in the anterior abdominal wall, other than the prestomal loop itself, makes the diagnosis self-evident.

Kock introduced the continent ileostomy in 1969 [109]. He fashioned a low pressure, highly compliant reservoir to be used in postprocto-colectomy patients. By leaving the patient with a noneverted flat stoma and eliminating the need for a collection bag for waste products, the patient was afforded an improved body image and could pursue a more active lifestyle.

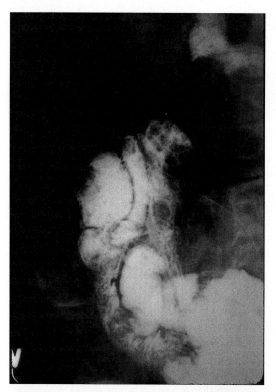

A

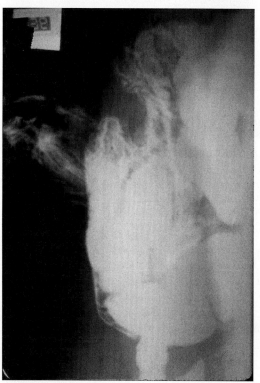

B

FIGURE 5.36. Parastomal hernia (and the value of a steep oblique film). (A) Frontal film from a small-bowel series shows multiple small-bowel loops in the right midabdomen without evidence of a hernia. They have lost their usual serpentine arrangement. (B) Spot film in a steep right posterior oblique position shows a knuckle of small bowel in the anterior abdominal wall, a parastomal hernia.

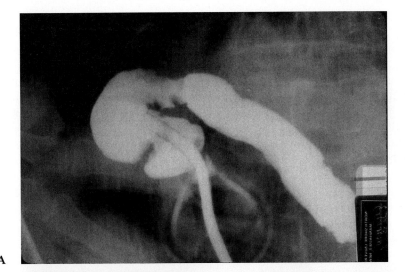

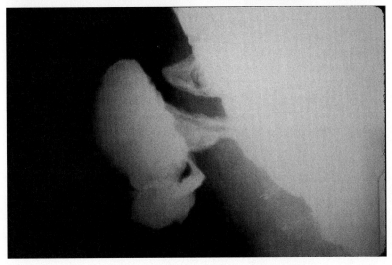

FIGURE 5.37. **Parastomal hernia.** (A) Frontal film from a retrograde small-bowel study performed through an ileostomy shows what appears to be normal anatomy at the stomal site. Note the use of a cone ostomy device rather than a catheter to cannulate the stoma. (B) Steep oblique film not only reveals a large parastomal hernia, but a second loop of herniated bowel superiorly.

The pouch comprises of three loops of ileum that are configured in an "S" shape. The bowel is opened along its antimesenteric border and then the contiguous portions of two loops are sutured together, creating a large saccular reservoir. The opposed nature of the loops prevents peristalsis from emptying the pouch [110,111]. Instead of an everted stoma, the terminal end of the pouch is retrograde intussuscepted into the pouch, creating a valve that further prevents inadvertent emptying of the pouch [110] (Figs. 5.38 and 5.39). Emptying is performed by intermittent catheterization. The entire pouch is anchored to the anterior abdominal wall.

Lycke and colleagues have noted that the radiological evaluation of the normal pouch includes examining the pouch (or reservoir) itself, the valve, and both the afferent and efferent ileal loops [110]. Over time, the reservoir gradually increases in capacity from 100 ml to 700 ml. On

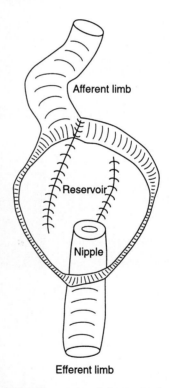

FIGURE 5.38. Kock contintent ileostomy. Schematic drawing reveals details of the construction of a Kock pouch. In this example, three loops of bowel have been brought together to form a large reservoir. The efferent limb has been retrograde intussuscepted into the pouch to form a nipple, which maintains continency.

FIGURE 5.39. **Kock pouch.** (A) Supine film of
the abdomen shows a large air collection in
the right lower quadrant. Some bowel mark-
ings are present. Within the air collection is
a round soft tissue density representing the
intussuscepted nipple within the pouch.
A catheter can be seen entering the nipple.
(B) Upright abdominal film on the same
patient reveals the large saccular configuration of the pouch brought about by uniting
multiple small-bowel loops to form a large
reservoir.

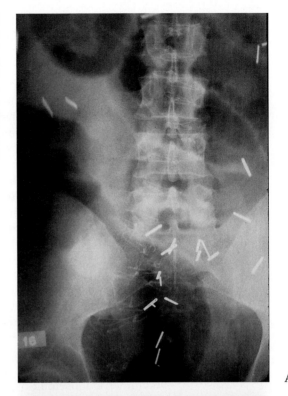

A

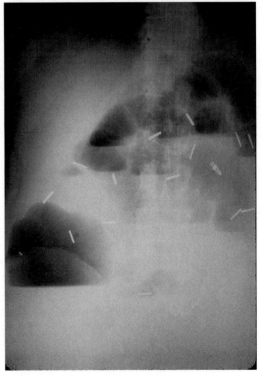

B

double-contrast studies, the suture lines interrupt the mucosal folds where the segments were joined. Again over time, the fold pattern inside the pouch becomes less distinct.

The valve that allows the patient to remain continent is seen as an intussuscepted segment, 3 to 5 cm long and usually 2.5 to 4 cm in diameter, that protrudes into the reservoir. It is best seen in profile, utilizing a steep oblique or lateral projection. The valve should be examined while the patient is catheterized as well as after catheter removal. In the latter circumstance, films should be obtained both at rest and while the patient is straining.

The afferent limb is usually slightly greater in diameter than the more proximal ileum; it is otherwise indistinguishable from the rest of the ileum. The efferent limb is that short segment of small bowel that begins at the base of the continence-producing valve and transits the anterior abdominal wall to end at the stoma. This segment may make a large angle with the lumen of the valve when the patient is examined in the upright position. However, this may be normal.

Again, Lycke and colleagues have written a detailed analysis of the radiographic findings of complications of Kock pouches [112]. Abnormalities of the Kock pouch may be grouped according to the segment of the pouch that is affected by mechanical problems, recurrent inflammatory disease, or "pouchitis," a nonspecific inflammation of the reservoir.

Asymmetric loosening of the staples that help form the valve may lead to sliding, with a reduction of length along the mesenteric side of the valve. This can result in both incontinence and difficulty in catheterization. This loosening may eventually result in loosening of the antimesenteric side as well. This leads to a tortuous elongated efferent limb that actually replaces the valve.

If the opening in the inner aspect of the anterior abdominal wall enlarges, the base of the valve may become everted. Folding of the staple lines along the valve itself best depicts this [112]. With contrast studies, the efferent limb and valve take on an "ace of spades" configuration in either eversion or sliding.

Detachment of the reservoir from the anterior abdominal wall is difficult to detect and often overlooked on contrast studies [112]. A "cul-de-sac" in the efferent limb can be seen in cases of incomplete detachment [112].

Fistulae may be secondary to recurrent Crohn's disease or may be mechanical in origin. They may involve the walls of the valve itself; they may be between the afferent limb and the reservoir (internal fistula); or they may connect the reservoir to the skin (external fistula).

Recurrent Crohn's disease in the reservoir and/or afferent limb resembles that seen in preoperative patients. A cobblestoned mucosa may be seen along with areas of stenosis [112]. The reservoir may also be affected by nonspecific painful inflammation characterized by increased discharge of fluid and gas (Fig. 5.40). Double-contrast studies may reveal a granular mucosa in mild disease, which may progress to ulceration and edema in severe cases of ileitis or "pouchitis" [112].

FIGURE 5.40. Kock "pouchitis." (A) Retrograde "pouchgram" study shows the large saccular reservoir of a Kock pouch. Some of the contrast has refluxed into the afferent loop of ileum, which shows thickened folds consistent with ileitis. (B) Another film from the same study shows that the folds within the pouch itself are severely thickened and distorted, consistent with so-called pouchitis.

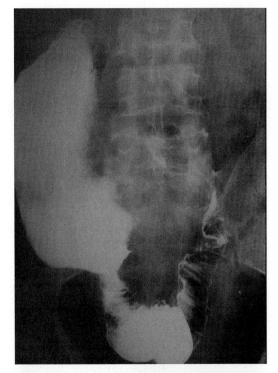

A

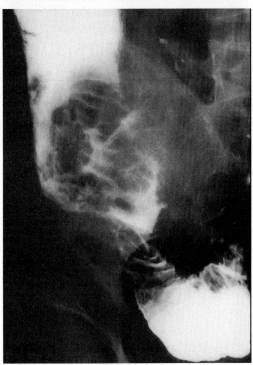

B

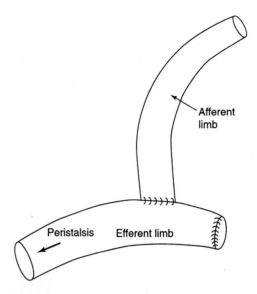

FIGURE 5.41. **End-to-side anastomosis.** Schematic drawing of a properly performed end-to-side anastomosis.

Enteroenteric Anastomoses

Following removal of a segment of small intestine, reestablishment of the continuity of the GI tract may be performed by means of an end-to-end anastomosis, a side-to-side or an end-to-side technique. The first allows reestablishment of antegrade flow without a blind-ending pouch or interruption of the circular muscle fibers, which could result in diminished antegrade flow. The end-to-side technique allows the union of two segments of bowel with disproportionate diameters [111] (Fig. 5.41). It should be performed with the end of the proximal loop anastomosed to the side of the distal limb. This promotes drainage of the blind pouch of the distal limb. A side-to-side technique is more often utilized in cases of widespread disease or when surgery must be performed expeditiously [111] (Fig. 5.42). Any of these techniques is subject to the usual complications of dehiscence and suture line leakage. The factors affecting the integrity of the anastomosis include sepsis, tissue oxygenation, and the general nutritional and health status of the patient [111].

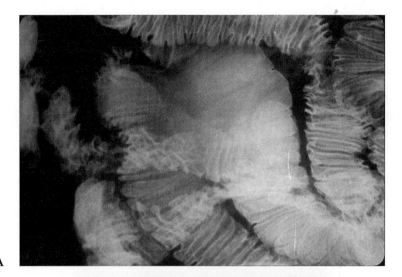

A

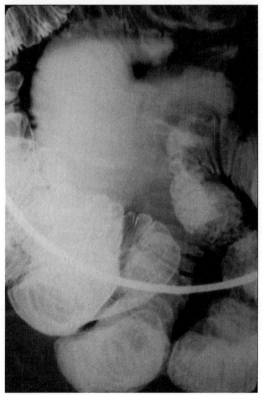

B

FIGURE 5.42. **Side-to-side enteroenterostomy.** (A, B) Spot films from a double-contrast small-bowel enema reveal a broad lumen formed by two separate loops of small bowel brought together in a side-to-side manner. (A) Small blind-ending pouch lies just superior to the anastomotic line. (B) The anastomotic seam is well demonstrated. Films are from the same patient in whom a metastatic melanoma resection resulted in a blind-ending jejunal loop (see Fig. 5.44).

Blind pouches may occur following side-to-side anastomoses (Fig. 5.32) [113]. The dilatation occurs 5 to 15 years postoperatively because of the interruption of a significant length of circular muscle fibers in creating the anastomosis [111]. Usually the loop proximal to the anastomosis dilates, although occasionally both proximal and distal limbs are involved. Inadvertent side-to-end anastomoses, rather than end-to-side ones, may also result in blind pouch formation (Figs. 5.43 and 5.44).

Supine roentgenograms of the abdomen reveal a soft tissue mass or air and fluid-filled masses of varying sizes and configurations [111,113]. Contrast studies, including enteroclysis, can readily demonstrate the etiology of such unusual masses or fluid collections. Clinically a blind pouch may present with enterolith formation, diarrhea, and malabsorption secondary to bacterial overgrowth, abdominal pain, weight loss, and GI bleeding.

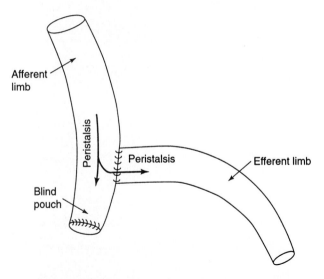

FIGURE 5.43. **Blind pouch formation.** Schematic drawing shows how a blind pouch forms following an improperly performed end-to-side anastomosis.

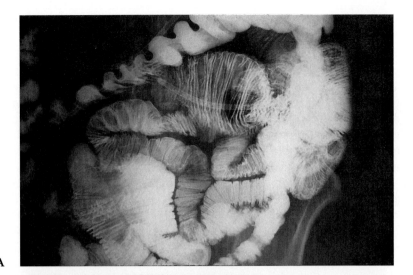

A

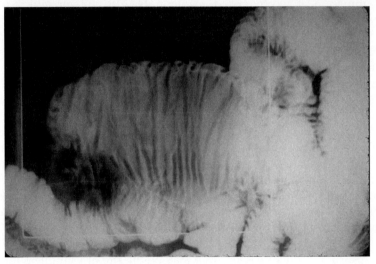

B

FIGURE 5.44. **Blind-ending jejunal loop.** (A) Supine film of the upper abdomen from a double-contrast enteroclysis reveals a blind-ending loop of jejunum in the left upper quadrant with the enteroclysis catheter inside it. (B) Spot film of the same area shows the blind pouch to better effect. This patient had had a previous resection of a jejunal metastasis from malignant melanoma with an end-to-side anastomosis. Preferential flow from the duodenum entered and enlarged the blind sac.

Bariatric Surgery

The use of surgical procedures to control morbid obesity, a condition that affects more than 5 million Americans [114], has been around for a long time. Currently, interest is focused on the stomach and various procedures to control its capacity and absorptive ability. Previously, a not uncommon procedure was jejunoileal bypass [115]. This was introduced in 1963 but is no longer performed. However, it is possible that one will be called upon to examine the abdomen and GI tract of an individual who has undergone the procedure.

Jejunoileal bypass consists of bypassing most of the length of the small intestine, thereby limiting the amount of mucosa available for absorption. A variable amount of jejunum is anastomosed either to the distal or terminal ileum [115] or to the right colon [116]. The bypassed portion of small bowel is then anastomosed either to the terminal ileum or to the colon [115,116]. Various complications may ensue, including inflammation of the bypassed segment [117,118], hyperoxaluria and renal lithiasis [119,120], and cholelithiasis [120].

Wade and his colleagues reported that during the first postoperative year both the length of the small bowel and its caliber will increase compared with baseline studies [115]. This most likely represents an adaptive mechanism in response to the surgery. Because of the limited amount of mucosa available for water resorption, air–fluid levels are commonly seen postoperatively on horizontal beam radiographs [115]. In addition most patients will show an increase in the thickness of the valvulae conniventes [115]. In the distal ileum this may become so marked that the bowel resembles the more proximal jejunum, so-called jejunization of the ileum [121]. The colon likewise dilates. Occasionally diffuse dilatation of the colon may be seen with the appearance of a so-called megacolon [115,122]. Another plain radiographic finding is that of pneumatosis intestinalis [118,123]. Besides being the location for bacterial overgrowth with resultant enteritis and malabsorption, the bypassed limb may be the site of jejunoileal intussusception [124–126]. Both CT and ultrasound scans have been reported to detect this complication. Routine contrast studies would not be expected to reflux into the bypassed loop to detect an intussusception. On ultrasound, an echogenic mass with a hyperechoic center and sonolucent rim may be seen [125]. On CT images, the typical findings of an intussusception, with a target or doughnut configuration, have been described [126].

Contrast studies of the small bowel will demonstrate the increased diameter (Fig. 5.45) as well as the thickened valvulae conniventes (Fig. 5.46). More than 80% of patients will demonstrate reflux of the contrast medium into the bypassed segment of small bowel [115] (Fig. 5.46). The jejunoileal anastomosis is readily seen on contrast studies (Figs. 5.45 and 5.46). The distance refluxed into the bypassed limb is usually less than 30 cm and does not correlate with the amount of weight loss [115].

FIGURE 5.45. **Jejunoileal bypass for obesity.** Over-head film from a small-bowel series reveals a very short segment of opacified jejunum with consider-able filling of the right colon with barium. Note the compensatory dilatation of the jejunum.

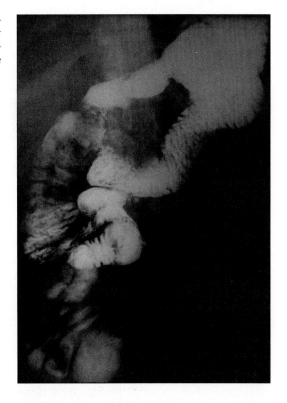

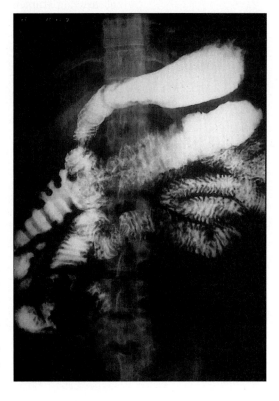

FIGURE 5.46. **Jejunoileal bypass for obesity.** Over-head film from a small-bowel series shows limi-ted opacification of the jejunum secondary to a jejunoileal bypass. A small amount of contrast has refluxed into the bypassed segment of ileum in the right lower quadrant. Also evident is dilation and fold thickening with the jejunum, presumably an adaptive change following the bowel short-circuiting.

References

1. Wilson MS, Ellis H, Menzies, et al. A review of the management of small bowel obstruction. Ann R Coll Surg Engl 1999;81:320–328.
2. Wurster SH, Bonet V, Mayberry A, et al. Intraperitoneal sodium carboxymethylcellulose administration prevents reformation of peritoneal adhesions following surgical lysis. J Surg Res 1995;59:97–102.
3. Baker SR, Cho KC. The Abdominal Plain Film with Correlative Imaging, 2nd ed. Stamford, CT: Appleton & Lange; 1999:217–359.
4. Pickleman J. Small bowel obstruction. In: Zinner MJ, ed. Maingot's Abdominal Operations, 10th ed. London: Prentice Hall; 1997:1159–1172.
5. Mucha P. Small intestinal obstruction. Surg Clin North Am 1987; 67:597–620.
6. Ellis H. The causes and preventions of intestinal adhesions. Br J Surg 1982;69:241–243.
7. Cox MR, Gunn IF. Operative aetiology and types of adhesions causing small bowel obstruction. Aust N Z J Surg 1993;63:848–852.
8. Menzies D, Ellis H. Intestinal obstruction from adhesions—How big is the problem? Ann R Coll Surg Engl 1990;72:60–63.
9. Wilson MS, Ellis H, Parker MC, et al. Adhesion related hospital readmissions following abdominal and pelvic surgery—A major healthcare problem. Lancet 1999;353:1476–1480.
10. Turner DM, Croom RD. Acute adhesive obstruction of the small intestine. Arch Surg 1982;117:334–337.
11. Landercasper J, Cogbill T, Merry W. Longterm outcome after hospitalisation for small bowel obstruction. Arch Surg 1993;128:765–770.
12. Montefusco RP, Ward RJ, Geiss AC. Recurrent adhesive small bowel obstruction. Contemp Surg 1985;27:98–101.
13. Graves EJ. 1992 summary: National Hospital Discharge Survey. Adv Data 1994;249:1–12.
14. Wilson MS, Hawkswell J, McCloy RF. The natural history of adhesional small bowel obstruction: Counting the cost. Br J Surg 1998;85:1294–1298.
15. Zbar RI, Crede WB, McKhann CF, Jekel JF. Postoperative incidence of small bowel obstruction after appendicectomy and cholecystectomy—6 year retrospective cohort study. Conn Med 1993;57:123–127.
16. Fazio VW, Ziv Y, Church JM, et al. Ileal pouch–anal anastomoses; complications and function in 1005 patients. Ann Surg 1995;222:120–127.
17. Buckman RF, Buckman PD, Hufnagel HV, Gervin AS. A physiologic basis for the adhesion-free healing of deperitonealized surfaces. J Surg Res 1976; 21:67–76.
18. Buckman RF, Wjoods M, Sargent L, Gervin AS. A unifying mechanism in the etiology of intraperitoneal adhesions. J Surg Res 1976;20:1–5.
19. Milligan DW, Rafferty AT. Observations on the pathogenesis of peritoneal adhesions: A light and electron microscopical study. Br J Surg 1974;61: 274–280.
20. Adoni A, Adatto-Levy R, Mogel P, et al. Postoperative pleural effusion caused by Dextran. Int J Gynaecol Obstet 1980;18:243–244.
21. Borten M, Seibert C, Taymor M. Recurrent anaphylactic reaction to intraperitoneal Dextran 75 used for prevention of postsurgical adhesions. Obstet Gynecol 1983;61:755–757.
22. Pear BL, Boyden FM. Intraperitoneal lipid granuloma. Radiology 1967; 89:47–51.
23. Blake JB. The use of sterile oil to prevent intraperitoneal adhesions. Surg Gynec Obst 1908;6:667–670.

24. Norris JC, Davison TC. Peritoneal reaction to liquid petrolatum. JAMA 1934;103:1846–1847.
25. Boyers S, Diamond MP, DeCherney AH. Reduction of postoperative pelvic adhesion in the rabbit with Gore-Tex surgical membrane. Fertil Steril 1989;51:509–512.
26. March CM, Boyers S, Franklin R. Prevention of adhesion formation/ reformation with the Gore-Tex surgical membrane. Prog Clin Biol Res 1993;381:253–259.
27. Becker JM, Dayton MT, Fazio VW, et al. Prevention of postoperative abdominal adhesions by a sodium hyaluronate–based bioresorbable membrane: A prospective, randomised, double-blinded multicentre study. J Am Coll Surg 1996;183:297–306.
28. Diamond MP. Reduction of adhesions after uterine myomectomy by Seprafilm membrane. A blinded, randomised, multicentre study. Fertil Steril 1996;66:904–910.
29. Frager D, Medwid SE, Baer JW, et al. CT of small bowel obstruction: Value in establishing the diagnosis and determining the degree and cause. AJR Am J Roentgenol 1994;162:37–41.
30. Frager D, Baer JW, Medwid SW, Rothpearl A, Bossart P. Detection of intestinal ischemia in patients with acute small-bowel obstruction due to adhesions or hernia: Efficacy of CT. AJR Am J Roentgenol 1996;166:67–71.
31. Shrake PD, Rex DK, Lappas JL, et al. Radiographic evaluation of suspected small bowel obstruction. Am J Gastroenterol 1991;88:175–178.
32. Maglinte DDT, Reyes BL, Harmon BH, et al. Reliability and role of plain film radiography and CT in the diagnosis of small-bowel obstruction. AJR Am J Roentgenol 1996;167:1451–1455.
33. Frimann-Dahl J. Roentgen Examinations In Acute Abdominal Diseases, 2nd ed. Springfield, IL: CC Thomas; 1960.
34. Harlow CL, Stears RLG, Zeligman BE, et al. Diagnosis of bowel obstruction on plain abdominal radiographs: Significance of air–fluid levels at different heights in the same loop of bowel. AJR Am J Roentgenol 1993; 161:291–295.
35. The Royal College of Radiologists. Making the Best Use of a Department of Clinical Radiology: Guidelines for Doctors, 2nd ed. London: Royal College of Radiologists; 1993.
36. Patel NH, Lauber PR. The meaning of a nonspecific abdominal gas pattern. Acad Radiol 1995;2:667–669.
37. Suh RS, Maglinte DDT, Lavonas EJ, et al. Emergency abdominal radiography: Discrepancies of preliminary and final interpretation and management relevance. Emerg Radiol 1995;2:1–4.
38. Brolin RE, Krasna MJ, Mast BA. Use of tubes and radiographs in the management of small-bowel obstruction. Ann Surg 1987;206:126–133.
39. Wolfson PH, Bauer JJ, Gelernt IM, et al. Use of the long tube in the management of patients with small bowel obstruction due to adhesions. Arch Surg 1985;120:1001–1006.
40. Williams JL. Fluid-filled loops in intestinal obstruction. AJR Am J Roentgenol 1962;88:677–686.
41. Mellins HZ, Rigler LG. The Roentgen findings in strangulating obstructions of the small intestine. AJR Am J Roentgenol 1954;71:404–416.
42. Maglinte DDT, Balthazar EJ, Kelvin FM, Megibow AJ. The role of radiology in the diagnosis of small-bowel obstruction. AJR Am J Roentgenol 1997; 168:1171–1180.

43. Birnbaum BA, Maglinte DDT. Small bowel obstruction. In: Maglinte DDT, Herlinger H, Birnbaum BA, eds. Clinical Imaging of the Small Intestine, 2nd ed. New York: Springer-Verlag; 1998:467–506.

44. Davidson JC, Einstein DM, Herts BR, et al. Comparison of two barium suspensions for dedicated small-bowel series. AJR Am J Roentgenol 1999; 172:379–382.

45. Makanjuola D. Computed tomography compared with small bowel enema in clinically equivocal intestinal obstruction. Clin Radiol 1998;53: 203–208.

46. Donckier V, Closset J, van Gansbeke D, et al. Contribution of computed tomography to decision making in the management of adhesive small bowel obstruction. Br J Surg 1998;85:1071–1074.

47. Balthazar EJ, Liebeskind ME, Macari M. Intestinal ischemia in patients in whom small bowel obstruction is suspected: Evaluation of accuracy, limitations, and clinical implications of CT in diagnosis. Radiology 1997; 205:519–522.

48. Ha HK, Kim JS, Lee MSL, et al. Differentiation of simple and strangulated small-bowel obstructions: Usefulness of known CT criteria. Radiology 1997;204:507–512.

49. Laufman H, Nora PF. Physiological problems underlying intestinal strangulation obstruction. Surg Clin North Am 1966;42:219–229.

50. Leffall Jr LD, Quander J, Syphax B. Strangulation intestinal obstruction: A clinical appraisal. Arch Surg 1965;91:592–596.

51. Makita O, Ikushima I, Matsumoto N, et al. CT differentiation between necrotic and nonnecrotic small bowel in closed loop and strangulating obstruction. Abdom Imaging 1999;24:120–124.

52. Pickleman J, Lee RM. Management of patients with suspected early post-operative small bowel obstruction. Ann Surg 1989;210:216–219.

53. Sannella NA. Early and late obstruction of the small bowel after abdominoperineal resection. Am J Surg 1975;130:270–272.

54. Lee JKT, Marcos HB, Semelka RC. MR imaging of the small bowel using the HASTE sequence. AJR Am J Roentgenol 1998;170:1457–1463.

55. Regan F, Beall DP, Bohlman ME, et al. Fast MR imaging and the detection of small-bowel obstruction. AJR Am J Roentgenol 1998;170:1465–1469.

56. Dubois A, Weise VK, Kopin IJ. Postoperative ileus in the rat: Physiopathology, etiology and treatment. Ann Surg 1973;178:781–786.

57. Tinckler LF. Surgery and intestinal motility. Br J Surg 1965;52:140–150.

58. Smith J, Kelly KA, Weinshilboum RM. Pathophysiology of postoperative ileus. Arch Surg 1977;112:203–209.

59. Nachlas MM, Younis MT, Roda CP, et al. Gastrointestinal motility studies as a guide to postoperative management. Ann Surg 1972;175: 510–522.

60. Wells C, Tinckler L, Rawlinson K, et al. Postoperative gastrointestinal motility. Lancet 1964;1:4–10.

61. McPhail JL, Hardy JD, Conn JH, et al. Studies in postoperative ileus: Intestinal motility as reflected in the propulsion of radiopaque materials. Surg Forum 1958;9:471–472.

62. Noer T. Roentgenological transit time through the small intestine in the immediate postoperative period. Acta Chir Scand 1968;134:577–580.

63. Wilson JP. Postoperative motility of the large intestine in man. Gut 1975; 16:689–692.

64. Dauchel J, Schang JC, Kachelhoffer J, et al. Gastrointestinal myoelectrical activity during the postoperative period in man. Digestion 1976;14: 293–303.

65. Frykberg ER, Phillips JW. Obstruction of the small bowel in the early post-operative period. South Med J 1989;82:169–173.

66. Epstein BS. Nonabsorbable water-soluble contrast studies. JAMA 1957; 165:44–46.

67. Rubin RJ, Ostrum BJ, Dex WJ. Water-soluble contrast media. Arch Surg 1960;80:151–156.

68. Vest B, Margulis AR. The Roentgen diagnosis of postoperative ileus-obstruction. Surg Gynecol Obstet 1962;115:421–427.

69. Finan MA, Barton KPJ, Fiorica JV, et al. Ileus following gynecologic surgery: Management with water-soluble hyperosmolar radiocontrast material. South Med J 1995;88:539–542.

70. Chen SC, Chang KJ, Lee PH, Wang SM, Chen KM, Lin FY. Oral Urografin in postoperative small bowel obstruction. World J Surg 1999;23:1051–1054.

71. Feigin E, Seror D, Szold A, et al. Water-soluble contrast material has no therapeutic effect on postoperative small-bowel obstruction: Results of a prospective, randomized clinical trial. Am J Surg 1996;171:227–229.

72. Assalia A, Schein M, Kopelman D, Hirshberg A, Hashmonai M. Thera-peutic effect of oral Gastrografin in adhesive, partial small-bowel obstruc-tion: A prospective randomized trial. Surgery 1994;115:433–437.

73. Ott DJ, Gelfand DW. Gastrointestinal contrast agents. Indications, uses, and risks. JAMA 1983;249:2380–2384.

74. Dunn JT, Halls JM, Bern TV. Roentgenographic contrast studies in acute small-bowel obstruction. Arch Surg 1984;119:1305–1308.

75. Stordahl A, Laerum F, Gjolberg T, et al. Water-soluble contrast media in radiography of small bowel obstruction. Acta Radiol 1988;29:53–56.

76. Mekhijian HS, Seitz DM, Watts D, et al. National Cooperative Crohn's Disease Study: Factors determing recurrence of Crohn's disease after surgery. Gastroenterology 1979;77:907–913.

77. Greenstein AJ, Sachar DB, Paternack BS, Janowitz HD. Reoperation and recurrence in Crohn's colitis and ileocolitis, crude and cumulative rates. N Engl J Med 1975;293:685–690.

78. Shivananda S, Hordijk ML, Pena AS, Mayberry JF. Crohn's disease: Risk of recurrence and reoperation in a defined population. Gut 1989;30:990–995.

79. Whelan G, Farmer RG, Fazio VW, Goormastic M. Recurrence after surgery in Crohn's disease. Relationship to location of disease (clinical pattern) and surgical indication. Gastroenterology 1985;88:1826–1833.

80. Sachar DB, Wolfson DM, Greenstein AJ, et al. Risk factors for postopera-tive recurrence of Crohn's disease. Gastroenterology 1983;85:917–921.

81. Ni X-Y, Goldberg HI. Aphthoid ulcers in Crohn disease: Radiographic course and relationship to bowel appearance. Radiology 1986;158:589–596.

82. Ekberg O, Fork FT, Hildell J. Predictive value of small bowel radiography for recurrent Crohn disease. AJR Am J Roentgenol 1980;135:1051–1055.

83. Hildell J, Lindstrom C, Wenckert A. Radiographic appearance in Crohn's disease: II. The course as reflected at repeat radiography. Acta Radiol Diagn 1979;20:933–944.

84. D'Haens GR, Gasparaitis AE, Hanauer SB. Duration of recurrent ileitis after ileocolonic resection correlates with presurgical extent of Crohn's disease. Gut 1995;36:715–717.

85. Lock MR, Fazio VW, Farmer RG, et al. Proximal recurrence and the fate of the rectum following excisional surgery for Crohn's disease of the large bowel. Ann Surg 1981;194:754–760.

86. Softley A, Myren J, Clamp SE, et al. Factors affecting recurrence after surgery for Crohn's disease. Scand J Gastroenterol Suppl 1988;144:31–34.
87. Ellis L, Calhoun P, Kaiser DL, Rudolf LE, Hanks JB. Postoperative recurrence in Crohn's disease. The effect of the intial length of bowel resection and operative procedure. Ann Surg 1984;199:340–347.
88. Lindhagen T, Ekelund G, Leandoer L, et al. Recurrence rate after surgical treatment of Crohn's disease. Scand J Gastroenterol 1983;18:1037–1044.
89. Pennington L, Hamilton SR, Bayless TM, Cameron JL. Surgical management of Crohn's disease. Influence of disease at margin of resection. Ann Surg 1980;192:311–318.
90. Holzheimer RG, Molloy RG, Wittmann DH. Postoperative complications predict recurrence of Crohn's disease. Eur J Surg 1995;161:129–135.
91. Sayfan J, Wilson DAL, Allan A, Andrews H, Alexander-Williams J. Recurrence after strictureplasty or resection for Crohn's disease. Br J Surg 1989;76:335–338.
92. Marshak RH, Wolf BS. Roentgen findings in regional enteritis. AJR Am J Roentgenol 1955;74:1000–1014.
93. Marshak RH, Lindner AH. Radiology of the Small Bowel, 2nd ed. Philadelphia: WB Saunders; 1976:226–228.
94. Marshak RH. Granulomatous disease of the intestinal tract (Crohn's disease). Radiology 1975;114:3–23.
95. Chérigié E, Monnier JP, Donelli G. Les aspects radiologues des recidives de l'iléo-colite granulomatouse. Ann Radiol 1973;16:433–447.
96. Morson BC. Histopathology of Crohn's disease. Scand J Gastroenterol 1971;6:573–576.
97. Solvig J, Ekberg O, Lindgren S, Floren CH, Nilsson P. Ultrasound examination of the small bowel: Comparison with enteroclysis in patients with Crohn disease. Abdom Imaging 1995;20:323–326.
98. Sheridan MB, Nicholson DA, Martin DF. Transabdominal ultrasonography as the primary investigation in patients with suspected Crohn's disease or recurrence: A prospective study. Clin Radiol 1993;48:402–404.
99. DiCandio G, Mosca F, Campatelli A, et al. Sonographic detection of postsurgical recurrence of Crohn disease. AJR Am J Roentgenol 1986;146:523–526.
100. Gore RM, Balthazar EJ, Ghahremani GG, Miller FH. CT features of ulcerative colitis and Crohn's disease. AJR Am J Roentgenol 1996;167:3–15.
101. Limberg B, Osswald B. Diagnosis and differential diagnosis of ulcerative colitis and Crohn's disease by hydrocolonic sonography. Am J Gastroenterol 1994;89:1051–1057.
102. Schwerk WB, Beck K, Raith M, et al. A prospective evaluation of high resolution sonography in the differential diagnosis of inflammatory bowel disease. Eur J Gastroenterol Hepatol 1992;4:173–182.
103. Gossios KJ, Tsianos EV. Crohn disease: CT findings after treatment. Abdom Imaging 1997;22:160–163.
104. Michelassi F. Crohn's disease. In: Bell Jr RH, Rikkers LF, Mulholland MW, eds. Digestive Tract Surgery. A Text and Atlas. Philadelphia: Lippincott-Raven; 1996:1201–1228.
105. Feczko PJ. Malignancy complicating inflammatory bowel disease. Radiol Clin N Am 1987;25:157–174.
106. Stahl D, Tyler G, Fischer JE. Inflammatory bowel disease—Relationship to carcinoma. Curr Probl Cancer 1981;5:1–72.
107. Greenstein AJ, Sachar D, Pucillo A, et al. Cancer in Crohn's disease after diversionary surgery. Am J Surg 1978;135:86–90.
108. Javors BR. Manual of GI Fluoroscopy. New York: Thieme;1996:139–140.

109. Kock NG. Continent ileostomy. Progr Surg 1973;12:180–201.
110. Lycke KG, Gothlin JH, Jensen JK, Philipson BM, Kock NG. Radiology of the continent ileostomy reservoir: I. Method of examination and normal findings. Abdom Imaging 1994;19:116–123.
111. Lappas JC, Campbell WL. Postsurgical small bowel. In: Maglinte DDT, Herlinger H, Birnbaum BA, eds. Clinical Imaging of the Small Intestine, 2nd ed. New York: Springer-Verlag; 1998:507–526.
112. Lycke KG, Gothlin JH, Jensen JK, Philipson BM, Kock NG. Radiology of the continent ileostomy reservoir: II. Findings in patients with late complications. Abdom Imaging 1994;19:124–131.
113. LeVine M, Katz I, Lampros PJ. Blind pouch formation secondary to side-to-side intestinal anastamosis. AJR Am J Roentgenol 1963;89:706–719.
114. Ghassemian AJ, MacDonald KG, Cunningham PG, et al. The workup for bariatric surgery does not require a routine upper gastrointestinal series. Obes Surg 1997;7:16–18.
115. Wade DH, Richards V, Burhenne HJ. Radiographic changes after small bowel bypass for morbid obesity. Radiol Clin North Am 1976;14:493–498.
116. Buchwald H. Intestinal bypass for hypercholesterolemia. In: Nyhus LM, Baker RJ, Fischer JE, eds. Mastery of Surgery, 3rd ed. Boston: Little, Brown; 1996:1358–1365.
117. Drenick EJ, Ament ME, Finegold SM, Corridi P, Passaro E. Bypass enteropathy. Intestinal and systemic manifestations following small-bowel bypass. JAMA 1976;236:269–272.
118. Passaro Jr E, Drenick E, Wilson SE. Bypass enteritis. A new complication of jejunoileal bypass for obesity. Am J Surg 1976;131:169–174.
119. Vainder M, Kelly J. Renal tubular dysfunction secondary to jejunoileal bypass. JAMA 1976;235:1257–1258.
120. Wise L, Stein T. Biliary and urinary calculi. Pathogenesis following small bowel bypass for obesity. Arch Surg 1975;110:1043–1047.
121. Balthazar EJ, Goldfine S. Jejunoileal bypass. Roentgenographic observations. AJR Am J Roentgenol 1975;125:138–142.
122. Moss AA, Goldberg HI, Koehler RE. The roentgenographic evaluation of complications occurring after jejunoileal bypass. AJR Am J Roentgenol 1976;127:737–741.
123. Martyak SN, Curtis LE. Pneumatosis intestinalis. A complication of jejunoileal bypass. JAMA 1976;235:1038–1039.
124. Kruse-Andersen S, Jessen G. Intussusception of the mid-jejunum after small intestinal bypass operation for obesity: Case report. Am J Gastroenterol 1982;77:554–555.
125. Sarti DA, Zablen MA. The ultrasonic findings in intussusception of the blind loop in jejunoileal bypass for morbid obesity. J Clin Ultrasound 1979; 7:50–52.
126. Lo G, Fish AK, Brodey PA. CT of the intussuscepted excluded loop after intestinal bypass. AJR Am J Roentgenol 1981;137:157–159.

6

The Colon

Colonic resections are commonly performed procedures for both malignant and benign disease. To perform the appropriate study, and to be able to properly evaluate the normal and abnormal radiographic findings, radiologists must be familiar with the terminology and types of surgery done. The terminology of colonic resections generally correlates with the portion of the colon removed.

Types of Colonic Resection

Segmental resection refers to removal of a short portion of the colon, such as a sigmoid resection, with continuity of the colon usually reestablished at the time of resection. When performed for carcinoma, wide margins should be obtained.

Anterior resection entails resection of the rectosigmoid and proximal rectum. **Low anterior resection** refers to resection of the rectosigmoid and distal rectum below the peritoneal reflection. Radiographically, an anastomosis is considered to be "low" if it is situated below the lower border of S2 on the lateral view [1]. This level corresponds to the lower limit of the peritoneal reflection on the anterior rectal wall. Improved technology associated with automatic stapling devices now allows some low rectal tumors formerly treated by abdominoperineal (AP) resection to be treated with low anterior resection. Some surgeons will also perform a temporary colostomy at the time of low anterior resection to protect the rectal anastomosis. After anterior resection, the retrorectal (presacral) space will appear widened (Fig. 6.1).

Right hemicolectomy refers to resection of the terminal ileum, cecum, ascending colon, and a portion of proximal transverse colon (Fig. 6.2). The resection generally extends to the middle third of the transverse colon to provide wide margins for tumor resection and to obtain a well-vascularized incision line. An extended right hemicolectomy, which includes resection of the splenic flexure and proximal descending colon, is performed to treat tumors in the hepatic flexure and proximal transverse colon. When one is performing a contrast enema on patients who have had bowel resections including the

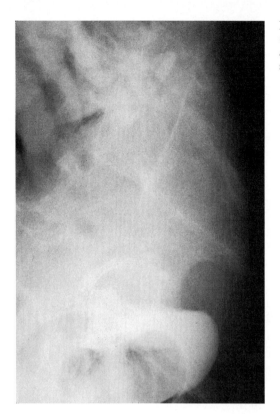

FIGURE 6.1. Anterior resection; widened retrorectal (presacral) space. Lateral postoperative view from a barium enema after an anterior resection demonstrates expected widening of the retrorectal space.

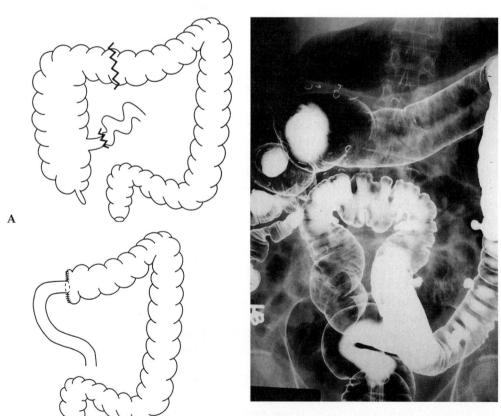

A

B

C

FIGURE 6.2. Right hemicolectomy. (A) Diagram of the colon depicting the resection margins (jagged lines) of a right hemicolectomy. (B) Diagram of the colon after resection. (C) Supine film from a double-contrast barium enema after right hemicolectomy.

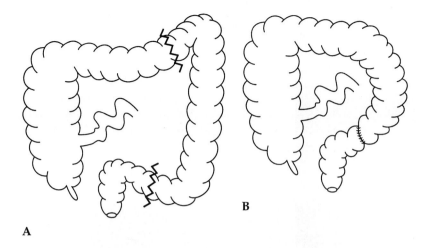

FIGURE **6.3. Left hemicolectomy.** (A) Diagram of the colon showing the resection margins (jagged lines) of a left hemicolectomy. (B) Diagram of the colon after resection.

ileocecal valve, such as a right hemicolectomy, care must be taken not to use so much barium that the small bowel is flooded with contrast medium, obscuring the colon.

A **left hemicolectomy** involves resection of the splenic flexure, descending colon, and sigmoid with anastomosis of the distal transverse colon to the rectosigmoid (Fig. 6.3).

Total colectomy refers to resection of the entire colon; the rectum remains, and continuity is usually established with an anastomosis from the ileum to the remaining rectum (Fig. 6.4).

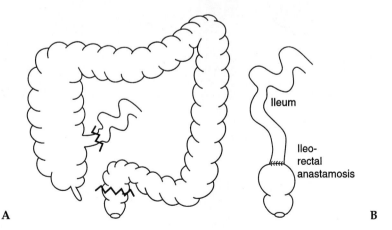

FIGURE **6.4. Total colectomy.** (A) Diagram depicting the resection margins (jagged arrows) of a total colectomy. (B) Diagram after resection.

Total proctocolectomy refers to resection of the entire colon and rectum. In this circumstance, a permanent ileostomy must be performed. **Subtotal colectomy** refers to resection of the entire colon proximal to the distal sigmoid (Fig. 6.5). Generally, an anastomosis is created between the ileum and the remaining sigmoid to establish continuity. In some patients after significant colonic resection (subtotal colectomy, right hemicolectomy, etc.), the small bowel proximal to the anastomotic site will develop an appearance of pseudohaustration and dilatation termed colonization.

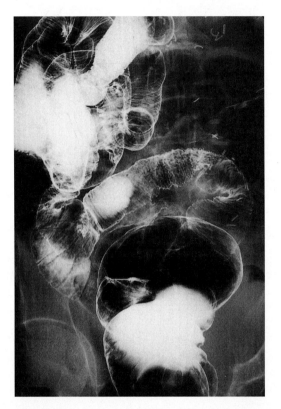

FIGURE **6.5. Subtotal colectomy.** Supine view from a double-contrast barium enema demonstrates only the rectum and a portion of the sigmoid to be present, with an anastomosis to the ileum. The ileum proximal to the anastomosis is dilated, with pseudohaustrations, due to colonization of the ileum.

Abdominoperineal resection (AP resection) is generally performed for tumors below the levator ani muscle. The rectum is removed, and a permanent colostomy is created at the distal descending colon (Fig. 6.6).

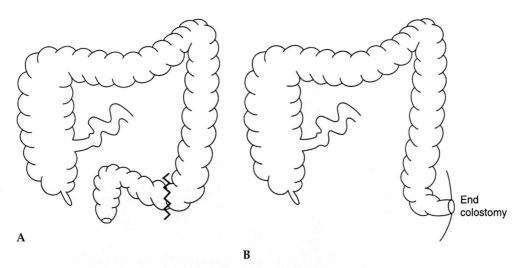

A

B

FIGURE 6.6. **Abdominoperineal resection.** (A) Diagram of the colon showing the resection margins (jagged line) of an AP resection. (B) Diagram of the colon after resection.

Hartmann's procedure, generally performed for diverticulitis, consists of resection of the sigmoid colon, closure of the rectal stump, and an end colostomy. Usually, the bowel continuity is reestablished later, after inflammatory changes have subsided. This procedure and the ileal pouch–anal anastomosis (IPAA) are discussed in more detail shortly. Other operations are fairly self-explanatory, including ileocecal resection and transverse colectomy.

The automatic stapling device is now used frequently for the creation of colonic anastomoses. These devices reduce operative time and permit lower rectal anastomoses than hand-sewn anastomoses. In patients who have undergone rectal or rectosigmoid resection, it has been suggested that a baseline plain film of the abdomen be obtained in the early postoperative period to evaluate the integrity of the staple ring (Fig. 6.7). In the early postoperative period a disrupted staple ring

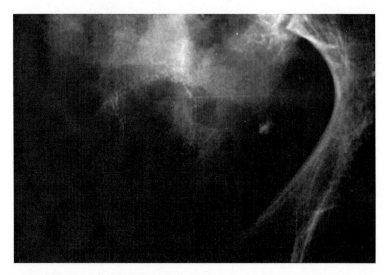

FIGURE 6.7. Intact staple ring. Plain film of the abdomen showing a typical intact staple ring anastomosis.

is suggestive of anastomotic dehiscence (Fig. 6.8) [2]. Animal studies have shown that the staple ring should remain intact for at least 4 weeks, but after that time migration of staples may occur as a result of healing with fibrosis [3]. To evaluate for disruption of the ring, the staple line must be viewed clearly en face, and additional films at different angles may therefore be necessary [4].

Now being increasingly performed by laparoscopy, colonic resection is considered to be a well-tolerated and safe procedure for benign disease. Although laparoscopic surgery is also being increasingly performed for malignant disease, there is some concern about the adequacy of resection with this technique, as well as the possibility of spread of cancer to the port site and long-term survival [5,6].

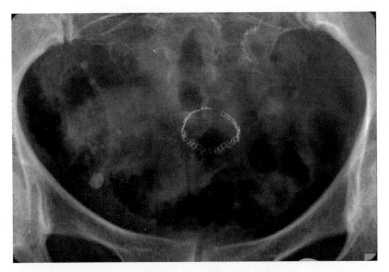

FIGURE 6.8. **Disrupted staple ring.** Plain film of the abdomen demonstrating a disrupted staple ring one week after sigmoid resection.

Types of Anastomosis

A colocolic or ileocolic anastomosis may be constructed in a side-to-side, end-to-side, or end-to-end fashion (Fig. 6.9). The choice will depend on the size of the bowel lumina to be connected and surgeon preference. The end to end is the most physiologic, but requires the two

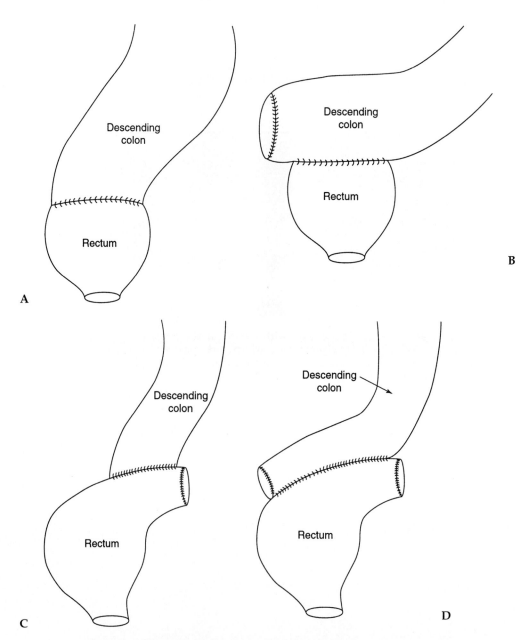

FIGURE 6.9. **Types of anastomosis.** (A) End-to-end anastomosis. (B) End-to-side anastomosis: the end of the rectum is anastomosed to the side of the descending colon. (C) End-to-side anastomosis: the end of the descending colon is anastomosed to the side of the rectum. (D) Side-to-side anastomosis.

segments of the bowel to have the same diameter. The end to side is usually used when the lumens are of different sizes (i.e., ileocolostomy) or for bypass with exclusion. The side to side is the least likely to leak, but is the least physiologic and may lead to the formation of a blind loop. In the early postoperative period, edema at the anastomotic site is expected (Fig. 6.10). In the later postoperative period, the end-to-end anastomotic site is often identified on barium enema as an area of mild

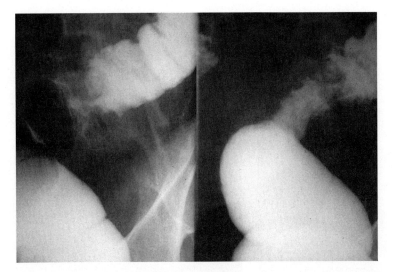

FIGURE 6.10. End-to-end anastomosis with edema at the anastomotic site. Oblique view from a water-soluble enema in the early postoperative period shows narrowing at the anastomotic site from edema.

narrowing (Fig. 6.11). If staples have been used, they will be apparent as well. The normal end-to-end colonic anastomosis should be pliable and distensible. An end-to-side anastomosis can be a source of confusion and may lead to an erroneous diagnosis of anastomotic leak (Fig. 6.12). A long side segment of bowel should generally be avoided, since it might act as a blind loop. Side-to-side anastomoses are usually easily identified (Fig. 6.13).

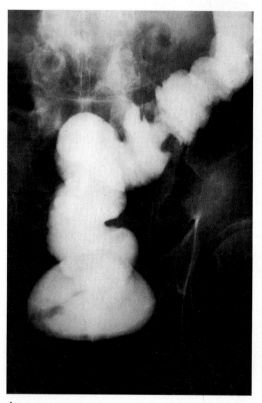

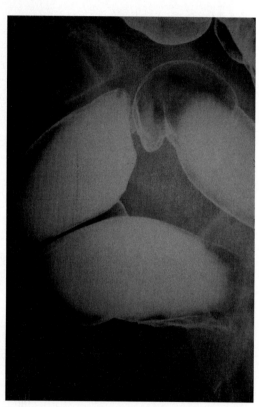

A   B

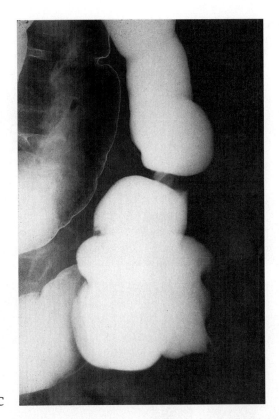

C

FIGURE 6.11. Normal end-to-end anastomosis. Films from single-contrast barium enema in three different patients (A–C) after colon resections, demonstrating normal area of mild narrowing at the anastomotic sites.

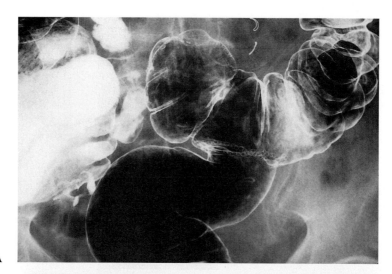

A

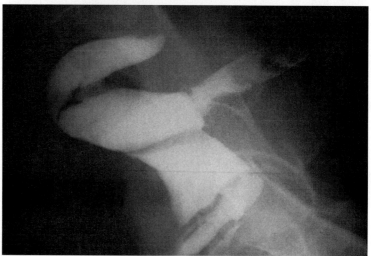

B

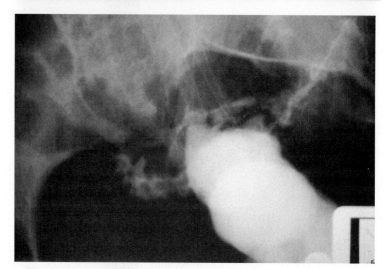

C

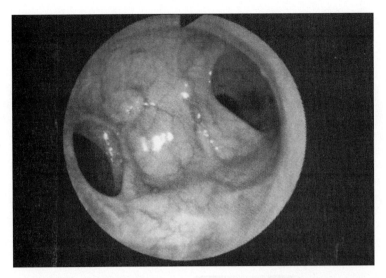

D

FIGURE **6.12. End-to-side anastomosis.** (A) Film from a double-contrast barium enema demonstrates a normal end-to-side rectosigmoid anastomosis. (B) Lateral film from a single-contrast barium enema shows an end-to-side anastomosis with a long closed-off side. A long side pouch can be confused with a leak, or may act as a blind loop. (C) Another postoperative patient with an end-to-side anastomosis with a long closed-off side pouch. (D) Endoscopic view in the same patient.

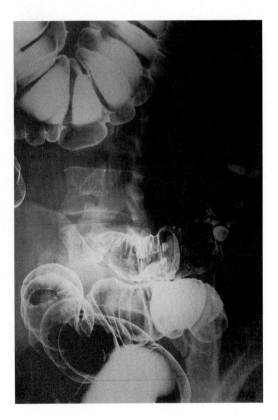

FIGURE **6.13. Side-to-side anastomosis.** Double-contrast barium enema after colonic resection showing a side-to-side anastomosis.

Hartmann's Procedure

Hartmann's procedure was described in 1923 as a technique for the treatment of rectal cancer. It is now frequently performed when primary bowel reanastomosis is deemed unsafe, as in obstructing or perforated diverticular disease, some cases of colon cancer, inflammatory bowel disease, and colorectal trauma. In this procedure, the diseased sigmoid is resected, an end colostomy is created, and the rectal stump is closed off (Fig. 6.14). The Hartmann pouch is a blind segment, which is generally reattached to the proximal colon at a later date, usually within 3 to 6 months after the initial surgery. In some cases, reanastomosis is never performed; for example, it may be thought to be unsafe because of high surgical risk due to poor medical condition,

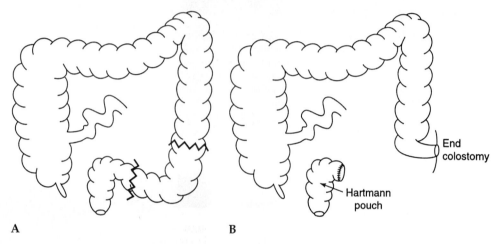

A   B

FIGURE **6.14. Hartmann's procedure.** (A) Diagram of the colon showing the margins of resection (jagged arrows). (B) Diagram of the colon after resection.

technical difficulty, or patient noncompliance. The classic pouch contains only the rectum, however in reality, the pouch may be substantially longer, and may include the entire sigmoid colon and may even extend to the transverse colon. If the pouch has been closed by stapling, the length of the pouch can be estimated by examination of the scout film of the abdomen. Generally, the pouch is "dropped" into peritoneal cavity, but it may be sutured to the anterior abdominal wall (Fig. 6.15).

Radiographic assessment after Hartmann's procedure may be necessary in the early postoperative period to assess for complications. In the early postoperative period, the most common complication

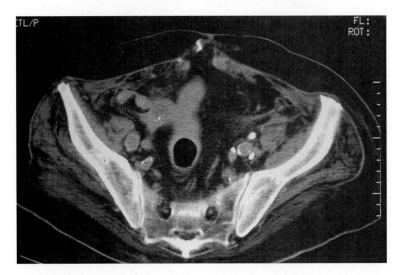

FIGURE 6.15. **Hartmann's procedure.** CT scan through the pelvis after Hartmann's procedure reveals the pouch to be anchored to the anterior abdominal wall, rather than "dropped" into the pelvis.

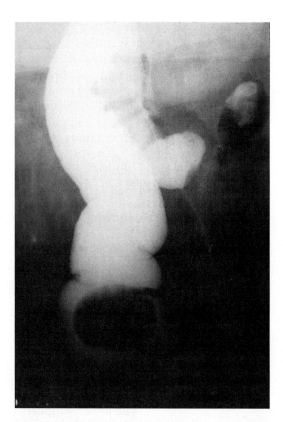

FIGURE 6.16. Hartmann's procedure with leak from the pouch. Film from a water-soluble contrast enema shows contrast medium and air extending beyond the staple line at the closed-off Hartmann pouch due to leak.

is breakdown and leakage from the rectal stump (Fig. 6.16). Leakage may be intraperitoneal or extraperitoneal, depending on the location of the stump. The reported leakage rate has ranged from 2 to 9% [7]. Leakage from the rectal stump is the cause of the highest morbidity and mortality after the first stage of this procedure [8]. Water-soluble contrast medium should be used to assess for leaks in the early post-operative period. When one is performing these studies, care must be taken not to inflate the balloon unless absolutely necessary, since high pressure may be produced in the rectum proximal to the balloon could lead to bowel perforation. CT imaging can identify a pelvic abscess as a further complication (Fig. 6.17). Routine contrast studies of the pouch and proximal colon via the colostomy are usually performed before

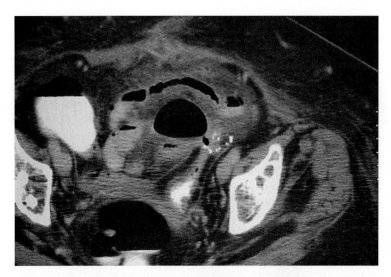

FIGURE 6.17. **Hartmann's procedure with leak from the pouch.** CT scan through the pelvis after oral and rectal administration of contrast medium shows an abscess containing air adjacent to the closed-off rectal stump. The abscess is due to a leak.

takedown of the colostomy and reanastomosis of bowel. The purpose of this is to assess the colonic anatomy and the length and integrity of the pouch. It is important to determine the length of the pouch and its relation to the colostomy, which will affect surgical planning. The pouch can slowly shorten over time, thereby changing its original relationship to the proximal diverted colon [9].

Complications involving the pouch in the later postoperative period include leakage, diversion colitis, stricture, fistula, pelvic adhesions, and recurrent carcinoma. Unexpected, asymptomatic leaks were identified in two patients, 3 and 7 months after creation of a Hartmann's pouch in one series of 84 patients [7]. For this reason, Cherukuri et al. advocate the use of water-soluble contrast medium rather than barium for study of the pouch, even months after surgery [7].

Diversion colitis, which can occur in any portion of the colon diverted from the fecal stream, is discussed in the section on colostomy. Fistulas have been reported from the rectal stump to the ileum and anterior abdominal wall. Pelvic adhesions may cause deformity of the proximal end of the pouch, simulating a leak or stricture, or they may interfere with complete filling of the pouch and lead to the erroneous interpretation, namely, that the pouch is shorter than its actual size. In patients who have had surgery for carcinoma of the colon, recurrence tumor may be detected in the pouch or pelvis. Primary carcinoma may develop in the rectal stump in patients who have had surgery for benign disease [10,11]. Since this is an "unused" segment and the pouch is diverted from the fecal stream, such tumors may grow to a large size without producing symptoms. For this reason, routine study of the pouch in patients with long-term Hartmann's procedures is advocated. The blind pouch may also contain polyps, fecal debris, and inspissated mucus.

Ileal Pouch–Anal Anastomosis (IPAA)

The ileal pouch–anal anastomosis (IPAA) (also called ileoanal anasto-mosis, ileoanal reservoir, and ileoanal pull-through) is a technique originally described by Ravich and Sabiston in 1948. It was devised to remove the entire colon while maintaining intestinal continuity, avoid-ing a permanent ileostomy, and maintaining continence. The operation is usually performed in patients with ulcerative colitis or familial ade-nomatous polyposis syndrome (FAPS). Patients with Crohn's disease are not good candidates for IPAA because of the potential for recurrent disease, including fistulas, strictures, and abscesses, and a subsequent higher incidence of pouch failure. A proctocolectomy is performed to about 8 cm above the peritoneal reflection with a rectal mucosectomy. The terminal ileum is used to construct an ileal reservoir or pouch to maintain continence. Various ileal pouch configurations have been used, including J, S, W, and lateral isoperistaltic (side-to-side) types. Straight ileal pull-throughs are generally not performed because of excessive stool frequency. The J and S shapes are currently the most widely used configurations (Fig. 6.18). The two-limbed J-shaped pouch is relatively simple to construct, is adaptable to stapling techniques, and is easily emptied. The three-limbed S-shaped pouch has a larger reservoir than the J-shaped pouch, but 40 to 50% of patients experience

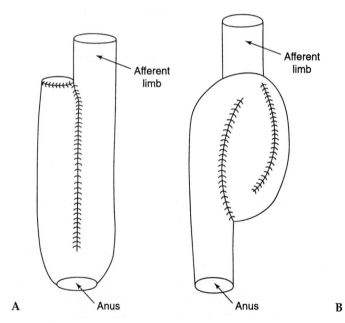

FIGURE 6.18. Pouch configurations for IPAA. (A) J pouch. (B) S pouch.

spontaneous defecation and incomplete evacuation [12]. After the reservoir has been constructed, the mucosa is dissected from the retained rectum, and an ileoanal anastomosis is created with the efferent limb of the reservoir. A temporary loop ileostomy, performed to allow healing of the anastomosis and suture lines, is generally closed after 6 to 8 weeks.

Radiographic examination of the pouch, by pouchography, CT imaging, and/or ^{111}In-labeled leukocyte scintigraphy, is necessary before closure of the ileostomy to exclude postoperative complications. Kremers et al. advocate studying the pouch by means of a 16 to 20F Foley catheter introduced through the anus [13]. Barium is administered under fluoroscopic guidance and anteroposterior, lateral, and oblique views are obtained in full distention. These authors advocate the use of barium rather than water-soluble contrast medium because barium permits detection of smaller leaks. Additional views are then obtained after catheter removal and spontaneous evacuation of the reservoir to identify leakage, which may not be identified on the filled films, and to evaluate the emptying function of the reservoir. On the other hand, Thoeni et al. advocate antegrade filling of the pouch via the ileostomy, since they feel that this technique better distends the pouch [14]. Thoeni et al. also suggest that CT imaging should be the initial examination; if an abscess is identified then, no other radiographic examination need be performed.

On pouchography, the normal S pouch has a globular appearance with an efferent limb (Fig. 6.19). The J pouch characteristically has a raphe corresponding to the suture lines between the two segments of the pouch (Fig. 6.20). J pouches can vary in size, shape, and pattern of external impressions [12]. In most patients, spiral folds run from the main portion of the pouch to the pectinate line. A lucency resembling a polyp may be identified at the lower edge of the interpouch suture. An impression from the mesentery is another variant that may be confused with a mass.

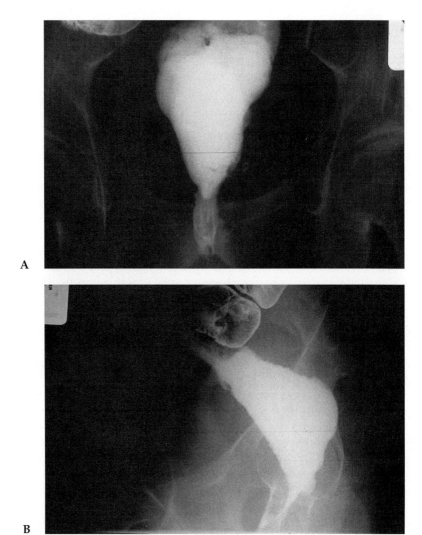

A

B

FIGURE **6.19. S pouch.** Contrast examination via the rectum after IPAA shows the normal globular appearance of the S pouch (A) in the anteroposterior projection and (B) in the lateral projection.

FIGURE 6.20. **J pouch.** (A) Contrast examination via the rectum after IPAA demonstrates the normal appearance of the J pouch in the anteroposterior projection with the characteristic raphe corresponding to the suture line. (B) Lateral view.

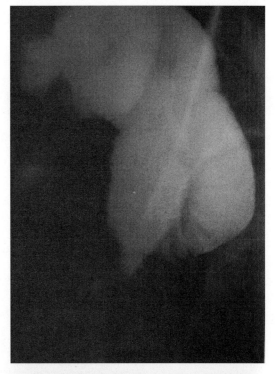

A

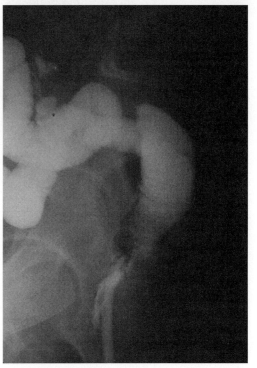

B

TABLE 6.1. Complications of ileoanal anastomosis.

Leak
Pouchitis
Small-bowel obstruction
Abscess
Stenosis
Fistula (perirectal, rectovaginal, rectovesical)
Superior mesenteric artery syndrome
Adenocarcinoma
Reservoir outlet obstruction (S pouch)

Various complications requiring radiologic evaluation may develop with this procedure (Table 6.1). Small-bowel obstruction, usually due to adhesions, may occur in the immediate postoperative period or anytime thereafter. Small-bowel obstruction may be simulated by normally dilated nonobstructed small bowel, however, because the small bowel may dilate with time as an accommodation to increased capacity.

Leakage most often occurs at the pouch–anal anastomosis. Less commonly, leakage may develop at the pouch suture lines. Most leaks will be small and can be treated conservatively. With the J-pouch configuration, a small amount of closed reflected ileum is often not incorporated into the pouch, which is termed the J-pouch appendage (Fig. 6.21). This appendage may leak, simulate a leak, twist, or become necrotic [13,15,16].

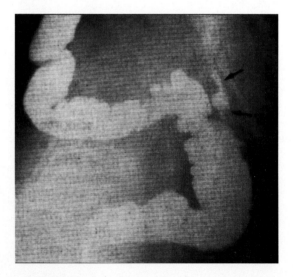

FIGURE 6.21. J-pouch appendage ("pseudoleak"). Lateral view after IPAA and J pouch shows the normal J pouch appendage extending from the posterior superior aspect of the pouch. This finding should not be confused with a leak. [Reprinted with permission from Kremers PW, Scholz FJ, Shoetz DJ. Radiology of the ileoanal reservoir. AJR Am J Roentgenol 145, (3):559–567, 1985, copyright by American Roentgen Ray Society.]

Pouchitis, a fairly common problem encountered after ileoanal anastomosis, occurs in up to half of patients [17]. It is a clinical condition of tenesmus and diarrhea, rarely accompanied by bleeding, fever, arthralgias, and other systemic symptoms. Pouchitis usually responds to medical therapy (antibiotics), but chronic pouchitis may lead to pouch failure. Hyperemia and ulceration may be identified endoscopically. The cause of pouchitis is unknown, although it is more common in patients who have had surgery for ulcerative colitis than for FAPS and is more common in patients with extracolonic manifestations of ulcerative colitis [18]. No consistent radiographic findings have been found on contrast examination, although abnormal mucosal patterns with fold thickening and spiculation have been reported [19]. On CT imaging, pouchitis may be diagnosed in some cases by identification of a thickened pouch wall (>3 mm) with or without adjacent wispy densities [14]. Increased uptake in the location of the pouch may be demonstrated on ^{111}In-labeled leukocyte scintigraphy although abscesses will have a similar pattern [14].

Stricture at the anastomotic site is the most common complication after IPAA [15]. The diagnosis can be made by digital examination or barium enema and generally can be easily treated by dilatation. Rectovaginal, perirectal, and rectovesical fistulas are other complications, reported in 6% of patients after IPAA in one series, although some of these patients later proved to have Crohn's disease [17]. Fistulas can generally be repaired surgically, although fistula formation may lead to pouch failure.

The S pouch may become obstructed and markedly enlarged secondary to stricture, kinking, or the weight of the superiorly placed reservoir on the efferent segment [13]. Surgical revision of the pouch with shortening of the efferent limb may be necessary in this circumstance. This complication appears to be unique to the S-shaped pouch.

Rarely, adenocarcinoma may develop in the retained rectal mucosa or the anal transition zone, with five cases reported on the literature [17]. One case of primary B-cell lymphoma has been reported, arising in an S pouch 8 years after IPAA [20].

The superior mesenteric artery (SMA) syndrome, an occasional complication of IPAA, has been attributed to the combination of weight loss and the reduction of the angle of origin of the SMA due to pulling of the terminal ileum down to the anus, leading to vascular compression of the duodenum [21].

Fibrous tumors, including desmoid tumors of the abdominal wall and mesenteric fibromatosis, may develop in patients with FAPS (Figs. 6.22 and 6.23). These tumors usually develop postoperatively, tend to recur locally after resection, and commonly invade bowel.

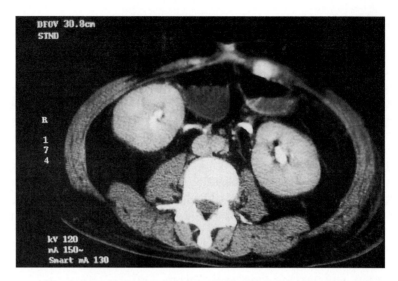

FIGURE **6.22. Desmoid tumor.** CT scan of the abdomen after colectomy and small-bowel resection for FAPS reveals an enhancing lesion in the left rectus muscle due to a desmoid tumor.

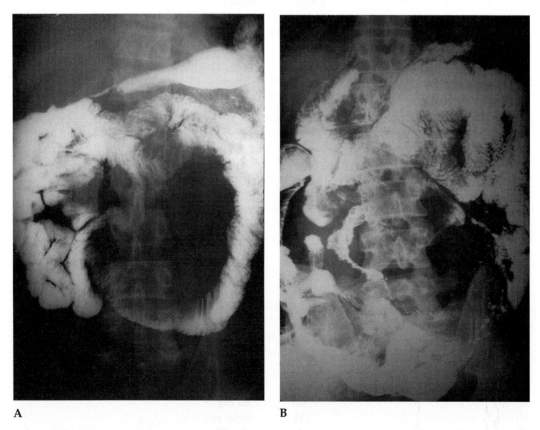

A   B

FIGURE **6.23. Mesenteric fibromatosis.** Films from small-bowel series in two different patients with FAPS demonstrating displacement of bowel. Invasion of bowel from fibrous tumors after colonic resection can be seen in (B).

Complications of Colonic Resection

Leakage

Leakage at the anastomotic site is the most common complication of colonic resection in the early postoperative period, and the cause of the highest morbidity and mortality. The rate of leakage is highest with low anterior resection, with clinically significant leaks reported in 5 to 10% of cases. A mortality rate of up to 50% may be expected if a leak is not promptly recognized [22]. Leaks usually develop 1 to 2 weeks after surgery but may be clinically silent and not apparent until up to months after surgery [23]. Leaks are often due to devascularization and necrosis of bowel at the anastomotic site. In some cases, plain films may reveal pneumoperitoneum, increasing over time, or obstruction or abscess. There is some evidence to suggest that the development of an anastomotic leak is associated with an increased incidence of tumor recurrence and poorer long-term outcome [24].

Controversy has existed with regard to the performance of a water-soluble enema as a routine procedure after colorectal surgery [1,4,25]. Although some surgeons request water-soluble enemas as a routine study after surgery, most surgeons and radiologists generally feel that since the procedure provides little information of diagnostic value, it should not be routinely performed. Contrast studies in the early post-operative period may demonstrate leaks in a high percentage of patients who are and remain clinically asymptomatic and indeed go on to an uneventful recovery [1]. Leaks may be manifested by extralumi-nal tracts, collections, or free intraperitoneal contrast. Leakage is often posterior in location, and since small leaks may be obscured on antero-posterior and oblique views, it is therefore necessary to obtain good lateral projections in this setting (Fig. 6.24). Postevacuation films should be obtained, since a leak that could not be detected on the filled examination may be identified after evacuation. In patients with low anastomoses, care must be used in rectal tube insertion, to prevent disruption of the anastomosis. A Foley catheter of approximately 16F should be utilized and the balloon should generally not be inflated. Another potential problem is insertion of the catheter through a dehisced anastomosis.

CT imaging may also be useful in the evaluation of postoperative leaks. In addition to demonstration of extraluminal contrast, associated abscesses may be identified. Contrast medium and/or air in the rectum and in a collection posterior to it has been termed the "double-rectum" sign (Fig. 6.25). More precise identification of the site of leakage is gene-rally determined with a water-soluble enema than with CT imaging, however. The retrorectal space typically widens after anterior resection; however, undue widening may suggest an anastomotic leak. In one study, CT images showed the retrorectal space to be 2 cm or more in patients without anastomotic leaks [23]. The same authors reported that the retrorectal space was greater than 5 cm in 70% of cases with acute leaks. Presacral fluid can often be identified normally in the post-operative period and can be distinguished from a leak by the absence

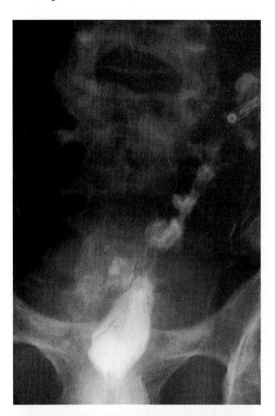

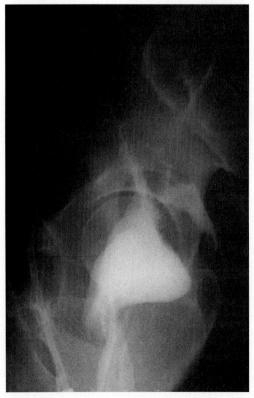

FIGURE 6.24. **Leak after anterior resection; value of the lateral view.** (A) Supine view from a water-soluble contrast enema after anterior resection showing no definite leak. (B) Lateral view in the same patient shows extraluminal contrast, due to leakage extending posteriorly from the region of the anastomosis.

A

B

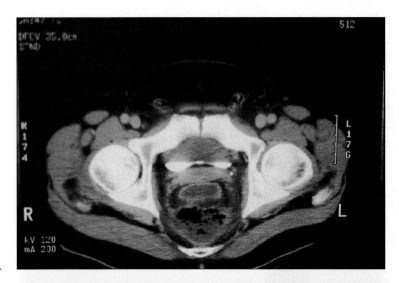

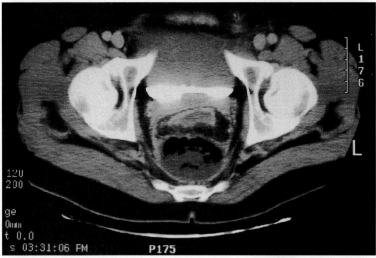

FIGURE 6.25. "Double-rectum" sign due to leak. (A,B) CT scan through the inferior pelvis demonstrates fluid in the rectum and an abscess containing fluid and air posterior to the rectum.

of contrast medium and/or air. In some cases, a collection may be the cause of anastomotic dehiscence rather than its result [1]. The identification of air in the presacral space for longer than 6 months after surgery is also an indication of leak [23].

Anastomotic Stricture

Anastomotic stricture may develop after any bowel anastomosis. If the surgery was performed for malignancy, the differentiation from recurrent tumor is necessary. Benign strictures may be treated by stricturoplasty or in some cases by endoscopic dilatation. In the colon, enteroliths may develop proximal to a stricture secondary to stasis (Fig. 6.26). Another potential complication is the development of proximal ischemia (Fig. 6.27). The etiology of colonic ischemia proximal to an obstructing lesion is thought to be increased intraluminal pressure, which leads to decreased mucosal perfusion.

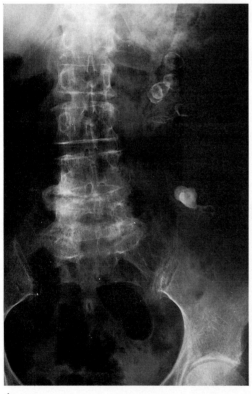

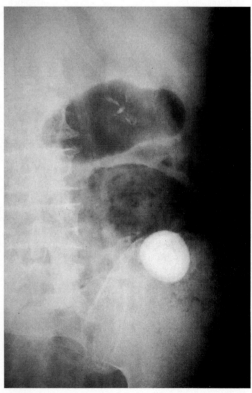

A   B

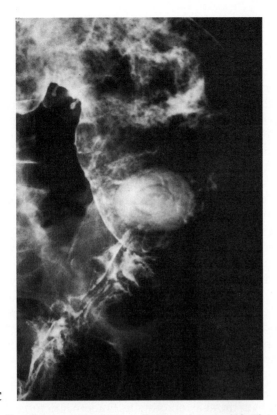

C

FIGURE **6.26. Fecaliths proximal to colonic stricture.** (A) Plain film of the abdomen shows multiple enteroliths in the colon after a left colectomy with an anastomotic stricture. (B) Coned-down view from a plain film of the abdomen reveals a laminated fecalith. (C) Postevacuation film from a barium enema showed a stricture at the anastomotic site after sigmoid resection with a fecalith proximal to the anastomosis.

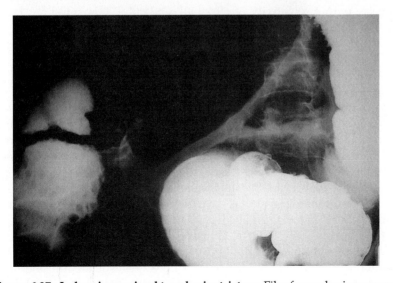

FIGURE 6.27. **Ischemia proximal to colonic stricture.** Film from a barium enema after anterior resection demonstrates a urticarial pattern due to ischemia proximal to a stricture at the anastomotic site.

Recurrent Tumor

Local recurrence after colonic resection for tumor is a catastrophic occurrence with an average survival time of 11 months if untreated [26]. The recurrence rate is related to the tumor stage and the histological grade at the time of diagnosis. The majority of recurrences occur in the first and second years after surgery [27]. Although the prognosis for recurrent disease is poor, early detection of recurrent tumor has been shown to improve the prospect for survival [28]. Postoperative assessment of the colon and abdomen is necessary to evaluate for locally recurrent disease at or near the anastomosis, for the detection of metachronous neoplasm, which occurs in 7 to 10% of patients, and to identify distant metastases, most frequently involving the liver. Local recurrence or metastatic disease develops in up to 40% of patients after curative resection of primary tumors [29]. If the recurrent tumor is localized, curative resection may be performed.

Traditionally, the postoperative evaluation of the colon in the later postoperative period was with barium enema and/or colonoscopy. CT and MR imaging, intrarectal ultrasound, radionuclide-labeled monoclonal antibody studies a carcinoembryonic antigen (CEA) levels, and positron emission tomography (PET) now play contributory roles. The barium enema findings in locally recurrent colorectal carcinoma include anastomotic narrowing (which may be irregular, eccentric, or smooth), mass effect adjacent to or removed from the anastomosis, and obstruction at the anastomotic site. Smooth strictures due to recurrent tumor may be difficult to differentiate from benign strictures on barium enema. The sensitivity of the barium enema in detecting locally recurrent disease is one study was 88% [30]. The CT diagnosis of anastomotic recurrence can be made by the identification of a soft tissue mass or obliteration of adjacent fat planes. In one study CT images were less sensitive than barium enema in identifying locally recurrent disease, with a sensitivity of 69% [30]. Overall, CT imaging has been shown to be fairly insensitive and nonspecific in the evaluation of recurrent tumor [31,32]. The barium enema is limited because of its inability to detect pelvic recurrence after AP resection, difficulty in determining the extent of recurrent disease, and inability to assess distant metastases.

In patients with rectal cancer after AP resection it is difficult to differentiate fibrosis from recurrent tumor [27]. If baseline studies have been obtained, an increase in soft tissue in the rectal bed over time would favor recurrent tumor. Nodularity at the anastomotic site, enlarged nodes, and evidence of tumor elsewhere also favor malignancy. Early reports advocated magnetic resonance imaging as a more specific examination than CT in differentiating tumor from fibrosis. Initial reports showed higher signal intensity on T2-weighted images in tumor recurrence than in fibrosis with scar formation [33]. These findings proved to be unreliable, however, in part because tumor with desmoplastic reaction or inflammatory changes, such as those occurring after radiation therapy, may not demonstrate the typical T2 intensity. The use of contrast-enhanced dynamic MRI has been reported to increase accuracy, with malignant lesions showing greater and faster enhancement than benign lesions, although this technique is still of limited diagnostic value in some cases [34]. Recently PET scanning with [^{18}F]fluorescein digalactopyranoside has been employed for the detection of postoperative recurrence of colorectal cancer. Since PET technology relies on the abnormal metabolic activity of tumor cells, it has the potential to identify the presence of tumor before structural changes may be seen on CT or MR imaging. PET scanning also has the capacity to differentiate recurrent tumor from fibrosis on this basis as well. Early experience has demonstrated the superiority of PET over CT and MR scanning in detecting and staging recurrent colorectal carcinoma, except in cases of mucinous adenocarcinoma [35–39].

Colostomy

A colostomy is generally performed to decompress an obstructed colon, or to divert the fecal stream away from the distal colon. Colostomies may be temporary or permanent. There are four types: end colostomy, loop colostomy, double-barreled colostomy, and end colostomy with a mucous fistula (Fig. 6.28). The type performed will

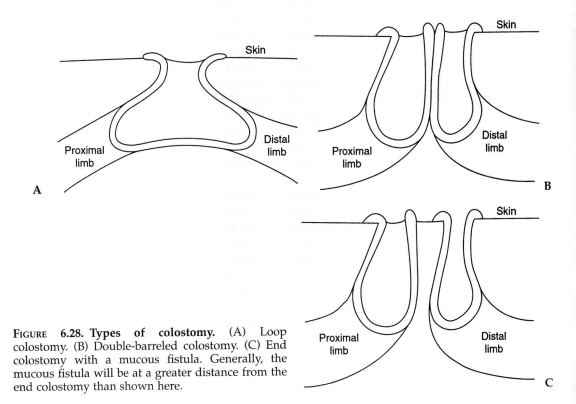

FIGURE 6.28. Types of colostomy. (A) Loop colostomy. (B) Double-barreled colostomy. (C) End colostomy with a mucous fistula. Generally, the mucous fistula will be at a greater distance from the end colostomy than shown here.

depend on the clinical circumstances, the patient's body habitus, previous abdominal surgery, and the surgeon's preference. A loop colostomy is usually performed as a temporary procedure in acute obstruction or to protect a distal anastomosis from the fecal stream. It is considered easier to construct than the other types of colostomy, although complete diversion of the fecal stream may not be achieved with this technique. A loop of colon is brought to the anterior abdominal wall, sutured on the outside, and then opened. This creates an afferent and efferent stoma with the posterior wall of the colon in continuity. In a double-barreled (end loop) colostomy, the colon is divided completely and the limbs are placed side by side. In a divided (end) colostomy with a mucous fistula, two separate colostomies are formed, so that no fecal stream enters the distal colon and only mucous is carried to the rectum.

Prior to closure of the colostomy, it may be necessary to study the distal limb to assess for leakage at the anastomotic site. The afferent limb may be studied as well, especially if it has not been examined preoperatively, to identify concurrent lesions such as polyps or carcinoma, and to assess anatomy.

The utility of contrast studies before colostomy closure has been questioned, however, particularly in trauma patients. Some research has shown that preoperative studies did not alter operative plans or yield unexpected findings and concluded that such studies were unnecessary in many instances [40,41]. Examination of the distal limb via the rectum is feasible in some cases. If there is a low rectal anastomosis, however, it may be dangerous to insert a rectal catheter. Examination of the colon via the colostomy may be performed by a variety of methods. A Foley catheter can be employed with the balloon inflated outside the stoma, although there may be leakage of contrast medium onto the abdominal wall with this technique. Inflation of the balloon inside the colon can lead to bowel perforation and generally is not recommended [42]. Special catheters with nipples or cones that create seals at the colostomy site, allow passage of a catheter into the colon, and prevent leakage onto the abdominal wall have been devised [43–45].

The type of contrast to employ to study the distal limb to evaluate for a leak before colostomy closure is somewhat controversial. In the asymptomatic patient being examined weeks or months after surgery, it is generally considered safe to use barium, since if a leak is present, it will have been sealed off, preventing the entrance of free barium into the peritoneal cavity [46]. Barium is denser than water-soluble contrast medium and is therefore a better contrast agent for visualizing and identifying leaks. Water-soluble agents are less dense, may be diluted in a tract or collection, and are also rapidly resorbed.

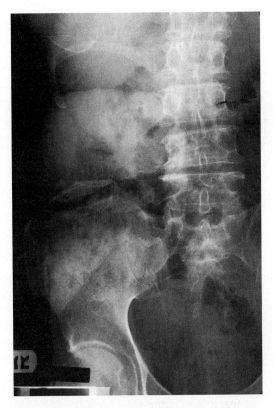

FIGURE **6.29. Prolapsed colostomy.** Plain films of the abdomen reveal a large soft tissue density extending from the colostomy as a result of prolapsed bowel.

Complications of stoma surgery include ischemic necrosis, retraction, peristomal abscess, stenosis, prolapse (Fig. 6.29), parastomal hernia (Fig. 6.30), peristomal fistula, opening the wrong (distal) end of a divided loop (Fig. 6.31), small-bowel obstruction, diversion colitis, and cancer at the stoma site. Prolapse is more common with loop colostomy than with end colostomy. Although prolapse is generally not of any clinical significance, occasionally it may lead to incarceration and strangulation. Parastomal hernias may contain large or small bowel and may remain in the subcutaneous tissues or herniate completely externally adjacent to the stoma. These hernias are readily demonstrated on CT imaging. Large parastomal hernias may require

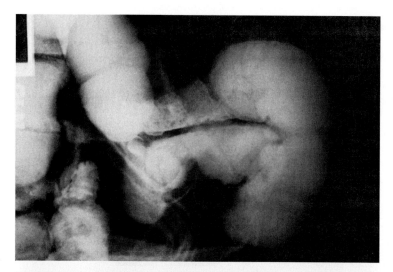

A

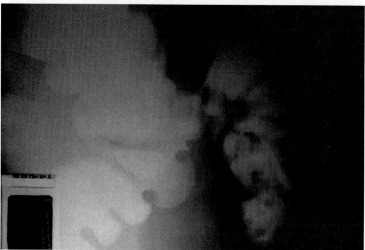

B

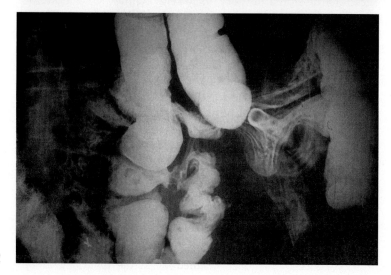

C

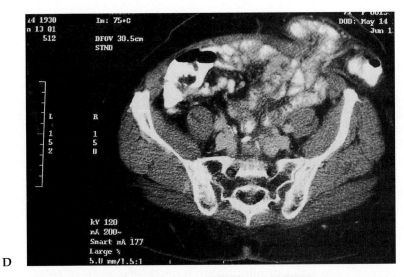

FIGURE 6.30. **Parastomal hernias.** (A–C) Contrast studies on three different patient demonstrating bowel extending out from the abdominal cavity into parastomal hernias. (D) CT scan through the upper pelvis demonstrating herniated small-bowel adjacent to the patient's colostomy.

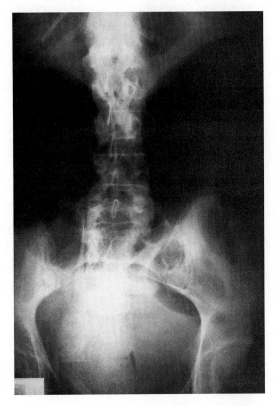

FIGURE 6.31. **Surgical error: opening the wrong (distal) end of a divided colostomy.** Large-bowel obstruction resulted when the distal end of the colostomy rather than the proximal limb was opened.

revision if they are associated with a permanent colostomy. The long-term incidence of parastomal hernia after colostomy is 37% [47]. Most hernias develop by 2 years after surgery, although some may not appear until 20 to 30 years later. The incidence increases in the elderly and in those with other abdominal wall hernias, obesity, malnourishment, steroid use, chronic cough, and wound sepsis.

Diversion colitis is a nonspecific colitis that has been shown to be present on biopsy in the majority of postcolostomy patients, although it is generally an asymptomatic condition [48]. Symptomatic patients may develop crampy abdominal pain, mucous discharge, and rectal bleeding, which may occur at any time after surgery. The etiology of diversion colitis is unclear; it is hypothesized to be due either to bacterial overgrowth of normal flora or pathogenic organisms or to a nutritional deficiency of short-chain fatty acids in the bowel lumen [49]. A spectrum of radiographic findings has been reported, including ulceration, a nodular mucosal pattern, pseudopolyposis, and nondistensibility [50]. Nondistensibility, also termed disuse microcolon, is probably due to chronic lack of distention (Fig. 6.32). All findings resolve with closure of the colostomy and reconstitution of the fecal stream.

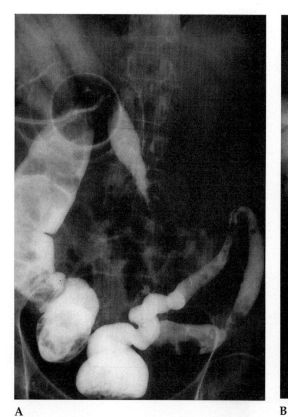 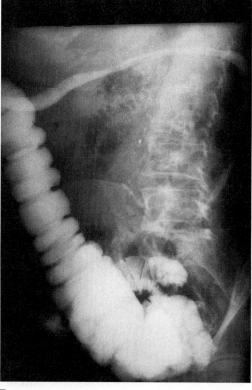

A   B

FIGURE 6.32. **Disuse microcolon.** (A, B) Colostomy studies on two different patients showing distal limbs of the colon markedly narrowed as a result of disuse microcolon.

Complications of colostomy closure include anastomotic stricture and leakage at the anastomotic site, in addition to enterocutaneous fistula, obstruction, and infection [51]. Dehiscence of the anastomosis may be more likely if an unrecognized distal stricture is present. In some cases after colostomy closure, a deformity may be identified in the colon at the site of the previous colostomy. This may appear as an annular or asymmetric short segment area of narrowing with intact mucosa.

Cecostomy

Now infrequently performed, cecostomy is used as a temporary treatment for distal colonic obstruction, usually carcinoma, or severe colonic ileus in patients deemed to be poor surgical candidates for colostomy or more definitive procedures. Traditionally, a tube is placed in the cecum and brought to the surface of the anterior abdominal wall under local or general anesthesia. The gastroenterologist and interventional radiologist are now performing this procedure as well. Mortality in a series of 113 patients who underwent cecostomy for obstructing colon cancer, was found to be comparable to that for patients undergoing diverting loop colostomy, but there was a decrease in mortality for the second operation [52]. Complications from the procedure include displacement of the catheter out of the cecum (Fig. 6.33).

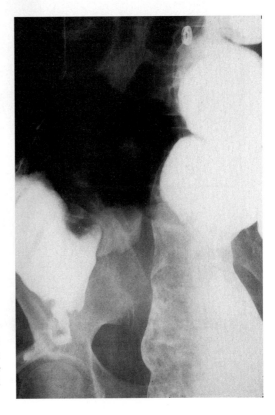

FIGURE 6.33. **Cecostomy with displacement of the tube outside the cecum.** Coned-down view from a contrast enema showing the cecostomy tube to be displaced outside the cecum in a tract connected with it.

Appendectomy

Appendectomy is a simple operation in uncomplicated cases. The appendix is ligated, and the stump is often inverted. The McBurney incision, described in 1894, has been the conventional traditional approach; however others, including the transverse incision, the paramedian incision, and the "bikini" incision may also be employed. Laparoscopic appendectomy is now being routinely performed and has been shown to decrease the length of hospital stay [53].

The postappendectomy barium enema appearance will depend on whether the appendiceal stump has been inverted, and if so, to what degree. If inversion of the stump has not been performed, the length of the appendiceal stump left behind will be variable (ideally it should not be visible, but if visible, very short) (Figs. 6.34 and 6.35). The inverted appendiceal stump may produce a polypoid mass in the apex of the cecum that may be several millimeters to 3 cm in size (Fig. 6.36). The stump may be especially prominent shortly after surgery owing to edema and/or inflammation. The surface may be smooth, lobulated,

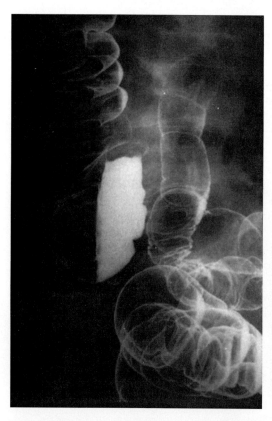

FIGURE 6.34. **Short appendiceal stump after appendectomy.** Decubitus view from a double contrast barium enema after appendectomy.

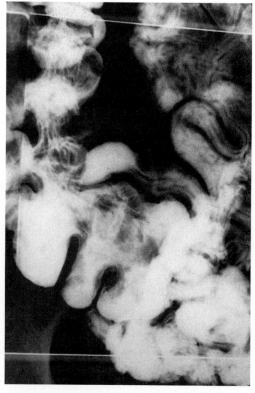

FIGURE 6.35. **Long appendiceal stump.** Supine film from a small-bowel series with filling of the right colon after appendectomy shows a very long appendiceal stump, which is generally undesirable.

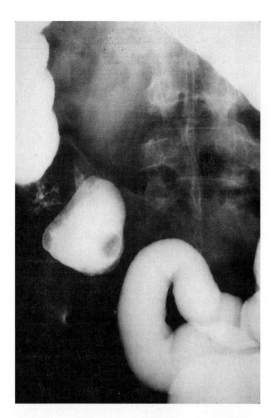

FIGURE 6.36. **Inverted appendiceal stump.** Film from a single-contrast barium enema demonstrating a small, smooth, polypoid defect in the cecum from inversion of the appendiceal stump at the time of appendectomy.

or irregular. The irregularities may be the result of the purse-string sutures, often used for this procedure [54]. In some cases endoscopy may be required to differentiate an inverted appendiceal stump from an adenomatous polyp.

The most common postoperative complications after appendectomy are wound infections and abscesses. These complications are observed twice as commonly in cases of perforated appendicitis than in nonperforated cases [55]. The rate of pelvic abscess after perforated appendicitis is 1.4 to 18% [56]. Fecal fistula is a rare complication, usually related to an inflamed or gangrenous appendiceal stump.

Intussusception is an unusual complication of appendectomy, resulting from the appendiceal stump serving as a lead point [57,58]. The reported time interval between appendectomy and intussusception has varied between 3 days to 4.5 years [57,59]. The diagnosis of intussusception can be made by CT or ultrasound imaging, or by barium enema.

Rarely, recurrent appendicitis will develop in a long appendiceal stump [60–62]. Cases have been reported to occur from 4 weeks to 10 years after appendectomy. It is important to amputate the appendix as closely as possible to the cecum to avoid this complication. Incomplete removal of the appendix is usually the result of failure to locate the appendiceal–cecal junction. The potential for appendicitis to recur is increased with laparoscopic appendectomy, since it may be more difficult to visualize the base of the appendix with this technique. If the base of the appendix is not visualized laparoscopically, it may be necessary to convert to the standard open method.

The incidence of right inguinal hernia is increased after traditional appendectomy. In one study, the incidence of right inguinal hernia was approximately three times greater than in the general population [63]. The theory is that damage to the hypogastric nerve from the incision leads to weakening of the transversus abduminus muscle and the transversalis fascia. This presumably leads to damage of the "shutter mechanism," which closes the internal ring when intra-abdominal pressure rises. For this reason, the appendectomy incision should be placed above the anterior superior iliac spine to avoid the hypogastric nerve [63].

Stents

Expandible metallic stents may be used in the treatment of left-sided colonic obstruction as an alternative to emergency colostomy. These devices have been shown to effectively produce rapid decompression of the colon, with a decrease in morbidity and mortality over conventional surgical therapy [64–67]. Stent placements may be performed for palliation in patients with metastatic disease or unresectable tumors and in those who are poor surgical candidates. Stenting may also be a temporary measure: to provide immediate bowel decompression or to allow for bowel preparation, tumor staging, and improvement in the patient's general condition, thus permitting a one-stage procedure (with primary anastomosis and avoidance of a colostomy) rather than a two- or three-stage procedure. Stents may also be used for the treatment of benign colonic strictures and colovesical fistulas. Perforation at the time of presentation is a contraindication to stent placement.

Colonic stents may be placed endoscopically or with fluoroscopic guidance alone by the interventional radiologist [64]. Uncovered stents are usually used. Before stent placement, it is helpful to obtain a contrast enema to determine the location, caliber, and length of the obstructing lesion [65]. Water-soluble contrast media is preferable to barium because barium may interfere with visualization during endoscopy, and it is not necessary to demonstrate mucosal detail. After stent placement, plain films and a water-soluble contrast enema may be obtained to confirm stent position and patency. Plain films may serve as a baseline to evaluate for stent migration in the future (Fig. 6.37). Complications include stent malposition, stent migration (including spontaneous expulsion of the stent), stent obstruction (from tumor ingrowth or fecal impaction), and colonic perforation. Colonic perforation may not require surgery in all cases. Stent obstruction by tumor growth can be avoided by using covered stents; however stent migra-

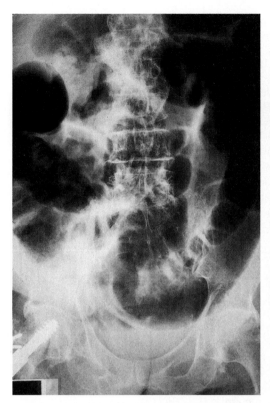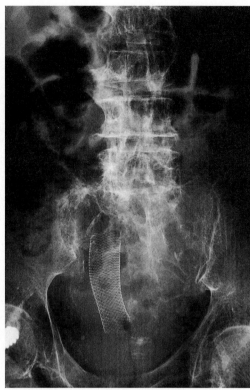

A   B

FIGURE 6.37. **Large-bowel obstruction secondary to colon cancer treated with metallic stent.** (A) Plain film of the abdomen showing large-bowel obstruction due to sigmoid carcinoma. (B) After stent placement, bowel decompression has been achieved.

tion is more likely to occur with covered stents. In some cases, stent migration may be secondary to tumor shrinkage, as the result of adjuvant chemotherapy. In these circumstances, stent extraction may be advisable.

References

1. Shorthouse AJ, Bartram CI, Eyers AA, Thomson JP. The water-soluble contrast enema after rectal anastomosis. Br J Surg 1982;69(12):714–717.
2. Daly BD, Crowley BM. Radiological appearances of colonic ring staple anastomoses. Br J Radiol 1989;62(735):256–259.
3. Fain SN, Patin CS, Morgenstern L. Use of a mechanical suturing apparatus in low colorectal anastomosis. Arch Surg 1975;110(9):1079–1082.
4. Williams CE, Makin CA, Reeve RG, Ellenbogen SB. Over-utilisation of radiography in the assessment of stapled colonic anastomoses. Eur J Radiol 1991;12(1):35–37.
5. Gibson M, Byrd C, Pierce C, Wright F, Norwood W, Gibson T, et al. Laparoscopic colon resections: A five-year retrospective review. Am Surg 2000;66(3):245–248.
6. Wexner SD, Cohen SM. Port site metastases after laparoscopic colorectal surgery for cure of malignancy. Br J Surg 1995;82(3):295–298.

7. Cherukuri R, Levine MS, Maki DD, Rubesin SE, Laufer I, Rosato EF. Hartmann's pouch: Radiographic evaluation of postoperative findings. AJR Am J Roentgenol 1998;171(6):1577–1582.

8. Lubbers EJ, de Boer HH. Inherent complications of Hartmann's operation. Surg Gynecol Obstet 1982;155(5):717–721.

9. Chua CL. Surgical considerations in the Hartmann's procedure. Aust N Z J Surg 1996;66(10):676–679.

10. Thaemert BC, Kisken WA. Neoplasms in long-term Hartmann's pouches. Wis Med J 1996;95(2):105–107.

11. Haas PA, Fox Jr TA. The fate of the forgotten rectal pouch after Hartmann's procedure without reconstruction. Am J Surg 1990;159(1):106–110.

12. Hillard AE, Mann FA, Becker JM, Nelson JA. The ileoanal J pouch: Radiographic evaluation. Radiology 1985;155(3):591–594.

13. Kremers PW, Scholz FJ, Schoetz Jr DJ, Veidenheimer MC, Coller JA. Radiology of the ileoanal reservoir. AJR Am J Roentgenol 1985;145(3):559–567.

14. Thoeni RF, Fell SC, Engelstad B, Schrock TB. Ileoanal pouches: Comparison of CT, scintigraphy, and contrast enemas for diagnosing postsurgical complications. AJR Am J Roentgenol 1990;154(1):73–78.

15. Hagen G, Kolmannskog F, Aasen S, Bakka A, Lotveit T, Mathisen O. Radiology of the ileal J-pouch–anal anastomosis (IPAA). Acta Radiol 1993;34(6):563–568.

16. Alfisher MM, Scholz FJ, Roberts PL, Counihan T. Radiology of ileal pouch–anal anastomosis: Normal findings, examination pitfalls, and complications. Radiographics 1997;17(1):81–98.

17. Stein RB, Lichtenstein GR. Complications after ileal pouch–anal anastomosis. Semin Gastrointest Dis 2000;11(1):2–9.

18. Dozois RR, Kelly KA, Welling DR, Gordon H, Beart Jr RW, Wolff BG, et al. Ileal pouch–anal anastomosis: Comparison of results in familial adenomatous polyposis and chronic ulcerative colitis. Ann Surg 1989;210(3):268–271.

19. Brown JJ, Balfe DM, Heiken JP, Becker JM, Soper NJ. Ileal J pouch: Radiologic evaluation in patients with and without postoperative infectious complications. Radiology 1990;174(1):115–120.

20. Frizzi JD, Rivera DE, Harris JA, Hamill RL. Lymphoma arising in an S-pouch after total proctocolectomy for ulcerative colitis: Report of a case. Dis Colon Rectum 2000;43(4):540–543.

21. Ballantyne GH, Graham SM, Hammers L, Modlin IM. Superior mesenteric artery syndrome following ileal J-pouch anal anastomosis. An iatrogenic cause of early postoperative obstruction. Dis Colon Rectum 1987;30(6):472–474.

22. Ghahremani GG, Gore RM. CT diagnosis of postoperative abdominal complications. Radiol Clin North Am 1989;27(4):787–804.

23. DuBrow RA, David CL, Curley SA. Anastomotic leaks after low anterior resection for rectal carcinoma: Evaluation with CT and barium enema. AJR Am J Roentgenol 1995;165(3):567–571.

24. Akyol AM, McGregor JR, Galloway DJ, Murray GD, George WD. Anastomotic leaks in colorectal cancer surgery: A risk factor for recurrence? Int J Colorectal Dis 1991;6(4):179–183.

25. Akyol AM, McGregor JR, Galloway DJ, George WD. Early postoperative contrast radiology in the assessment of colorectal anastomotic integrity. Int J Colorectal Dis 1992;7(3):141–143.

26. Welch JP, Donaldson GA. Detection and treatment of recurrent cancer of the colon and rectum. Am J Surg 1978;135(4):505–511.

27. Krestin GP. Is magnetic resonance imaging the method of choice in the diagnosis of recurrent rectal carcinoma? Abdom Imaging 1997;22(3):343–345.

28. Quentmeier A, Schlag P, Smok M, Herfarth C. Re-operation for recurrent colorectal cancer: The importance of early diagnosis for resectability and survival. Eur J Surg Oncol 1990;16(4):319–325.

29. Bruinvels DJ, Stiggelbout AM, Kievit J, van Houwelingen HC, Habbema JD, van de Velde CJ. Follow-up of patients with colorectal cancer. A meta-analysis. Ann Surg 1994;219(2):174–182.

30. Chen YM, Ott DJ, Wolfman NT, Gelfand DW, Karsteadt N, Bechtold RE. Recurrent colorectal carcinoma: Evaluation with barium enema examination and CT. Radiology 1987;163(2):307–310.

31. Balthazar EJ. CT of the gastrointestinal tract: Principles and interpretation. AJR Am J Roentgenol 1991;156(1):23–32.

32. Freeny PC, Marks WM, Ryan JA, Bolen JW. Colorectal carcinoma evaluation with CT: Preoperative staging and detection of postoperative recurrence. Radiology 1986;158(2):347–353.

33. Krestin GP, Steinbrich W, Friedmann G. Recurrent rectal cancer: Diagnosis with MR imaging versus CT. Radiology 1988;168(2):307–311.

34. Muller-Schimpfle M, Brix G, Layer G, Schlag P, Engenhart R, Frohmuller S, et al. Recurrent rectal cancer: Diagnosis with dynamic MR imaging. Radiology 1993;189(3):881–889.

35. Whiteford MH, Whiteford HM, Yee LF, Ogunbiyi OA, Dehdashti F, Siegel BA, et al. Usefulness of FDG-PET scan in the assessment of suspected metastatic or recurrent adenocarcinoma of the colon and rectum. Dis Colon Rectum 2000;43(6):759–767.

36. Arulampalam TH, Costa DC, Loizidou M, Visvikis D, Ell PJ, Taylor I. Positron emission tomography and colorectal cancer. Br J Surg 2001;88(2):176–189.

37. Keogan MT, Lowe VJ, Baker ME, McDermott VG, Lyerly HK, Coleman RE. Local recurrence of rectal cancer: Evaluation with F-18 fluorodeoxyglucose PET imaging. Abdom Imaging 1997;22(3):332–337.

38. Ito K, Kato T, Tadokoro M, Ishiguchi T, Oshima M, Ishigaki T, et al. Recurrent rectal cancer and scar: Differentiation with PET and MR imaging. Radiology 1992;182(2):549–552.

39. Schiepers C, Penninckx F, De Vadder N, Merckx E, Mortelmans L, Bormans G, et al. Contribution of PET in the diagnosis of recurrent colorectal cancer: Comparison with conventional imaging. Eur J Surg Oncol 1995;21(5):517–522.

40. Pokorny RM, Heniford T, Allen JW, Tuckson WB, Galandiuk S. Limited utility of preoperative studies in preparation for colostomy closure. Am Surg 1999;65(4):338–340.

41. Swenson K, Stamos M, Klein S. The role of barium enema in colostomy closure in trauma patients. Am Surg 1997;63(10):893–895.

42. Spiro RH, Hertz RE. Colostomy perforation. Surgery 1966;60(3):590–597.

43. Pochaczevsky R. A colostomy device for barium enema examinations. Radiology 1982;143(2):565.

44. Goldstein HM, Miller MH. Air contrast colon examination in patients with colostomies. AJR Am J Roentgenol 1976;127(4):607–610.

45. Burhenne HJ. Technique of colostomy examination. Radiology 1970;97(1):183–185.

46. Scholz FJ, Jakomin BV. Postoperative colon. In: Gore RM, Levine MS, eds. Textbook of Gastrointestinal Radiology. Philadelphia: WB Saunders; 2000:1151–1158.

47. Shellito PC. Complications of abdominal stoma surgery. Dis Colon Rectum 1998;41(12):1562–1572.
48. Ferguson CM, Siegel RJ. A prospective evaluation of diversion colitis. Am Surg 1991;57(1):46–49.
49. Harig JM, Soergel KH, Komorowski RA, Wood CM. Treatment of diversion colitis with short-chain-fatty acid irrigation. N Engl J Med 1989;320(1):23–28.
50. Scott RL, Pinstein ML. Diversion colitis demonstrated by double-contrast barium enema. AJR Am J Roentgenol 1984;143(4):767–768.
51. Parks SE, Hastings PR. Complications of colostomy closure. Am J Surg 1985;149(5):672–675.
52. Perrier G, Peillon C, Liberge N, Steinmetz L, Boyet L, Testart J. Cecostomy is a useful surgical procedure: Study of 113 colonic obstructions caused by cancer. Dis Colon Rectum 2000;43(1):50–54.
53. Vallina VL, Velasco JM, McCulloch CS. Laparoscopic versus conventional appendectomy. Ann Surg 1993;218(5):685–692.
54. Freedman E, Rabwin MH, Linsman JF. Roentgen simulation of polypoid neoplasms by invaginated appendiceal stumps. AJR Am J Roentgenol 1956;75(2):380–385.
55. Cooperman M. Complications of appendectomy. Surg Clin North Am 1983;63(6):1233–1247.
56. Silen W, Cope Z. Cope's Early Diagnosis of the Acute Abdomen, 17 ed. New York: Oxford University Press; 1987.
57. O'Brien SE. Intussusception complicating appendectomy: A case report. Can J Surg 1966;9(3):278–279.
58. Wolfson S, Shachor D, Freund U. Ileocolic intussusception in an adult. A postoperative complication of appendectomy. Dis Colon Rectum 1984;27(4):265–266.
59. Fraser K. Intussusception of appendix. Br J Surg 1943;31:23.
60. Devereaux DA, McDermott JP, Caushaj PF. Recurrent appendicitis following laparoscopic appendectomy. Report of a case. Dis Colon Rectum 1994;37(7):719–720.
61. Harris CR. Appendiceal stump abscess ten years after appendectomy. Am J Emerg Med 1989;7(4):411–412.
62. Rose TF. Recurrent appendiceal abscess. Med J Aust 1945;32:659–662.
63. Arnbjornsson E. Development of right inguinal hernia after appendectomy. Am J Surg 1982;143(1):174–175.
64. Camunez F, Echenagusia A, Simo G, Turegano F, Vazquez J, Barreiro-Meiro I. Malignant colorectal obstruction treated by means of self-expanding metallic stents: Effectiveness before surgery and in palliation. Radiology 2000;216(2):492–497.
65. Canon CL, Baron TH, Morgan DE, Dean PA, Koehler RE. Treatment of colonic obstruction with expandable metal stents: Radiologic features. Am J Roentgenol 1997;168(1):199–205.
66. de Gregorio MA, Mainar A, Tejero E, Tobio R, Alfonso E, Pinto I, et al. Acute colorectal obstruction: Stent placement for palliative treatment—Results of a multicenter study. Radiology 1998;209(1):117–120.
67. Mainar A, Tejero E, Maynar M, Ferral H, Castaneda-Zuniga W. Colorectal obstruction: Treatment with metallic stents. Radiology 1996;198(3):761–764.

Index